Antibiotic Manual

A Guide to Commonly Used Antimicrobials

Antibiotic Manual

A Guide to Commonly Used Antimicrobials

David Schlossberg MD, FACP, FIDSA
Professor of Medicine
Temple University School of Medicine
Philadelphia, Pennsylvania
Medical Director, Tuberculosis Control Program
Philadelphia Department of Public Health
Philadelphia, Pennsylvania

Rafik Samuel MD, FACP, FIDSA
Associate Professor of Medicine
Director Infectious Diseases Fellowship Program
Temple University School of Medicine
Philadelphia, Pennsylvania

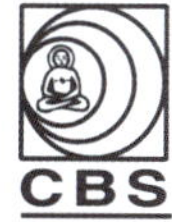

CBS Publishers & Distributors Pvt Ltd

New Delhi • Bengaluru • Pune • Kochi • Chennai
Mumbai • Kolkata • Hyderabad • Patna • Manipal

PEOPLE'S MEDICAL PUBLISHING HOUSE—USA, Shelton, Connecticut

People's Medical Publishing House–USA
2 Enterprise Drive, Suite 509
Shelton, CT 06484
Tel: 203-402-0646; Fax: 203-402-0854
E-mail: info@pmph-usa.com

09 10 11 12 13/PMPH/9 8 7 6 5 4 3 2 1

ISBN 13: 978-1-60795-084-4
ISBN 10: 1-60795-084-7

Editor: Linda H. Mehta, Copyeditor/Typesetter: Spearhead Global, Inc.; Cover Designer: Mary McKeon

This Edition has been published by special arrangement with PMPH-USA, Ltd

CBS ISBN: 978-81-239-2231-7

Special Indian Edition: 2012

Published by Satish Kumar Jain and produced by Vinod K. Jain for

CBS Publishers & Distributors Pvt Ltd
4819/XI Prahlad Street, 24 Ansari Road, Daryaganj, New Delhi 110 002, India.
Ph: 23289259, 23266861, 23266867 Fax: 011-23243014 Website: www.cbspd.com
e-mail:delhi@cbspd.com; cbspubs@airtelmail.in.

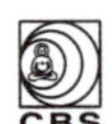

Corporate Office: 204 FIE, Industrial Area, Patparganj, Delhi 110 092
Ph: 4934 4934 Fax: 4934 4935

Branches

- **Bengaluru:** Seema House 2975, 17th Cross, K.R. Road, Banasankari 2nd Stage, Bengaluru 560 070, Karnataka
  Ph: +91-80-26771678/79 Fax: +91-80-26771680 e-mail: bangalore@cbspd.com
- **Pune:** Bhuruk Prestige, Sr. No. 52/12/2+1+3/2 Narhe, Haveli (Near Katraj-Dehu Road Bypass), Pune 411 041, Maharashtra
  Ph: +91-20-64704058, 64704059, 32392277 Fax: +91-20-24300160 e-mail: pune@cbspd.com
- **Kochi:** 36/14 Kalluvilakam, Lissie Hospital Road, Kochi 682 018, Kerala
  Ph: +91-484-4059061-65 Fax: +91-484-4059065 e-mail: cochin@cbspd.com
- **Chennai:** 20, West Park Road, Shenoy Nagar, Chennai 600 030, Tamil Nadu
  Ph: +91-44-26260666, 26208620 Fax: +91-44-45530020 e-mail: chennai@cbspd.com

Representatives

- **Mumbai** 0-9833017933
- **Kolkata** 0-9831437309
- **Hyderabad** 0-9885175004
- **Patna** 0-9334159340
- **Manipal** 0-9742022075

Printed at Manipal Technologies Limited

Canada
McGraw-Hill Ryerson Education
Customer Care
300 Water St
Whitby, Ontario L1N 9B6
Canada
Tel: 1-800-565-5758
Fax: 1-800-463-5885
www.mcgrawhill.ca

Foreign Rights
People's Medical Publishing House
Suzanne Robidoux, Copyright Sales Manager
International Trade Department
No. 19, Pan Jia Yuan Nan Li
Chaoyang District
Beijing 100021
P.R. China
Tel: 8610-59787337
Fax: 8610-59787336
www.pmph.com/en/

Japan
United Publishers Services Limited
1-32-5 Higashi-Shinagawa
Shinagawa-ku, Tokyo 140-0002
Japan
Tel: 03-5479-7251
Fax: 03-5479-7307
Email: kakimoto@ups.co.jp

United Kingdom, Europe, Middle East, Africa
McGraw Hill Education
Shoppenhangers Road
Maidenhead
Berkshire, SL6 2QL
England
Tel: 44-0-1628-502500
Fax: 44-0-1628-635895
www.mcgraw-hill.co.uk

Singapore, Thailand, Philippines, Indonesia, Vietnam, Pacific Rim, Korea
McGraw-Hill Education
60 Tuas Basin Link
Singapore 638775
Tel: 65-6863-1580
Fax: 65-6862-3354
www.mcgraw-hill.com.sg

Australia, New Zealand
Elsevier Australia
Locked Bag 7500
Chatswood DC NSW 2067
Australia
Tel: 161 (2) 9422-8500
Fax: 161 (2) 9422-8562
www.elsevier.com.au

Brazil
SuperPedido Tecmedd
Beatriz Alves, Foreign Trade Department
R. Sansao Alves dos Santos, 102 | 7th floor
Brooklin Novo
Sao Paolo 04571-090
Brazil
Tel: 55-16-3512-5539
www.superpedidotecmedd.com.br

India, Bangladesh, Pakistan, Sri Lanka, Malaysia
CBS Publishers
4819/X1 Prahlad Street 24
Ansari Road, Darya Ganj, New Delhi-110002
India
Tel: 91-11-23266861/67
Fax: 91-11-23266818
Email:cbspubs@vsnl.com

People's Republic of China
People's Medical Publishing House
International Trade Department
No. 19, Pan Jia Yuan Nan Li
Chaoyang District
Beijing 100021
P.R. China
Tel: 8610-67653342
Fax: 8610-67691034
www.pmph.com/en/

This book is dedicated to my grandsons, Nathan and Adam.
"The world endures only for the sake of the breath of schoolchildren."

- Babylonian Talmud, Shabbat, 119

—DS

The book is dedicated to my parents, Farid and Leila. Thanks for all the love, support, and understanding through the years.

—RS

TABLE OF CONTENTS

Preface xv

Abacavir (Ziagen) 1
Acyclovir (Zovirax) 3
Adefovir (Hepsera) 6
Albendazole (Albenza) 8
Amantadine (Symmetrel) 10
Amikacin (Amikin) 12
Amoxicillin (Amoxil) 15
Amoxicillin plus Clavulanate Potassium (Augmentin, Augmentin ES-600, Augmentin XR) 18
Amphotericin B, Liposomal (Ambisome) 22
Amphotericin B Colloidal Dispersion (Amphotec) 25
Amphotericin B Deoxycholate (Fungizone) 27
Amphotericin B Lipid Complex (Abelcet) 30
Ampicillin 32
Ampicillin plus Sulbactam (Unasyn) 35
Anidulafungin (Eraxis) 37
Artemether – see Artemisinin
Artemether plus Lumefantrine (Coartem) — see Artemisinin
Artemisinin and its Derivatives 39
Artesunate – see Artemisinin
Atazanavir (Reyataz) 44
Atovaquone (Mepron) 48
Atovaquone plus Proguanil (Malarone) 50
Azithromycin (Zithromax, Zmax) 53
Aztreonam (Azactam) 57

Benznidazole 59
Bithionol (Bitin) 60

Capreomycin (Capastat) 61
Caspofungin (Cancidas) 63
Cefaclor (Ceclor) 65
Cefadroxil (Duricef) 67
Cefamandole (Mandol, Mandokef) 69
Cefazolin (Ancef) 72
Cefdinir (Omnicef) 75
Cefditoren pivoxil (Spectracef) 78
Cefepime (Maxipime) 80

Table of Contents

Cefixime (Suprax) 83
Cefoperazone (Cefobid) 85
Cefotaxime (Claforan) 87
Cefotetan (Cefotan) 90
Cefoxitin (Mefoxin) 93
Cefpirome (Cefrom, Keiten, Broact, Cefir) 96
Cefpodoxime proxetil (Vantin) 98
Cefprozil (Cefzil) 101
Ceftazidime (Fortaz) 104
Ceftazidime (Tazicef) 104
Ceftibuten (Cedax) 107
Ceftizoxime (Cefizox) 109
Ceftriaxone (Rocephin) 112
Cefuroxime (Zinacef) 115
Cefuroxime axetil (Ceftin) 115
Cephalexin (Keflex) 119
Chloramphenicol (Chloromycetin) 121
Chloroquine phosphate (Aralen) 123
Cidofovir (Vistide) 126
Ciprofloxacin (Cipro) 129
Clarithromycin (Biaxin) 133
Clindamycin (Cleocin) 137
Clofazimine (Lamprene) 140
Colistimethate sodium (Coly-Mycin) 142
Cycloserine (Seromycin) 144

Dapsone 146
Daptomycin (Cubicin) 148
Darunavir (Prezista) 150
Delavirdine (Rescriptor) 153
Dicloxacillin 156
Didanosine (Videx EC) 158
Diethyl carbamazine (Hetrazan) 160
Dihydroartemisinin – see Artemisinin
Diloxanide furoate (Furamide) 162
Doripenem (Doribax) 163
Doxycycline (Vibramycin, Doryx) 165

Efavirenz (Sustiva) 168
Eflornithine (Ornidyl) 171

Emtricitabine (Emtriva) 173
Enfuvirtide (Fuzeon) 175
Entecavir (Baraclude) 177
Ertapenem (Invanz) 179
Erythromycin 182
Ethambutol (Myambutol) 185
Ethionamide (Trecator) 187
Etravirine (Intelence) 189

Famciclovir (Famvir) 192
Fluconazole (Diflucan) 194
Flucytosine (Ancobon) 197
Fosamprenavir (Lexiva) 199
Foscarnet (Foscavir) 203
Furazolidone (Furoxone) 206

Ganciclovir (Cytovene) 208
Gemifloxacin (Factive) 212
Gentamicin (Garamycin) 214
Griseofulvin (Grifulvin V, Gris-Peg) 217

Halofantrine (Halfan) 219
Hydroxychloroquine – see Chloroquine phosphate

Imipenem plus Cilastatin (Primaxin) 220
Indinavir (Crixivan) 223
Interferon alpha (Infergen, ROFERON-A) 226
Iodoquinol (Yodoxin) 228
Isoniazid 230
Itraconazole (Sporanox) 232
Ivermectin (Stromectol) 236

Kanamycin (Kantrex) 238
Ketoconazole 240

Lamivudine (Epivir) 243
Lamivudine plus Abacavir (Epzicom) 246
Lamivudine plus Zidovudine (Combivir) 249
Lamivudine plus Zidovudine plus Abacavir (Trizivir) 252
Levofloxacin (Levaquin) 255

Table of Contents

Linezolid (Zyvox) 259
Lopinavir plus Ritonavir (Kaletra) 262
Loracarbef (Lorabid) 265

Maraviroc (Selzentry) 268
Mebendazole (Vermox) 271
Mefloquine hydrochloride (Lariam) 273
Meglumine antimonite (Glucantime) 275
Melarsoprol B (Mel-B) 277
Meropenem (Merrem) 279
Metronidazole (Flagyl) 282
Micafungin (Mycamine) 285
Miltefosine (Impavido, Miltex) 287
Minocycline (Dynacin, Minocin) 289
Moxifloxacin (Avelox) 292

Nafcillin 295
Nelfinavir (Viracept) 297
Neomycin (Neo-Fradin) 300
Nevirapine (Viramune) 302
Niclosamide (Yomesan) 305
Nifurtimox (Lampit) 307
Nitazoxanide (Alinia) 308
Nitrofurantoin (Furadantin, Macrobid, Macrodantin) 310
Norfloxacin (Noroxin) 312

Ofloxacin (Floxin) 315
Oseltamivir (Tamiflu) 318
Oxacillin 320
Oxamniquine (Vansil) 322

Para-aminosalicylate Sodium (PASER) 323
Peginterferon α-2A (Pegasys) 325
Peginterferon α-2B (Pegintron) 328
Penicillin (Penicillin G, Penicillin V, Penicillin G procaine, Penicillin G benzathine [Bicillin L-A, Permapen]) 331
Pentamidine (NebuPent) 337
Pentamidine (Pentam) 337
Piperacillin (Pipracil) 339
Piperacillin plus Tazobactam (Zosyn) 342

Piperazine citrate 345
Posaconazole (Noxafil) 346
Praziquantel (Biltricide) 349
Primaquine phosphate (Primaquine) 351
Pyrantel pamoate (Antiminth) 353
Pyrazinamide 354
Pyrimethamine (Daraprim) 356

Quinacrine HCl (Atabrine) 358
Quinidine 359
Quinine sulfate (Qualaquin) 361
Quinupristin plus Dalfopristin (Synercid) 364

Raltegravir (Isentress) 366
Ribavirin (Copegus, Rebetol, Ribasphere, Virazole) 368
Rifabutin (Mycobutin) 372
Rifampin (Rifadin) 375
Rifampin plus Isoniazid (Rifamate) 378
Rifampin plus Isoniazid plus Pyrazinamide (Rifater) 381
Rifapentine (Priftin) 385
Rifaximin (Xifaxan) 388
Rimantadine (Flumadine) 390
Ritonavir (Norvir) 392

Saquinavir (Invirase) 396
Spectinomycin (Trobicin) 399
Spiramycin (Rovamycine) 401
Stavudine (Zerit) 404
Stibogluconate (Pentostam) 406
Streptomycin 408
Sulfadiazine 411
Suramin sodium (Germanin) 413

Teicoplanin (Targocid) 415
Telavancin (Vibativ) 417
Telbivudine (Tyzeka) 419
Tenofovir Disoproxil Fumarate (Viread) 421
Tenofovir plus Emtricitabine (Truvada) 423
Tenofovir plus Emtricitabine plus Efavirenz (Atripla) 425
Terbinafine (Lamisil) 428

Tetracycline Hydrochloride 430
Thiabendazole (Mintezole) 433
Ticarcillin (Ticar) 435
Ticarcillin plus Clavulanate (Timentin) 438
Tigecycline (Tygacil) 441
Tinidazole (Tindamax) 443
Tipranavir (Aptivus) 446
Tobramycin 450
Trimethoprim (Proloprim) 453
Trimethoprim plus Sulfamethoxazole (Bactrim, Septra) 455
Trimetrexate glucuronate (Neutrexin) 458

Valacyclovir Hydrochloride (Valtrex) 461
Valganciclovir (Valcyte) 464
Vancomycin, IV (Vancomycin) 467
Vancomycin PO (Vancocin) 470
Voriconazole (Vfend) 472

Zanamivir (Relenza) 476
Zidovudine (Retrovir) 478

Helpful Formulas, Equations, and Definitions 481
Bibliography and References 483
Brand Name Index 485

PREFACE

We intend this book to fill a particular niche in the clinician's arsenal: it is a compilation of 188 brief chapters, each dedicated to a specific antimicrobial. A final chapter includes formulas, equations, and definitions that are useful when prescribing these agents. Each antimicrobial chapter lists the drug's class, mechanism of action, mechanism of resistance, metabolic route, indications and off-label uses, pertinent toxicities, significant drug interactions, and dosage for routine and special populations. This book does not recommend individual drugs for specific organisms or clinical syndromes; rather, it is a reference for the clinician to consult once the decision to use a particular antimicrobial has already been made.

For many agents, the toxicities and drug interactions are numerous and complex; frequently, the clinician must research several sites or even multiple locations in the drug label itself to identify significant toxicities. We have tried to organize the most frequent and important toxicities and drug interactions in a convenient, user-friendly format.

Dosage information includes the special populations of renal failure, hepatic dysfunction, pediatrics, pregnancy, and breastfeeding, and each chapter concludes with a list of clinical pearls, adding practical tips to the preceding discussion. When possible, we have used the official drug label as a primary source of information, supplemented by the various print and electronic sources in the references; further details may be sought in these resources.

In addition to FDA-approved indications, we have also listed off-label uses of selected agents; further, since many of the anti-parasitic drugs are difficult to acquire in the USA, we have supplied relevant contact information for the CDC or compounding pharmacies, when appropriate.

The Table of Contents lists the antimicrobials alphabetically by generic name followed by the brand name; a supplementary list at the end of the book sorts the drugs by brand name for alternative access. The chapter on formulas, definitions, and equations provides classifications for pregnancy risk, liver disease, formulas for computing creatinine clearance and ideal body weight or body surface area, and a discussion of the varied terminology for continuous renal replacement therapy (CRRT).

We hope this book will help the clinician navigate — in a convenient and clinically oriented format — the increasingly complex details of antimicrobial prescribing.

We gratefully acknowledge the vision, wisdom, and expertise of Martin Wonsiewicz, Linda Mehta, Christine Dodd, Michelle Quirk, and Marc Strauss.

Note: Also available combined with lamivudine as Epzicom and with both lamivudine and zidovudine as Trizivir.

BASIC CHARACTERISTICS

Class: Nucleoside reverse transcriptase inhibitor (NRTI) with activity against HIV

Mechanism of Action: Converted by cellular enzymes to its active drug, carbovir triphosphate, an analogue of guanosine triphosphate. The carbovir triphosphate competes with the naturally occurring nucleotide for incorporation in newly forming HIV DNA. Because carbovir triphosphate does not have a terminal hydroxyl group, it halts transcription and replication of the virus.

Mechanism of Resistance: Changes in the structure of HIV reverse transcriptase lead to preferred incorporation of guanosine triphosphate and decreased incorporation of carbovir triphosphate, which allows transcription of DNA to continue. Resistance mutations include L74V, K65R, and 3 "TAMS" (41L, 67N, 70R, 210W, 215F, and 219E) + M184V.

Metabolic Route: Metabolized by alcohol dehydrogenase and glucuronyl transferase into inactive metabolites that are eliminated primarily in the feces.

FDA-APPROVED INDICATIONS

Abacavir is approved to be used in combination with other antiretrovirals for the treatment of HIV infection.

SIDE EFFECTS/TOXICITY

WARNING: Hypersensitivity to abacavir can be fatal. The hypersensitivity syndrome is a multiorgan clinical syndrome with 2 or more of the following: fever, rash, gastrointestinal symptoms, constitutional symptoms, and respiratory symptoms. If hypersensitivity develops, abacavir should be discontinued immediately and never restarted. Reintroduction can lead to serious or fatal reactions. Hypersensitivity occurs in up to 8% of patients and usually occurs within the first month of initiating therapy. Determining the patient's HLA-B5701 status may screen for the risk of reaction: if HLA-B5701 test is negative, the risk of hypersensitivity is near zero; if positive, the risk is 50%.

Lactic acidosis and hepatomegaly with steatosis have been reported with nucleoside analogues, including abacavir. If this syndrome occurs, the drug should be discontinued.

Other side effects: Immune reconstitution inflammatory syndrome, fat redistribution (including central obesity and dorsocervical fat enlargement, peripheral wasting, facial wasting, and breast enlargement), gamma-glutamyl transferase elevation, and pancreatitis.

DRUG INTERACTIONS/FOOD INTERACTIONS

Abacavir can be taken with or without food and is unaffected by pH. There are no drug interactions noted with abacavir.

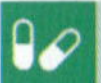

DOSING

Abacavir is administered in a 300-mg tablet or in a strawberry-banana–flavored liquid, which contains 20 mg/cc. The recommended adult dose is 300 mg twice daily or 600 mg once daily.

SPECIAL POPULATIONS

RENAL IMPAIRMENT: No dose adjustment is necessary.

HEPATIC DYSFUNCTION: Mild hepatic disease: 200 mg twice daily; avoid in patients with severe liver disease.

PEDIATRIC PATIENTS: The approved dose is 8 mg/kg twice daily up to 300 mg twice daily.

PREGNANCY: Category C.

BREASTFEEDING: It is recommended that mothers with HIV not breastfeed their children to decrease mother-to-child transmission of HIV.

THE ART OF ANTIMICROBIAL THERAPY

Clinical Pearls

1. Abacavir should be used in combination with other antiretroviral agents.
2. Abacavir is present in 3 different medications: Ziagen, Trizivir, and Epzicom.
3. An HLA-B5701 test should be done prior to starting abacavir; if positive, abacavir should be avoided.
4. If a person has suspected hypersensitivity, abacavir should not be used.

ACYCLOVIR (Zovirax)

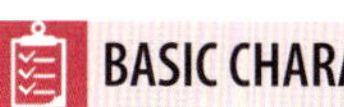

BASIC CHARACTERISTICS

Class: Nucleoside analogue

Mechanism of Action: Acyclovir is a nucleoside analogue that is phosphorylated by thymidine kinase to the active triphosphate form. Acyclovir triphosphate stops replication of herpes viral DNA in three ways:

1. competitively inhibits viral DNA polymerase,
2. incorporates into and terminates the growing viral DNA chain, and
3. inactivates the viral DNA polymerase. The greater antiviral activity of acyclovir against herpes simplex virus (HSV) compared with its activity against varicella zoster virus (VZV) is attributable to its more efficient phosphorylation by the viral thymidine kinase.

Mechanism of Resistance: Resistance of HSV and VZV to acyclovir can result from qualitative or quantitative changes in the viral thymidine kinase or DNA polymerase.

Metabolic Route: Acyclovir is metabolized to 9-[(carboxymethoxy)methyl]guanine and is excreted in the urine.

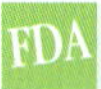

FDA-APPROVED INDICATIONS

FDA-Approved Indications: Oral acyclovir is indicated for the acute treatment of herpes zoster, initial and recurrent episodes of genital herpes, and the treatment of chickenpox.

Intravenous (IV) acyclovir is indicated for the treatment of initial and recurrent mucosal and cutaneous herpes simplex (HSV-1 and HSV-2) in immunocompromised patients, severe initial clinical episodes of herpes genitalis in immunocompetent patients, herpes simplex encephalitis, neonatal herpes infections, and VZV infections in immunocompromised patients.

SIDE EFFECTS/TOXICITY

Nausea, vomiting, and diarrhea are the most common side effects in those receiving oral acyclovir. Central nervous system side effects including confusion, ataxia, altered behavior, seizure, and coma have been seen, particularly in older adults or in patients with renal impairment. Precipitation of acyclovir in renal tubules may occur when the solubility (2.5 mg/mL) is exceeded in the intratubular fluid. This has resulted in elevated blood urea nitrogen and serum creatinine and subsequent renal failure.

Other reported adverse events include anaphylaxis, angioedema, rash including toxic epidermal necrolysis and Stevens-Johnson syndrome, fever, headache, hepatitis, diarrhea, peripheral edema, anemia, leukopenia, and thrombocytopenia.

ACYCLOVIR (Zovirax)

 DRUG INTERACTIONS/FOOD INTERACTIONS

Oral acyclovir can be administered with or without food. Coadministration of probenecid has been shown to reduce the urinary excretion and renal clearance of acyclovir.

 DOSING

Acyclovir is supplied in 200-mg capsules, 400-mg and 800-mg tablets, and a crystalline powder for solution for oral dosing and a white crystalline powder for injection.

Herpes zoster: 800 mg every 4 hours orally, five times daily for 7 to 10 days.

Genital herpes: 200 mg every 4 hours, five times daily for 10 days.

Chronic suppressive therapy for **herpes:** 400 mg twice daily or 200 mg three to five times daily.

Intermittent therapy of **HSV:** 200 mg five times daily for 5 days.

Treatment of **chickenpox:** 800 mg four times daily for 5 days.

Mucosal and cutaneous **herpes simplex:** 5 mg/kg IV every 8 hours for 7 days in immunocompromised patients.

Severe initial **herpes** genitalis: 5 mg/kg IV every 8 hours for 5 days.

Herpes simplex **encephalitis:** 10 mg/kg IV every 8 hours for 10 days.

Varicella zoster in immunocompromised patients: 10 mg/kg IV every 8 hours for 7 days.

 SPECIAL POPULATIONS

RENAL IMPAIRMENT:

For Oral Dose Adjustment

Normal Dosage/ Interval	*CrCl, mL/min*	*Adjusted Dosage/ Interval*
200 mg every 4 hours	0 to 10	200 mg every 12 hours
400 mg every 12 hrs	0 to 10	200 mg every 12 hours
800 mg five times a day	10 to 25	800 mg every 8 hours
800 mg five times a day	0 to <10	800 mg every 12 hours

For Intravenous Dose Adjustment

CrCl, mL/min	*% of Dose*	*Dosing Interval*
>50	100%	8 hours
25 to 50	100%	12 hours
10 to <25	100%	24 hours
0 to 10	50%	24 hours

Note: CrCl = Creatinine Clearance

Hemodialysis: An additional dose is administered after each dialysis.

Peritoneal dialysis: No supplemental dose appears necessary after adjustment of dosing interval.

Continuous renal replacement therapy: 5 mg/kg to 7.5 mg/kg daily.

HEPATIC DYSFUNCTION: No dosage adjustment is necessary.

PEDIATRIC PATIENTS:

- **Chickenpox:** Children aged 2 years and older: 20 mg/kg per dose orally four times daily (80 mg/kg/day) for 5 days. Children who weigh more than 40 kg should receive the adult dosage.
- Mucosal and cutaneous **herpes simplex:** 10 mg/kg IV every 8 hours for 7 days in immunocompromised patients (aged younger than 12 years).
- **Herpes simplex encephalitis:** Children aged 3 months to 12 years: 20 mg/kg IV every 8 hours for 10 days.
- **Neonatal herpes** (birth to age 3 months): 10 mg/kg IV up to 20 mg/kg every 8 hours for 10 days
- **Varicella zoster** in immunocompromised patients (aged younger than 12 years): 20 mg/kg IV every 8 hours for 7 days.

PREGNANCY: Category B.

BREASTFEEDING: Acyclovir may be administered with caution to breastfeeding mothers.

THE ART OF ANTIMICROBIAL THERAPY

Clinical Pearls

1. Acyclovir dosage should be based on ideal body weight.
2. Acyclovir is effective against HSV and VZV. It has no activity against the other herpesviruses.
3. Oral acyclovir is not recommended for children aged younger than 2 years; intravenous acyclovir is recommended in this age group.
4. Acyclovir can cause confusion or renal insufficiency.

BASIC CHARACTERISTICS

Class: Nucleotide reverse transcriptase inhibitor.

Mechanism of Action: Adefovir is an acyclic nucleotide analogue of adenosine monophosphate, which is phosphorylated to the active metabolite adefovir diphosphate by cellular kinases. Adefovir diphosphate inhibits hepatitis B virus (HBV) DNA polymerase by competing with the natural substrate deoxyadenosine triphosphate and by causing DNA chain termination after its incorporation into viral DNA.

Mechanism of Resistance: Amino acid substitutions rtN236T and rtA181T/V have been observed in association with adefovir resistance, leading to decreased incorporation of adefovir diphosphate.

Metabolic Route: Adefovir dipivoxil is rapidly converted to adefovir. Adefovir is renally excreted by a combination of glomerular filtration and active tubular secretion.

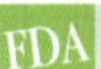

FDA-APPROVED INDICATIONS

FDA-Approved Indications: Treatment of chronic hepatitis B with evidence of active viral replication and either evidence of persistent elevations in serum aminotransferases (ALT or AST) or histologically active disease.

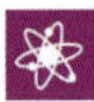

SIDE EFFECTS/TOXICITY

WARNING: Severe acute exacerbation of hepatitis has been reported in patients who have discontinued anti–hepatitis B therapy, including therapy with adefovir. Hepatic function should be monitored for at least several months in patients who discontinue adefovir. Chronic administration of adefovir may result in delayed **nephrotoxicity**. Prior to initiating adefovir therapy, HIV antibody testing should be offered. Treatment with adefovir may result in emergence of HIV resistance. **Lactic acidosis and severe hepatomegaly** with steatosis, including fatal cases, have been reported with the use of nucleoside analogues alone or in combination with antiretrovirals. Treatment with adefovir should be suspended in any patient who develops clinical or laboratory findings suggestive of lactic acidosis or pronounced hepatotoxicity (which may include hepatomegaly and steatosis even in the absence of marked transaminase elevations).

Other side effects: Possible additional adverse effects include hypophosphatemia, myopathy, osteomalacia, proximal renal tubulopathy, and Fanconi's syndrome.

DRUG INTERACTIONS/FOOD INTERACTIONS

Adefovir may be taken without regard to food. Patients should be monitored closely for adverse events when adefovir is coadministered with drugs that are excreted renally or with other drugs known to affect renal function.

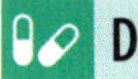

DOSING

Adefovir is available in a 10 mg tablet of adefovir dipivoxil. The recommended dose is 10 mg once daily.

SPECIAL POPULATIONS

RENAL IMPAIRMENT:

Creatinine Clearance, mL/min	*Dosage*
>50	10 mg daily
30–49	10 mg every 48 hours
10–29	10 mg every 72 hours

Hemodialysis (HD): 10 mg every week postdialysis.

HEPATIC DYSFUNCTION: Caution should be used when adefovir is administered to those with hepatic impairment.

PEDIATRIC PATIENTS: Adefovir is contraindicated in children aged younger than 12 years.

PREGNANCY: Category C.

BREASTFEEDING: It is not known whether adefovir is secreted in human milk or if it can harm a breastfeeding infant. Therefore, a decision should be made whether to discontinue breastfeeding or drug.

THE ART OF ANTIMICROBIAL THERAPY

Clinical Pearls

1. To reduce the risk of resistance in patients with lamivudine-resistant HBV, adefovir dipivoxil should be used in combination with lamivudine and not as adefovir dipivoxil monotherapy.
2. All patients should be tested for HIV before initiating adefovir.
3. Renal function must be monitored closely in those receiving adefovir.
4. Hepatic function should be monitored for at least several months after discontinuing adefovir.

ALBENDAZOLE (Albenza)

BASIC CHARACTERISTICS

Class: Broad-spectrum anthelminthic

Mechanism of Action: Inhibits tubulin polymerization, resulting in loss of cytoplasmic microtubules.

Metabolic Route: Albendazole is converted in the liver to albendazole sulfoxide and is excreted in the feces.

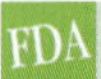

FDA-APPROVED INDICATIONS

FDA-Approved Indications: Treatment of the larval forms of *Echinococcus granulosus* and *Taenia solium.*

Also Used For: *Ancyclostomiasis,* ascariasis, cutaneous larva migrans, *Enterobius vermicularis, Clonorchis sinensis,* gnathostomiasis, hookworm, microsporidiosis, strongyloidiasis, trichinellosis, trichuriasis, and visceral larva migrans.

SIDE EFFECTS/TOXICITY

Side effects include granulocytopenia, agranulocytosis, and pancytopenia; increased hepatic enzymes in more than 15% of patients.

DRUG INTERACTIONS/FOOD INTERACTIONS

Albendazole should be administered with food.

Albendazole induces the cytochrome P450-1A enzymes and should be given with caution when used with theophylline, cimetidine, dexamethasone, and praziquantel.

DOSING

Albendazole is administered in 200-mg tablets.

Hydatid disease: 400 mg twice daily with meals for 28 days, followed by 14 days without treatment. This cycle is repeated twice to complete three cycles.

Neurocysticercosis: 400 mg twice daily with meals given for 8 to 30 days. For those who weigh less than 60 kg, the dose is 15 mg/kg/day in divided doses with a maximum of 800 mg daily dose.

***Ancyclostomiasis*:** 400 mg for 1 dose.

Ascariasis: 400 mg for 1 dose.

***Clonorchiasis*:** 10 mg/kg once daily for 7 days.

Cutaneous larva migrans: 400 mg once daily for 3 days.

Enterobiasis: 400 mg for 1 dose.

Gnathostomiasis: 400 mg twice daily for 21 days.

Hookworm: 400 mg for 1 dose.

Microsporidiosis: 400 mg twice in 1 day.

Strongyloidiasis: 400 mg for 1 dose.

Trichinellosis: 400 mg twice daily for 14 days.

Trichuriasis: 400 mg for 1 dose.

Visceral larva migrans: 400 mg twice daily for 5 days.

SPECIAL POPULATIONS

RENAL IMPAIRMENT: There is no dosage adjustment for patients with renal impairment.

HEPATIC DYSFUNCTION: There are increases in levels of albendazole in those with extrahepatic obstruction, though no dosage adjustment is necessary.

PEDIATRIC PATIENTS: 15 mg/kg/day, divided in two doses.

PREGNANCY: Category C.

BREASTFEEDING: Caution should be exercised when albendazole is given to breastfeeding mothers.

THE ART OF ANTIMICROBIAL THERAPY

Clinical Pearls

1. In the treatment of neurocysticercosis, steroids should be given before the albendazole is administered.
2. Albendazole should be given with food.
3. For children, the pill should be crushed because children often have trouble swallowing the tablet.
4. Complete blood count and liver function tests should be performed every 2 weeks while the patient is on therapy.

BASIC CHARACTERISTICS

Class: Adamantanamine

Mechanism of Action: Inhibits the ion channels of the M2 protein of influenza A, and inhibits viral uncoating during endocytosis.

Mechanism of Resistance: Mutations in the transmembrane region of the M2 protein lead to high-level resistance.

Metabolic Route: Amantadine is well absorbed orally and is excreted unchanged in the urine.

FDA-APPROVED INDICATIONS

FDA-Approved Indications: Prophylaxis and treatment of influenza A.

Also Used For: Parkinson's disease.

SIDE EFFECTS/TOXICITY

Most frequent: nausea, dizziness, and insomnia. Also: depression, anxiety, irritability, seizures, congestive heart failure, dry mouth, constipation, dry nose, blurred vision, and urinary retention.

Avoid in patients with angle closure glaucoma.

Neuroleptic malignant syndrome has been seen following dosage reduction.

DRUG INTERACTIONS/FOOD INTERACTIONS

Data are inadequate regarding effect of food. Other medications with anticholinergic effects should be used with caution with amantadine. Careful observation is required when amantadine is used with central nervous system stimulants; alcohol should be avoided. Quinine or quinidine reduces the renal clearance of amantadine.

DOSING

Recommended dosage is 200 mg daily.

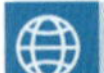

SPECIAL POPULATIONS

RENAL IMPAIRMENT:

CrCl Measurement/Hemodialysis	*Dosage*
30 mL/min to 50 mL/min	200 mg first day and 100 mg daily thereafter

CrCl Measurement/Hemodialysis	*Dosage*
15 mL/min to 29 mL/min	200 mg first day followed by 100 mg on alternate days
<15 mL/min	200 mg weekly
Hemodialysis	200 mg weekly

Note: CrCl = Creatinine Clearance

HEPATIC DYSFUNCTION: Caution should be used when amantadine is administered to those with hepatic impairment.

PEDIATRIC PATIENTS: Amantadine is not recommended for neonates or those aged younger than 1 year. After 1 year of age, amantadine is given 4.4 mg/kg/day, not to exceed 150 mg/day.

PREGNANCY: Category C.

BREASTFEEDING: The use of amantadine is not recommended for breastfeeding mothers.

THE ART OF ANTIMICROBIAL THERAPY

Clinical Pearls

1. Amantadine does not have activity against influenza B or novel H1N1 influenza.
2. Viruses resistant to amantadine are also resistant to rimantadine.
3. Amantadine may be effective in Parkinson's disease.
4. Amantidine should be avoided in patients with angle closure glaucoma.

 BASIC CHARACTERISTICS

Class: Aminoglycoside

Mechanisms of Action:

1. Rearranges lipopolysaccharide in the outer membrane of the bacterial cell wall, resulting in disruption of the cell wall, and
2. binds the 30S subunit of the bacterial ribosome, which terminates protein synthesis.

Mechanisms of Resistance:

1. Gram-negative bacteria inactivate aminoglycosides by acetylation,
2. some bacteria alter the 30S ribosomal subunit, which prevents amikacin's interference with protein synthesis, and
3. low-level resistance may result from inhibition of amikacin uptake by the bacteria.

Metabolic Route: Amikacin is excreted unchanged in the urine.

FDA FDA-APPROVED INDICATIONS

FDA-Approved Indications: Treatment of susceptible gram-negative bacteria causing bacteremia, pneumonia, osteomyelitis, arthritis, meningitis, skin and skin structure infection, intraabdominal infections, in burns and postoperative infections, and urinary tract infections.

Also Used For: *Mycobacterium tuberculosis, Mycobacterium avium intracellulare* lung disease, *Nocardia*, combination therapy with β-lactams for the treatment of gram-positive endovascular infections.

 SIDE EFFECTS/TOXICITY

WARNINGS: Ototoxicity: vestibular toxicity and auditory ototoxicity, especially in patients with renal damage, those treated with higher doses, and those with prolonged treatment. Avoid use with potent diuretics such as ethacrynic acid because of additive ototoxicity. **Nephrotoxicity**: especially in patients with impaired renal function and those treated with higher doses or prolonged treatment. Avoid concurrent use with other nephrotoxic agents and potent diuretics, which can cause dehydration. **Neuromuscular blockade**: especially in those receiving anesthetics, neuromuscular blocking agents, or massive transfusions.

Other side effects: Other adverse effects include rash, fever, headache, paresthesia, tremor, nausea and vomiting, eosinophilia, arthralgia, anemia, hypotension, and hypomagnesemia. Macular infarction sometimes leading to permanent loss of vision has been reported following intravitreous administration (injection into the eye) of amikacin.

DRUG INTERACTIONS

Amikacin should not be administered with other medications that are nephrotoxic or ototoxic.

DOSING

Total dose: 15 mg/kg/day intramuscularly or intravenously (IV), either once daily or in divided doses every 8 to 12 hours.

Intrathecal dose: 10 mg to 40 mg every 24 hours.

Dosing for treatment of tuberculosis (all doses once daily): Adults 15 mg/kg/day; 60 years and older 10 mg/kg/day, with maximum dose of 750 mg. Children 15-30 mg/kg/day.

Renal failure: 12-15 mg/kg/dose, 2-3 times per week.

SPECIAL POPULATIONS

RENAL IMPAIRMENT: Adjust dosage either by increased interval (serum creatinine multiplied by 9, based on every-12-hour dosing, or usual dose every 24 hours for CrCl 10-50 and every 48 hours for CrCl less than or equal to 10), or by lowering the dose by multiplying the dose by the ratio of observed creatinine clearance to normal creatinine clearance. With either approach, give initial dose as for normal renal function, and then adjust by following serum assays with the goal of peak 56 μg/mL to 64 μg/mL, and trough less than 1 μg/mL.

HEMODIALYSIS: One-half of normal renal function dose after hemodialysis, then adjust by serum levels.

PERITONEAL DIALYSIS: 15-20 mg/L lost in dialysate daily and should be replaced.

CONTINUOUS RENAL REPLACEMENT THERAPY: 10 mg/kg loading dose followed by 7.5 mg/kg every 24 to 48 hours.

HEPATIC DYSFUNCTION: No dosage adjustment necessary.

PEDIATRIC PATIENTS: 15 mg/kg/day, in divided doses every 8-12 hours. Amikacin should be used with caution in premature and neonatal infants because of renal immaturity and prolonged half-life.

PREGNANCY: Category D

BREASTFEEDING: It is not known if amikacin is secreted in human milk.

THE ART OF ANTIMICROBIAL THERAPY

Clinical Pearls

1. Amikacin is more likely to be active against gram-negative rods compared with the other aminoglycosides.
2. Aminoglycosides require oxygen to be active and thus are less effective in anaerobic environments such as an abscess or infected bone.
3. Aminoglycosides have decreased activity in low-pH environments such as respiratory secretions or abscesses.
4. When dosing aminoglycosides, use the ideal body weight, not true body weight.
5. Amikacin has a postantibiotic effect that allows it to be used once daily.
6. Aminoglycosides are concentration-dependent, and, therefore, are more effective if given at longer intervals and with higher doses. For example, giving amikacin at 15 mg/kg per day may be more effective than 5 mg/kg every 8 hours.
7. Intravenous dose should be infused over 60 minutes to avoid neuromuscular blockade.

AMOXICILLIN (Amoxil)

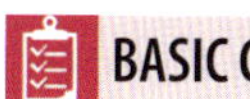

BASIC CHARACTERISTICS

Class: Aminopenicillin

Mechanism of Action: Binds penicillin-binding protein (PBP), disrupting cell wall synthesis.

Mechanisms of Resistance:

1. The PBP can be altered, with reduced affinity,
2. production of a β-lactamase resulting in hydrolysis of the β-lactam ring, and
3. decreased ability of the antibiotic to reach the penicillin-binding protein when bacteria decrease porin production, resulting in a decrease of the drug concentration within the cell.

Metabolic Route: Amoxicillin is excreted unchanged in urine.

FDA-APPROVED INDICATIONS

FDA-Approved Indications: Treatment of the following infections caused by susceptible (only β-lactamase–negative) strains of microorganisms: ear, nose, and throat; genitourinary tract, skin and skin structure, and lower respiratory tract.

Treatment of gonorrhea, acute uncomplicated (anogenital and urethral infections).

Helicobacter pylori eradication: triple therapy (amoxicillin plus clarithromycin plus lansoprazole); or dual therapy (amoxicillin plus lansoprazole).

SIDE EFFECTS/TOXICITY

A history of allergic reaction to any of the penicillins is a **contraindication.**

Side effects include *Clostridium difficile*–associated diarrhea; mucocutaneous candidiasis; nausea; vomiting; diarrhea; black hairy tongue; hypersensitivity reactions including rashes, erythema multiforme, and Stevens-Johnson syndrome; rise in aspartate transaminase (SGOT) and/or alanine transaminase (SGPT); crystalluria; anemia; thrombocytopenia; eosinophilia; leukopenia; hyperactivity; and convulsions.

DRUG INTERACTIONS/FOOD INTERACTIONS

Amoxicillin capsules, chewable tablets, and oral suspensions may be given without regard to meals. Concurrent use of amoxicillin and probenecid may result in increased and prolonged blood levels of amoxicillin. Chloramphenicol, macrolides, sulfonamides, and tetracyclines may interfere with the bactericidal effects of penicillins. High urine concentrations of amoxicillin may result in false-positive reactions when one is testing for the presence of glucose in urine with Clinitest; it is recommended that glucose tests based on enzymatic glucose oxidase reactions (such as Clinistix) be used instead.

AMOXICILLIN (Amoxil)

DOSING

Each capsule contains 250 mg or 500 mg; each tablet contains 500 mg or 875 mg; each chewable tablet contains 125 mg, 200 mg, 250 mg, or 400 mg; the oral suspension contains 200 mg/5 mL or 400 mg/5 mL.

Infection	*Dosage*
Ear/nose/throat (mild/moderate)	500 mg every 12 hours or 250 mg every 8 hours
Ear/nose/throat (severe)	875 mg every 12 hours or 500 mg every 8 hours
Lower respiratory tract	875 mg every 12 hours or 500 mg every 8 hours
Skin/skin structure (mild/moderate)	500 mg every 12 hours or 250 mg every 8 hours
Skin/skin structure (severe)	875 mg every 12 hours or 500 mg every 8 hours
Genitourinary (mild/moderate)	500 mg every 12 hours or 250 mg every 8 hours
Genitourinary (severe)	875 mg every 12 hours or 500 mg every 8 hours
H. pylori eradication	1 g amoxicillin, 500 mg clarithromycin, and 30 mg lansoprazole, all given twice daily (every 12 hours) for 14 days **or** 1 g amoxicillin and 30 mg lansoprazole, each given three times daily (every 8 hours) for 14 days

SPECIAL POPULATIONS

RENAL IMPAIRMENT:

Patients with a glomerular filtration rate of <30 mL/minute should not receive the 875-mg tablet.

Creatinine Clearance	*Dosage*
10 mL/min to 30 mL/min	250 mg to 500 mg every 12 hours
<10 mL/min	250 mg to 500 mg daily
Hemodialysis	250 mg to 500 mg every 24 hours and an additional dose after dialysis
Chronic ambulatory peritoneal dialysis	250 mg every 12 hours
Continuous renal replacement therapy	N/A

HEPATIC DYSFUNCTION: No dosage adjustment is necessary.

PEDIATRIC PATIENTS:

- **Neonates and infants aged 12 weeks or younger (3 months or younger):** The recommended upper dose of amoxicillin is 30 mg/kg/day in divided doses every 12 hours.
- **Pediatric patients aged older than 3 months:** 25 mg/kg/day to 45 mg/kg/day in divided doses every 12 hours **or** 20 mg/kg/day to 40 mg/kg/day in divided doses every 8 hours, depending on severity of infection.

PREGNANCY: Category B.

BREASTFEEDING: Amoxicillin should be used only with caution in breastfeeding mothers.

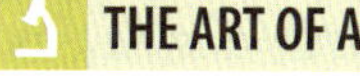

THE ART OF ANTIMICROBIAL THERAPY

Clinical Pearls

1. Dosage of amoxicillin needs to be adjusted for patients with renal dysfunction.
2. Patients with mononucleosis who receive amoxicillin may develop an erythematous rash.

AMOXICILLIN PLUS CLAVULANATE POTASSIUM (Augmentin, Augmentin ES-600, Augmentin XR)

BASIC CHARACTERISTICS

Class: Aminopenicillin plus a β-lactamase inhibitor

Mechanism of Action: Binds penicillin-binding protein, disrupting cell wall synthesis.

Mechanisms of Resistance:

1. The penicillin-binding protein (PBP) can be altered, with reduced affinity, and
2. decreased ability of the antibiotic to reach the PBP when bacteria decrease porin production, resulting in a decrease of the drug concentration within the cell.

Metabolic Route: Amoxicillin and clavulanate are excreted unchanged in the urine.

FDA FDA-APPROVED INDICATIONS

FDA-Approved Indications: (1) **Augmentin**: Treatment of infections caused by susceptible strains of microorganisms in lower respiratory tract infections, otitis media, sinusitis, skin and skin structure infections, and urinary tract infections. (2) **Augmentin ES-600**: Treatment of **pediatric patients** with recurrent or persistent acute otitis media. (3) **Augmentin XR:** Treatment of adults with community-acquired pneumonia or acute bacterial sinusitis.

SIDE EFFECTS/TOXICITY

A history of allergic reaction to any of the penicillins is a **contraindication.**

Side effects include *Clostridium difficile*–associated diarrhea; hypersensitivity reactions including rashes, erythema multiforme, toxic epidermal necrolysis, and Stevens-Johnson syndrome; nausea; vomiting; diarrhea; hepatic and renal dysfunction; crystalluria; anemia; thrombocytopenia; eosinophilia; leukopenia; hyperactivity; and seizures.

DRUG INTERACTIONS/FOOD INTERACTIONS

Augmentin capsules may be given without regard to meals. Augmentin XR should be taken at the start of the meal. Concurrent use of amoxicillin plus clavulanate potassium and probenecid may result in increased and prolonged blood levels of amoxicillin.

Chloramphenicol, macrolides, sulfonamides, and tetracyclines may interfere with the bactericidal effects of penicillins. Amoxicillin plus clavulanate potassium may reduce the efficacy of oral contraceptives. High urine concentrations of amoxicillin may result in false-positive reactions when one is testing for the presence of glucose in urine with Clinitest; it is recommended that glucose tests based on enzymatic glucose oxidase reactions (such as Clinistix) be used instead.

DOSING (Augmentin and Augmentin XR)

Augmentin

Augmentin is supplied in multiple formulations as follows:

Dosage and Formulation	*Amoxicillin*	*Clavulanate*
250-mg tablet	250 mg	125 mg
500-mg tablet	500 mg	125 mg
875-mg tablet	875 mg	125 mg
125-mg chewable tablet	125 mg	31.25 mg
200-mg chewable tablet	200 mg	28.5 mg
250-mg chewable tablet	250 mg	62.5 mg
400-mg chewable tablet	400 mg	57.0 mg
125 mg/5 mL	125 mg	31.25 mg
200 mg/5 mL	200 mg	28.5 mg
250 mg/5 mL	250 mg	62.5 mg
400 mg/5 mL	400 mg	57.0 mg

The usual adult dose is one 500-mg tablet every 12 hours or one 250-mg tablet every 8 hours.

For severe infections and infections of the respiratory tract, the dose should be one 875-mg tablet every 12 hours or one 500-mg tablet every 8 hours.

Augmentin XR

Augmentin XR is supplied as a 1-g/67.5-mg tablet and the recommended dose is two tablets every 12 hours.

SPECIAL POPULATIONS

RENAL IMPAIRMENT:

Augmentin

Creatinine Clearance	*Dosage*
10 mL/min to 30 mL/min	250 mg to 500 mg every 12 hours
<10 mL/min	250 mg to 500 mg every 24 hours
Hemodialysis	250 mg to 500 mg every 24 hours and an additional dose during and at the end of dialysis
Chronic ambulatory peritoneal dialysis	No recommendation

Augmentin XR and Augmentin 875 mg are contraindicated in patients with a creatinine clearance of less than 30 mL/min and in hemodialysis patients.

HEPATIC DYSFUNCTION: No dosage adjustment, but use with caution.

PEDIATRIC PATIENTS:

Augmentin: Neonates and infants aged younger than 12 weeks: 30 mg/kg/day in divided doses every 12 hours, based on the amoxicillin component. The 200 mg/5 mL formulation is not recommended in this age group.

Augmentin: Patients Aged 12 Weeks (3 Months) and Older:

Infection	*Dosage*[a,b]
Otitis media, sinusitis	45 mg/kg every 12 hours[c] or 40 mg/kg every 8 hours[d]
Lower respiratory infections	45 mg/kg every 12 hours[c] or 40 mg/kg every 8 hours[d]
Less severe infections	25 mg/kg every 12 hours[c] or 20 mg/kg every 8 hours[d]

[a]The every-12-hours regimen is associated with less diarrhea.

[b]Pediatric patients weighing 40 kg and more should be dosed following adult dosages.

[c]Use the 200 mg/5 mL or 400 mg/5 mL formulations for this dosage.

[d]Use the 125 mg/5 mL or 250 mg/5 mL formulations for this dosage.

Augmentin ES-600: Supplied as a suspension with 600 mg amoxicillin and 42.9 mg of clavulanate per 5 mL.

Pediatric patients aged 3 months and older: The recommended dosage is 45 mg/kg every 12 hours, administered for 10 days. For pediatric patients weighing 40 kg and more, follow the Augmentin adult dosing recommendation.

Augmentin XR: Safety and effectiveness in pediatric patients aged younger than 16 years have not been established.

PREGNANCY: Category B.

BREASTFEEDING: Amoxicillin plus clavulanate potassium should be used only with caution in breastfeeding mothers.

THE ART OF ANTIMICROBIAL THERAPY

Clinical Pearls

1. Dosage of amoxicillin plus clavulanate potassium needs to be adjusted for renal dysfunction.
2. Augmentin XR and Augmentin 875 mg are contraindicated in patients with a creatinine clearance of less than 30 mL/min and in hemodialysis patients.
3. Augmentin XR is not recommended for patients aged younger than 16 years.

4. Augmentin ES-600 is recommended only for children.
5. The 400- and 200-mg suspension formulations contain aspartame.
6. A high percentage of patients with mononucleosis who receive ampicillin develop an erythematous rash. Thus, ampicillin-class antibiotics (e.g., amoxicillin) should not be administered to patients with mononucleosis.
7. Amoxicillin plus clavulanate potassium should be used with caution in patients with evidence of hepatic dysfunction.

AMPHOTERICIN B, LIPOSOMAL (Ambisome)

BASIC CHARACTERISTICS

Class: Lyophilized polyene

Mechanisms of Action:

1. Inserts into the cytoplasmic membrane through ergosterol leading to increased permeability of the fungal membrane and loss of intracellular ions, and
2. affects oxidation and may cause fungal death in this manner.

Mechanism of Resistance: Resistance is rare, but is caused by changes in the cell membrane that prevent amphotericin B from inserting into the membrane.

Metabolic Route: Details of possible metabolic pathways are not known.

FDA FDA-APPROVED INDICATIONS

FDA-Approved Indications: Empirical therapy for presumed fungal infection in febrile, neutropenic patients.

Cryptococcal meningitis in HIV-infected patients; *Aspergillus, Candida,* or *Cryptococcus* species infections refractory to amphotericin B deoxycholate, or in patients where renal impairment or unacceptable toxicity precludes the use of amphotericin B deoxycholate; visceral leishmaniasis.

SIDE EFFECTS/TOXICITY

Side effects/toxicities are similar to those seen with amphotericin B deoxycholate but tend to be less frequent or less severe.

Contraindicated in patients who have shown hypersensitivity to amphotericin B or any other component in the formulation.

Acute reactions including fever, shaking chills, hypotension, anorexia, nausea, vomiting, headache, and tachypnea are common 1 to 3 hours after starting an intravenous infusion. Rapid intravenous infusion has been associated with hypotension, hypokalemia, arrhythmias, and shock and should, therefore, be avoided.

Amphotericin B should be used with care in patients with reduced renal function; frequent monitoring of renal function is recommended.

Because acute pulmonary reactions have been reported in patients given amphotericin B during or shortly after leukocyte transfusions, it is advisable to temporally separate these infusions as far as possible and to monitor pulmonary function.

Leukoencephalopathy has been reported following use of amphotericin B.

DRUG INTERACTIONS/FOOD INTERACTIONS

Antineoplastic agents may enhance the potential for renal toxicity, bronchospasm, and hypotension and should be given concomitantly only with great caution.

Corticosteroids and corticotropin (ACTH): Closely monitor serum electrolytes and cardiac function.

Digitalis glycosides: Amphotericin B–induced hypokalemia may potentiate digitalis toxicity.

Flucytosine: Concomitant use may increase the toxicity of flucytosine.

Imidazoles (e.g., fluconazole) may induce fungal resistance to amphotericin B. Combination therapy should be administered with caution.

Other nephrotoxic medications may enhance the potential for drug-induced renal toxicity, and should be used concomitantly only with great caution.

Skeletal muscle relaxants: Amphotericin B–induced hypokalemia may enhance the curariform effect of skeletal muscle relaxants.

Leukocyte transfusions: Acute pulmonary toxicity has been reported in patients receiving intravenous amphotericin B and leukocyte transfusions.

DOSING

Indication	*Dosage*
Empirical therapy	3 mg/kg/day
Systemic fungal infection	3 mg/kg/day to 5 mg/kg/day
Cryptococcal meningitis	6 mg/kg/day
Visceral leishmaniasis (immunocompetent)	3 mg/kg/day for 5 days, then again on days 14 and 21
Visceral leishmaniasis (immunocompromised)	4 mg/kg/day for 5 days, then again on days 10, 17, 24, 31, and 38

SPECIAL POPULATIONS

RENAL IMPAIRMENT: Monitor renal function closely. No dosage adjustment recommended for renal impairment or for dialysis.

HEPATIC IMPAIRMENT: Liver tests should be monitored routinely.

PEDIATRICS: Use similar dosage as adults.

PREGNANCY: Category B.

BREASTFEEDING: Discontinue breastfeeding or discontinue the drug.

THE ART OF ANTIMICROBIAL THERAPY

Clinical Pearls

1. There are various forms of amphotericin B with many important differences: amphotericin B deoxycholate, amphotericin B colloidal dispersion, amphotericin B lipid complex, and liposomal amphotericin B. This section pertains only to liposomal amphotericin B. **Side effects with liposomal amphotericin B are similar to those seen with amphotericin B deoxycholate but tend to be less frequent or less severe.**
2. Premedication with acetaminophen, diphenhydramine, meperidine, and even hydrocortisone can decrease infusion-related toxicity.
3. Hydration and sodium repletion prior to amphotericin B administration may reduce the risk of the patient developing nephrotoxicity.
4. *Candida lusitaniae, Pseudallescheria boydii,* and *Fusarium* species are often resistant to amphotericin B. Voriconazole is frequently used for these infections.
5. It is advisable to monitor on a regular basis liver function, serum electrolytes (particularly magnesium and potassium), blood counts, and hemoglobin concentrations.

AMPHOTERICIN B COLLOIDAL DISPERSION (Amphotec)

BASIC CHARACTERISTICS

Class: Polyene

Mechanisms of Action:

1. Inserts into the cytoplasmic membrane through ergosterol leading to increased permeability of the fungal membrane and loss of intracellular ions, and
2. affects oxidation and may cause fungal death in this manner.

Mechanism of Resistance: Resistance is rare, but is caused by changes in the cell membrane that prevent amphotericin B from inserting into the membrane.

Metabolic Route: Details of possible metabolic pathways are not known.

FDA-APPROVED INDICATIONS

FDA-Approved Indications: Treatment of invasive aspergillosis in patients where renal impairment or unacceptable toxicity precludes the use of amphotericin B deoxycholate in effective doses, and in patients with invasive aspergillosis where prior amphotericin B deoxycholate therapy has failed.

SIDE EFFECTS/TOXICITY

Contraindicated in patients who have shown hypersensitivity to amphotericin B or any other component in the formulation. Acute reactions including fever, shaking chills, hypotension, anorexia, nausea, vomiting, headache, and tachypnea are common 1 to 3 hours after starting an intravenous infusion. Rapid intravenous infusion has been associated with hypotension, hypokalemia, arrhythmias, and shock and should, therefore, be avoided.

Other side effects: Amphotericin B should be used with care in patients with reduced renal function; frequent monitoring of renal function is recommended.

Because acute pulmonary reactions have been reported in patients given amphotericin B during or shortly after leukocyte transfusions, it is advisable to temporally separate these infusions as far as possible and to monitor pulmonary function. Leukoencephalopathy has been reported following use of amphotericin B.

DRUG INTERACTIONS/FOOD INTERACTIONS

Antineoplastic agents may enhance the potential for renal toxicity, bronchospasm, and hypotension and should be given concomitantly only with great caution.

Corticosteroids and Corticotropin (ACTH): closely monitor serum electrolytes and cardiac function.

Digitalis glycosides: amphotericin B–induced hypokalemia may potentiate digitalis toxicity.

Flucytosine: concomitant use may increase the toxicity of flucytosine.

Imidazoles (e.g., fluconazole) may induce fungal resistance to amphotericin B. Combination therapy should be administered with caution.

Other nephrotoxic medications may enhance the potential for drug-induced renal toxicity, and should be used concomitantly only with great caution.

Skeletal muscle relaxants: amphotericin B–induced hypokalemia may enhance the curariform effect of skeletal muscle relaxants.

Leukocyte transfusions: acute pulmonary toxicity has been reported in patients receiving intravenous amphotericin B and leukocyte transfusions.

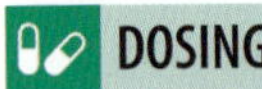

DOSING

Recommended dosage is 3 mg/kg to 4 mg/kg once a day IV.

SPECIAL POPULATIONS

RENAL IMPAIRMENT: Monitor renal function closely. No dosage adjustment recommended for renal impairment or for dialysis.

HEPATIC IMPAIRMENT: Liver tests should be monitored routinely.

PEDIATRIC PATIENTS: Doses (mg/kg) similar to those given to adults.

PREGNANCY: Category B.

BREASTFEEDING: Data insufficient; it is prudent to advise a breastfeeding mother to discontinue breastfeeding.

THE ART OF ANTIMICROBIAL THERAPY

Clinical Pearls

1. There are various forms of amphotericin B with many important differences: amphotericin B deoxycholate, amphotericin B colloidal dispersion, amphotericin B lipid complex, and liposomal amphotericin B. This section pertains only to amphotericin B colloidal dispersion.
2. Premedication with acetaminophen, diphenhydramine, meperidine, and even hydrocortisone can decrease infusion-related toxicity.
3. Hydration and sodium repletion prior to amphotericin B administration may reduce the risk of developing nephrotoxicity.
4. *Candida lusitaniae, Pseudallescheria boydii,* and *Fusarium* species are often resistant to amphotericin B. Voriconazole is frequently used for these infections.
5. It is advisable to monitor on a regular basis liver function, serum electrolytes (particularly magnesium and potassium), blood counts, and hemoglobin concentrations.

AMPHOTERICIN B DEOXYCHOLATE (Fungizone)

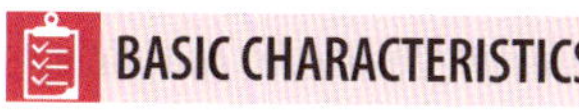

BASIC CHARACTERISTICS

Class: Polyene

Mechanism of Action:

1. Inserts into the cytoplasmic membrane through ergosterol leading to increased permeability of the fungal membrane and loss of intracellular ions, and
2. affects oxidation and may cause fungal death in this manner.

Mechanism of Resistance: Resistance is rare, but is caused by changes in the cell membrane that prevent amphotericin B from inserting into the membrane.

Metabolic Route: Amphotericin B is excreted very slowly by the kidneys. After discontinuation of treatment, amphotericin B is detectable in urine for at least 7 weeks.

FDA FDA-Approved Indications

Treatment of potentially life-threatening fungal infections: aspergillosis, cryptococcosis, blastomycosis, systemic candidiasis, coccidioidomycosis, histoplasmosis, zygomycosis, and sporotrichosis, and infections caused by related susceptible species of *Conidiobolus* and *Basidiobolus*.

Also Used for: Treatment of American mucocutaneous leishmaniasis, but it is not the drug of choice as primary therapy.

SIDE EFFECTS/TOXICITY

> **WARNING:** This drug should be used *primarily* for treatment of patients with progressive and potentially life-threatening fungal infections; it should not be used to treat noninvasive forms of fungal disease such as oral thrush, vaginal candidiasis, and esophageal candidiasis in patients with normal neutrophil counts.

Amphotericin B should not be given in doses greater than 1.5 mg/kg.

Exercise caution to prevent inadvertent overdosage, which may result in potentially fatal cardiac or cardiopulmonary arrest. Verify the product name and dosage if dose exceeds 1.5 mg/kg.

Contraindicated in patients who have shown hypersensitivity to amphotericin B or any other component in the formulation.

Acute reactions including fever, shaking chills, hypotension, anorexia, nausea, vomiting, headache, and tachypnea are common 1 to 3 hours after starting an intravenous infusion. Rapid intravenous infusion has been associated with hypotension, hypokalemia, arrhythmias, and shock and should, therefore, be avoided.

Amphotericin B should be used with care in patients with reduced renal function; frequent monitoring of renal function is recommended.

Other side effects: Because acute pulmonary reactions have been reported in patients given amphotericin B during or shortly after leukocyte transfusions, it is advisable to temporally separate these infusions as far as possible and to monitor pulmonary function. Leukoencephalopathy has been reported following use of amphotericin B.

DRUG INTERACTIONS

Antineoplastic agents may enhance the potential for renal toxicity, bronchospasm, and hypotension and should be given concomitantly only with great caution.

Corticosteroids and corticotropin (ACTH): closely monitor serum electrolytes and cardiac function.

Digitalis glycosides: amphotericin B–induced hypokalemia may potentiate digitalis toxicity.

Flucytosine: concomitant use may increase the toxicity of flucytosine.

Imidazoles (e.g., fluconazole) may induce fungal resistance to amphotericin B. Combination therapy should be administered with caution.

Other nephrotoxic medications may enhance the potential for drug-induced renal toxicity, and should be used concomitantly only with great caution.

Skeletal muscle relaxants: amphotericin B–induced hypokalemia may enhance the curariform effect of skeletal muscle relaxants.

Leukocyte transfusions: acute pulmonary toxicity has been reported in patients receiving intravenous amphotericin B and leukocyte transfusions.

DOSING

A single intravenous test dose (1 mg in 20 mL of 5% dextrose solution) administered over 20 to 30 minutes may be preferred. The patient's temperature, pulse, respiration, and blood pressure should be recorded every 30 minutes for 2 to 4 hours.

Therapy is usually initiated with a daily dose of 0.25 mg/kg of body weight and can be increased by 5 mg to 10 mg per day to final daily dosage of 0.5 mg/kg to 0.7 mg/kg. Total daily dosage may range from 1.0 mg/kg to 1.5 mg/kg when given on alternate days.

SPECIAL POPULATIONS

RENAL IMPAIRMENT: Technically not contraindicated; however, monitor renal function closely or use lipid formulation. No dosage adjustment recommended.

HEPATIC IMPAIRMENT: Liver tests should be monitored routinely.

PEDIATRIC PATIENTS: Safety and effectiveness in pediatric patients have not been established. Amphotericin B, when administered to pediatric patients, should be limited to the smallest dose compatible with an effective therapeutic regimen.

PREGNANCY: Category B.

BREASTFEEDING: Data insufficient; it is prudent to advise a breastfeeding mother to discontinue breastfeeding.

THE ART OF ANTIMICROBIAL THERAPY

Clinical Pearls

There are various forms of amphotericin B with many important differences: amphotericin B deoxycholate, amphotericin B colloidal dispersion, amphotericin B lipid complex, and liposomal amphotericin B. This chapter pertains only to amphotericin B deoxycholate.

1. Premedication with acetaminophen, diphenhydramine, meperidine, and even hydrocortisone can decrease infusion-related toxicity.
2. Hydration and sodium repletion prior to amphotericin B administration may reduce the risk of developing nephrotoxicity.
3. Under no circumstances should a total daily dose of 1.5 mg/kg be exceeded.
4. In patients with poor underlying renal function or those with worsening renal function, a lipid formulation of amphotericin B is preferred.
5. Some experts believe that mold infections should be treated with the lipid forms of amphotericin B to allow more drug delivery.
6. For *Candida* infections, the echinocandins and azoles may be preferred options for selected patients.
7. *Candida lusitaniae, Pseudallescheria boydii,* and *Fusarium* species are often resistant to amphotericin B. Voriconazole is frequently used for these infections.
8. It is advisable to monitor on a regular basis liver function, serum electrolytes (particularly magnesium and potassium), blood counts, and hemoglobin concentrations.

AMPHOTERICIN B LIPID COMPLEX (Abelcet)

BASIC CHARACTERISTICS

Class: Polyene

Mechanism of Action: Amphotericin B inserts into the cytoplasmic membrane through ergosterol leading to increased permeability of the fungal membrane and loss of intracellular ions. Amphotericin B also affects oxidation and may cause fungal death in this manner.

Mechanism of Resistance: Resistance is rare, but is caused by changes in the fungal cell membrane that prevent amphotericin B from inserting into the membrane.

Metabolic Route: Amphotericin B is excreted very slowly by the kidneys, with 2% to 5% of a given dose being excreted in the biologically active form. After discontinuation of treatment, amphotericin B is detectable in urine for at least 7 weeks. Details of possible metabolic pathways are not known.

FDA FDA-APPROVED INDICATIONS

Invasive fungal infections in patients who are refractory to or intolerant of conventional amphotericin B therapy.

SIDE EFFECTS/TOXICITY

Side effects are similar to those seen with Amphotericin B deoxycholate but tend to be less frequent or less severe.

Contraindicated in patients who have shown hypersensitivity to amphotericin B or any other component in the formulation.

Acute reactions including fever, shaking, chills, hypotension, anorexia, nausea, vomiting, headache, and tachypnea are common 1 to 3 hours after starting an intravenous infusion. Rapid intravenous infusion has been associated with hypotension, hypokalemia, arrhythmias, and shock, and should, therefore, be avoided.

Amphotericin B should be used with care in patients with reduced renal function; frequent monitoring of renal function is recommended.

Because acute pulmonary reactions have been reported in patients given amphotericin B during or shortly after leukocyte transfusions, it is advisable to temporally separate these infusions as far as possible and to monitor pulmonary function.

Leukoencephalopathy has been reported following use of amphotericin B.

DRUG INTERACTIONS/FOOD INTERACTIONS

Antineoplastic agents may enhance the potential for renal toxicity, bronchospasm, and hypotension and should be given concomitantly only with great caution.

Corticosteroids and corticotropin (ACTH): closely monitor serum electrolytes and cardiac function.

Digitalis glycosides: amphotericin B–induced hypokalemia may potentiate digitalis toxicity.

Flucytosine: concomitant use may increase the toxicity of flucytosine.

Imidazoles (e.g., fluconazole): imidazoles may induce fungal resistance to amphotericin B. Combination therapy should be administered with caution.

Other nephrotoxic medications: may enhance the potential for drug-induced renal toxicity, and should be used concomitantly only with great caution.

Skeletal muscle relaxants: amphotericin B–induced hypokalemia may enhance the curariform effect of skeletal muscle relaxants.

Leukocyte transfusions: acute pulmonary toxicity has been reported in patients receiving intravenous amphotericin B and leukocyte transfusions.

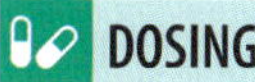

DOSING

Amphotericin B lipid complex is given 5 mg/kg/day as a single infusion.

SPECIAL POPULATIONS

RENAL IMPAIRMENT: Monitor renal function closely. No dosage adjustment is recommended for renal impairment or for dialysis.

HEPATIC IMPAIRMENT: Liver tests should be monitored routinely.

PEDIATRIC PATIENTS: As for adults.

PREGNANCY: Category B.

BREASTFEEDING: **Insufficient data;** it is prudent to advise a nursing mother to discontinue nursing.

THE ART OF ANTIMICROBIAL THERAPY

Clinical Pearls

There are various forms of amphotericin with many important differences: amphotericin B deoxycholate, amphotericin B lipid dispersion, amphotericin B lipid complex, and liposomal amphotericin B. This section pertains only to amphotericin B lipid complex. **Side effects of amphotericin B lipid complex are similar to those seen with amphotericin B deoxycholate but tend to be less frequent or less severe.**

1. Premedication with acetaminophen, diphenhydramine, meperidine, and even hydrocortisone can decrease infusion-related toxicity.
2. Hydration and sodium repletion prior to amphotericin B administration may reduce the patient's risk of developing nephrotoxicity.
3. *Candida lusitaniae*, *Pseudallescheria boydii*, and *Fusarium* sp. are often resistant to amphotericin B. Voriconazole is frequently used for these infections.

BASIC CHARACTERISTICS

Class: Aminopenicillin

Mechanism of Action: Binds penicillin-binding protein, disrupting cell wall synthesis.

Mechanisms of Resistance: (1) Alteration of the penicillin-binding protein, with reduced affinity. (2) Production of a β-lactamase resulting in hydrolysis of the β-lactam ring. (3) Decreased ability of the antibiotic to reach the penicillin-binding protein when bacteria decrease porin production resulting in a decrease of the drug concentration within the cell.

Metabolic Route: Ampicillin is excreted unchanged in the urine.

FDA FDA-APPROVED INDICATIONS

1. Ampicillin for **injection** is indicated in the treatment of infections caused by susceptible (only β-lactamase–negative) strains of microorganisms in respiratory tract infections, bacterial meningitis, septicemia, endocarditis, urinary tract infections, and gastrointestinal tract infections.
2. Ampicillin **capsules** are indicated in the treatment of infections caused by susceptible (only β-lactamase–negative) strains of microorganisms in genitourinary tract infections, respiratory tract infections, and gastrointestinal tract infections.

SIDE EFFECTS/TOXICITY

A history of allergic reaction to any of the penicillins is a **contraindication.**

Side effects include *Clostridium difficile*–associated diarrhea; hypersensitivity reactions, including rashes, erythema multiforme, toxic epidermal necrolysis, and Stevens-Johnson syndrome; nausea; vomiting; diarrhea; hepatic and renal dysfunction; crystalluria; anemia; thrombocytopenia; eosinophilia; and leukopenia.

DRUG INTERACTIONS/FOOD INTERACTIONS

Ampicillin capsules are stable in the presence of gastric acid.

The concurrent administration of allopurinol and ampicillin increases the incidence of rash.

Concurrent use of ampicillin and probenecid may result in increased and prolonged blood levels of ampicillin.

Chloramphenicol, macrolides, sulfonamides, and tetracyclines may interfere with the bactericidal effects of ampicillins.

High urine concentrations of ampicillin may result in false-positive reactions when one is testing for the presence of glucose in urine with Clinitest. It is recommended that glucose tests based on enzymatic glucose oxidase reactions (such as Clinistix) be used instead.

DOSING

AMPICILLIN FOR INJECTION:

Infection	*Dosage for Patients Weighing 40 kg or More*
Respiratory tract	250 mg to 500 mg every 6 hours IV or intramuscularly (IM)
Soft tissues	250 mg to 500 mg every 6 hours IV or IM
Gastrointestinal tract	500 mg every 6 hours IV or IM
Genitourinary tract	500 mg every 6 hours IV or IM
Bacterial meningitis	150 mg/kg/day to 200 mg/kg/day IV in divided doses every 3 to 4 hours
Septicemia	150 mg/kg/day to 200 mg/kg/day IV in divided doses every 3 to 4 hours

ORAL AMPICILLIN:

Ampicillin is supplied as 250-mg and 500-mg capsules. It is also supplied as an oral suspension with 2 concentrations: 125 mg/5 mL and 250 mg/5 mL.

Infection	*Dosage*
Genitourinary or gastrointestinal tract	500 mg 4 times daily
Respiratory tract	250 mg 4 times daily

SPECIAL POPULATIONS

Renal impairment	*Dosage*
Creatinine clearance 10 mL/min to 30 mL/min	500 mg or 250 mg every 12 hours
Creatinine clearance <10 mL/min	500 mg or 250 mg every 24 hours
Hemodialysis	500 mg or 250 mg every 24 hours; an additional dose should be administered during and at the end of dialysis
Chronic ambulatory peritoneal dialysis	250 mg every 12 hours
Continuous renal replacement therapy	1 gram every 8 hours

HEPATIC DYSFUNCTION: No dose adjustment is necessary.

PEDIATRIC PATIENTS:
AMPICILLIN FOR INJECTION:

Infection	*Dosage for Patients Weighing 40 kg or Less*
Respiratory tract	20 mg/kg/day to 50 mg/kg/day in divided doses every 6 to 8 hours IV or IM
Soft tissues	20 mg/kg/day to 50 mg/kg/day in divided doses every 6 to 8 hours IV or IM
Gastrointestinal tract	50 mg/kg/day in divided doses every 6 to 8 hours IV or IM
Genitourinary tract	50 mg/kg/day in divided doses every 6 to 8 hours IV or IM
Bacterial meningitis	150 mg/kg/day to 200 mg/kg/day IV in divided doses every 3 to 4 hours
Septicemia	150 mg/kg/day to 200 mg/kg/day IV in divided doses every 3 to 4 hours

ORAL AMPICILLIN:

Infection	*Dosage for Children Weighing 20 kg or Less*
Genitourinary or gastrointestinal tract	25 mg/kg 4 times daily
Respiratory tract	50 mg/kg/day in divided doses 3 to 4 times daily

PREGNANCY: Category B.

BREASTFEEDING: Ampicillin should be used only with caution.

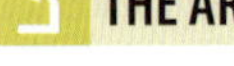

THE ART OF ANTIMICROBIAL THERAPY

Clinical Pearls

1. Ampicillin needs to be dose-adjusted for patients with renal dysfunction.
2. A high percentage (43% to 100%) of patients with infectious mononucleosis who receive ampicillin develop a skin rash.

AMPICILLIN SODIUM PLUS SULBACTAM SODIUM (Unasyn)

BASIC CHARACTERISTICS

Class: Aminopenicillin and β-lactamase–inhibitor combination

Mechanism of Action: Binds penicillin-binding protein (PBP), disrupting cell wall synthesis.

Mechanisms of Resistance:

1. The PBP can be altered, with reduced affinity,
2. production of a β-lactamase resulting in hydrolysis of the β-lactam ring, and
3. decreased ability of the antibiotic to reach the PBP when bacteria decrease porin production, resulting in a decrease of the drug concentration within the cell.

Metabolic Route: Ampicillin and sulbactam are excreted unchanged in the urine.

FDA-APPROVED INDICATIONS

FDA-Approved Indications: Treatment of infections caused by susceptible strains of microorganisms in skin and skin structure infections, intraabdominal infections, and gynecologic infections.

SIDE EFFECTS/TOXICITY

A history of allergic reaction to any of the penicillins is a **contraindication.**

Side effects include *Clostridium difficile*–associated diarrhea; hypersensitivity reactions, including rashes, erythema multiforme, toxic epidermal necrolysis, and Stevens-Johnson syndrome; mucocutaneous candidiasis; black hairy tongue; nausea; vomiting; diarrhea; hepatic and renal dysfunction; seizures with high central nervous system levels; crystalluria; anemia; thrombocytopenia; eosinophilia; and leukopenia.

DRUG INTERACTIONS/FOOD INTERACTIONS

Concurrent use of ampicillin sodium plus sulbactam sodium and probenecid may result in increased and prolonged blood levels of ampicillin and sulbactam. Chloramphenicol, macrolides, sulfonamides, and tetracyclines may interfere with the bactericidal effects of penicillins. High urine concentrations of ampicillin may result in false-positive reactions when one is testing for the presence of glucose in urine with Clinitest. It is recommended that glucose tests based on enzymatic glucose oxidase reactions (such as Clinistix) be used instead.

DOSING

Ampicillin plus sulbactam contains ampicillin to sulbactam in a 2:1 ratio.

AMPICILLIN SODIUM PLUS SULBACTAM SODIUM (Unasyn)

Ampicillin plus sulbactam may be administered by either the intravenous or the intramuscular routes.

The recommended adult dosage is 1.5 g to 3 g every 6 hours.

SPECIAL POPULATIONS

RENAL IMPAIRMENT:

CrCl Measurement or Treatment	*Dosage*
CrCl 10 mL/min to 50 mL/min	1.5 g every 12 hours
CrCl <10 mL/min	1.5 g every 24 hours
Hemodialysis	1.5 g every 24 hours and 1.5 g after hemodialysis
Chronic ambulatory peritoneal dialysis	1.5 g every 24 hours (no supplemental dose)
Continuous renal replacement therapy	1.5 g every 12 hours

Note: CrCl = Creatinine Clearance

HEPATIC DYSFUNCTION: No dosage adjustment necessary

PEDIATRIC PATIENTS:

Patients aged 1 year or older: Recommended daily dose is 75 mg/kg every 6 hours.

Patients weighing 40 kg or more: Dose according to adult recommendations.

PREGNANCY: Category B

BREASTFEEDING: Ampicillin plus sulbactam should be used only with caution in breastfeeding mothers.

THE ART OF ANTIMICROBIAL THERAPY

Clinical Pearls

1. Dosage of ampicillin plus sulbactam needs to be adjusted for patients with renal dysfunction.
2. A high percentage of patients with mononucleosis who receive ampicillin develop a skin rash.

ANIDULAFUNGIN (Eraxis)

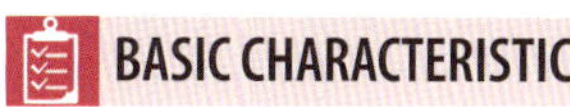

BASIC CHARACTERISTICS

Class: Echinocandin

Mechanism of Action: Inhibits synthesis of 1,3-β-D-glucan, an essential component of fungal cell walls.

Mechanism of Resistance: Data incomplete.

Metabolic Route: Anidulafungin undergoes slow chemical degradation to an open ring structure, which is then degraded to peptidic products and eliminated in the feces. It is not metabolized by the cytochrome P450 enzymes.

FDA-APPROVED INDICATIONS

FDA-Approved Indications: Candidemia, intraabdominal candidal infections, and esophageal candidiasis in HIV-infected patients.

Also Used for: *Aspergillus* infections, prevention of fungal infections in neutropenic patients, and other *Candida* infections such as endocarditis, osteomyelitis, or meningitis.

SIDE EFFECTS/TOXICITY

Hepatotoxicity; possible histamine-related syndrome characterized by rash, urticaria, flushing, pruritus, and hypotension. Also seen are diarrhea, thrombocytopenia, arrhythmia, QT prolongation, seizures, hypercalcemia, hyperglycemia, hypokalemia, hyperkalemia, hypernatremia, and hypomagnesemia.

DRUG INTERACTIONS

There are no significant drug interactions with anidulafungin.

DOSING

Candidemia or intraabdominal candidiasis: 200 mg intravenous (IV) loading dose and then 100 mg IV daily.

Esophageal candidiasis: 100 mg IV daily and then 50 mg daily.

SPECIAL POPULATIONS

RENAL OR HEPATIC IMPAIRMENT: There is no dosage adjustment needed.

PEDIATRIC PATIENTS: The loading dose of 3 mg/kg/day and then 1.5 mg/kg/day is equivalent to the 200-mg then 100-mg dosage recommendation for adults. For esophageal candidiasis, the recommended dosages are 1.5 mg/kg for the first dose, then 0.75 mg/kg/day.

PREGNANCY: Category C.

BREASTFEEDING: Anidulafungin should be used only if the benefit outweighs the risk in breastfeeding mothers.

THE ART OF ANTIMICROBIAL THERAPY

Clinical Pearls

1. Echinocandins have activity only against *Candida* species and *Aspergillus* species. They should not be used for any other fungal infections.
2. Anidulafungin is active against all pathogenic *Candida* species including those resistant to fluconazole.

ARTEMISININ AND ITS DERIVATIVES
ARTEMETHER PLUS LUMEFANTRINE (Coartem)

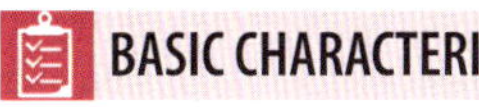

BASIC CHARACTERISTICS

Class: Fixed-dose combination of artemether and lumefantrine in the ratio of 1 to 6 is an antimalarial agent

Mechanisms of Action:

1. Lumefantrine inhibits the formation of β-hematin by forming a complex with hemin, and
2. both artemether and lumefantrine inhibit nucleic acid and protein synthesis.

Metabolic Route: Lumefantrine is excreted unchanged in feces and with traces only in urine. Metabolites of both drug components are eliminated in bile/feces and urine.

FDA FDA-APPROVED INDICATIONS

FDA-Approved Indications: Treatment of acute, uncomplicated malaria infections caused by *Plasmodium falciparum* in patients who weigh 5 kg or more.

SIDE EFFECTS/TOXICITY

Contraindicated in:

1. Patients hypersensitive to artemether, lumefantrine, or to any of the excipients of artemether plus lumefantrine,
2. patients with congenital prolongation of the QT interval (e.g., long QT syndrome) or any other clinical condition known to prolong the QTc interval such as patients with a history of symptomatic cardiac arrhythmias, clinically relevant bradycardia, or severe cardiac disease,
3. patients with a family history of congenital prolongation of the QT interval or sudden death, and
4. patients with known disturbances of electrolyte balance (e.g., hypokalemia or hypomagnesemia).

Frequently reported adverse reactions are headache, anorexia, dizziness, asthenia, pyrexia, cough, vomiting, and headache.

Other reported events include eosinophilia, tinnitus, conjunctivitis, constipation, dyspepsia, dysphagia, peptic ulcer, hepatitis, gait disturbance, hypokalemia, back pain, ataxia, clonus, fine motor delay, hyperreflexia, hypoaesthesia, nystagmus, tremor, agitation, mood swings, hematuria, proteinuria, asthma, pharyngo-laryngeal pain, urticaria, and angioedema.

DRUG INTERACTIONS/FOOD INTERACTIONS

Artemether plus lumefantrine tablets should be taken with food.

Contraindicated to administer artemether plus lumefantrine to:

1. patients receiving other medications that prolong the QT interval, such as class IA (quinidine, procainamide, disopyramide), or class III (amiodarone, pimozide, sotalol) antiarrhythmic agents; antipsychotics (ziprasidone); antidepressants; certain antimicrobials (macrolide antibiotics, fluoroquinolone antibiotics, imidazole, and triazole antifungal agents); certain nonsedating antihistaminics (terfenadine, astemizole); or cisapride; and
2. patients receiving medications that are metabolized by the cytochrome enzyme CYP2D6 that also have cardiac effects (e.g., flecainide, imipramine, amitriptyline, clomipramine).

When artemether plus lumefantrine is coadministered with an inhibitor of CYP3A4, including grapefruit juice, it may result in increased concentrations of artemether and/or lumefantrine and potentiate QT prolongation.

When artemether plus lumefantrine is coadministered with inducers of CYP3A4, it may result in decreased concentrations of artemether and/or lumefantrine and loss of antimalarial efficacy.

Drugs that have a mixed effect on CYP3A4, especially antiretroviral drugs and those that have an effect on the QT interval, should be used with caution in patients taking artemether plus lumefantrine; the result may be an increase in lumefantrine concentrations causing QT prolongation or a decrease in concentrations of the artemether resulting in loss of efficacy, or a decrease in artemether and/or lumefantrine concentrations resulting in loss of antimalarial efficacy of artemether plus lumefantrine. Artemether plus lumefantrine may reduce the effectiveness of hormonal contraceptives. Therefore, patients who are using oral, transdermal patch, or other systemic hormonal contraceptives should be advised to use an additional nonhormonal method of birth control.

DOSING

Coartem tablets contain 20 mg of artemether and 120 mg of lumefantrine.

Dosage is four tablets as a single initial dose, four tablets again after 8 hours, and then four tablets twice daily (morning and evening) for the following 2 days (total course of 24 tablets).

SPECIAL POPULATIONS

RENAL IMPAIRMENT: There is no dosage adjustment for renal insufficiency.

HEPATIC DYSFUNCTION: No dosage adjustment for mild-to-moderate hepatic dysfunction.

PEDIATRICS: A 3-day treatment schedule with a total of six doses is recommended:

*Weight**	*Regimen*
5 kg to 15 kg	One tablet, then one tablet 8 hours later, then one tablet twice daily for 2 days
>15 kg to 25 kg	Two tablets, then two tablets 8 hours later, then two tablets twice daily for 2 days
>25 kg to 35 kg	Three tablets, then three tablets 8 hours later, then three tablets twice daily for 2 days
>35 kg	Four tablets, then four tablets 8 hours later, then four tablets twice daily for 2 days

*The safety and efficacy have not been established in pediatric patients who weigh less than 5 kg.

PREGNANCY: Category C.

BREASTFEEDING: The benefits of breastfeeding to mother and infant should be weighed against potential risk from infant exposure to artemether and lumefantrine through breastmilk.

THE ART OF ANTIMICROBIAL THERAPY

Clinical Pearls

1. Artemether plus lumefantrine has been shown to be effective in geographical regions where resistance to chloroquine has been reported.
2. Artemether plus lumefantrine is not approved for patients with severe or complicated *P falciparum* malaria.
3. Artemether plus lumefantrine is not approved for the prevention of malaria.
4. Artemether plus lumefantrine tablets may be crushed and mixed with a small amount of water.

Addendum: Other artemisinin derivatives are not approved in the United States, but are used globally. They should not be used as monotherapy and are commonly combined with atovaquone plus proguanil, doxycycline, clindamycin, or mefloquine in adults, and with atovaquone plus proguanil, clindamycin, or mefloquine in children.

Artesunate may be available through the Centers for Disease Control and Prevention Parasitic Diseases Drug Service, 770-488-7775.

	Artemisinin (QHS)	*Artesunate (ARTS)*
Used for	Severe and uncomplicated *P falciparum* and *P vivax* malaria	Severe and uncomplicated *P falciparum* and *P vivax* malaria
Routes	Oral, rectal	Oral, IV, IM, rectal
Dosage	Oral: 500 mg to 1000 mg orally (10-20 mg/kg) on first day, followed by 500 mg daily for 4 days. Suppositories: 600 mg to 1200 mg initially, followed by 400 mg to 600 mg 4 hours later and 400-800 mg daily for 3 days. **Not recommended as monotherapy**	IV/IM: 120 mg initially, followed by 60 mg at 4, 24, and 48 hours, continued for up to 5 days. Oral: 100 mg to 200 mg initially, then 100 mg daily for 2 to 4 days. Rectal: 10-20 mg/kg/day **Not recommended as monotherapy**
Toxicity	Rare bradycardia and prolonged QT	Nausea, vomiting, diarrhea, seizures, tinnitus, rash, sinus bradycardia, and first-degree heart block, potential cerebellar toxicity
Drug interactions		Mefloquine clearance is increased and mefloquine should be given at least 24 hours after ARTS

	Dihydroartemisinin (DHA)	*Artemether*
Used for	Severe and uncomplicated *P. falciparum* malaria	Severe and uncomplicated *P. falciparum* malaria
Routes	Oral, rectal	IM, oral
Dosage	DHA-orally: 120 mg initially, followed by 60 mg daily for 4 to 6 days. A fixed combination (Artekin) contains 40 mg DHA and 320 mg piperaquine and is given as 1.6/12.8 mg/kg/dose at 0, 8, 24, and 48 hours. **Not recommended as monotherapy**	IM: 3.2 mg/kg day one, 1.6 mg/kg daily for up to 7 days Oral: 2 mg/kg/day for up to 7 days **Not recommended as monotherapy**
Toxicity	Similar to other artemisinin derivatives	Mild QTc prolongation
Drug interactions		Ketoconazole and grapefruit juice may increase the area under the curve; clinical significance is unclear

Note: IM = intramuscular; IV = intravenous

ATAZANAVIR (Reyataz)

BASIC CHARACTERISTICS

Class: Protease inhibitor

Mechanism of Action: Reversibly binds the active site of the enzyme protease. Inhibition of protease prevents cleavage of the *gag* and *gag-pol* polyprotein resulting in the production of immature, noninfectious virus.

Mechanism of Resistance: Development of mutations on the enzyme protease causes a conformational change that prevents atazanavir from binding the active site, allowing protease activity to continue. The most frequent resistance mutations include I50L.

Metabolic Route: Atazanavir is mostly excreted in the feces.

FDA FDA-APPROVED INDICATIONS

FDA-Approved Indications: Treatment of HIV-1 in combination with other antiretroviral agents.

SIDE EFFECTS/TOXICITY

Side effects include new-onset diabetes mellitus; exacerbation of preexisting diabetes mellitus; hyperglycemia; increased bleeding, including spontaneous skin hematomas and hemarthrosis, in patients with hemophilia type A and B; redistribution or accumulation of body fat including central obesity, dorsocervical fat enlargement (buffalo hump), peripheral wasting, facial wasting, and breast enlargement; "cushingoid appearance"; immune reconstitution syndrome; rash; nephrolithiasis; prolongation of PR interval; QTc prolongation; torsade de pointes; abdominal pain; headache; anorexia; dyspepsia; epigastric pain; hepatitis; mouth ulceration; pancreatitis; vomiting; anemia; leukopenia; thrombocytopenia; increases in alkaline phosphatase, amylase, creatine phosphokinase, lactic dehydrogenase, SGOT, SGPT, indirect bilirubin, and gamma glutamyl transpeptidase; hyperlipemia; hyperuricemia; hyperglycemia; hypoglycemia; and dehydration.

DRUG INTERACTIONS/FOOD INTERACTIONS

Atazanavir should be taken with a meal, even when given with ritonavir.

Drugs that should not be coadministered with atazanavir include amiodarone, quinidine, rifampin, ergot derivatives, Saint John's wort, HMG-CoA reductase inhibitors simvastatin and lovastatin, pimozide, benzodiazepines, irinotecan, etravirine, nevirapine, fluticasone, salmeterol, indinavir, and rifampin.

Atazanavir is an inhibitor of the CYP3A enzyme and UGT1A1; coadministration of atazanavir and drugs primarily metabolized by CYP3A or UGT1A1 may result in increased plasma concentrations of the other drug that could increase or prolong its therapeutic and adverse effects.

Atazanavir is metabolized by CYP3A; coadministration of atazanavir and drugs that induce CYP3A may decrease atazanavir plasma concentrations and reduce its therapeutic effect. Coadministration of atazanavir and drugs that inhibit CYP3A may increase atazanavir plasma concentrations. Because of these metabolic effects, potential drug interactions may require dosage change or clinical or laboratory monitoring, including:

Medication	*Adjustment or Action*
Itraconzole	Monitor for toxicity
Voriconazole	Monitor for toxicity
Rifabutin	Decrease rifabutin to 150 mg every other day or three times weekly
Contraceptives	Use lowest effective dose
Atorvastatin	Use lowest possible dose with close monitoring
Phenobarbital, phenytoin, or carbamazepine	Monitor anticonvulsant level; consider alternative
Sildenafil	25 mg every 48 hours
Tadalafil	5 mg in 24 hours, no more than 10 mg in 72 hours
Vardenafil	2.5 mg in 24 hours
Diltiazem	Electrocardiogram monitoring recommended
H2 receptors	Not recommended with unboosted (without ritonavir) atazanavir Dosage should not exceed 40 mg twice daily equivalent of famotidine if ritonavir-boosted atazanavir is used
Proton pump inhibitors	Not recommended with unboosted (without ritonavir) atazanavir Dosage should not exceed 20 mg equivalent of omeprazole and should be given 12 hours before ritonavir-boosted atazanavir
Antacids	Administer 2 hours apart
Didanosine	Administer separately from atazanavir
Tenofovir	Not recommended with unboosted (without ritonavir) atazanavir
Efavirenz	Not recommended with unboosted (without ritonavir) atazanavir
Maraviroc	Maraviroc dosage is 150 mg twice daily

DOSING

Atazanavir is available in 100-mg, 150-mg, 200-mg, and 300-mg capsules. For treatment-naive patients, the recommended dosage is atazanavir 300 mg with ritonavir 100 mg once daily (all as a single dose with food).

For treatment-naive patients who are unable to tolerate ritonavir, the recommended dosage is atazanavir 400 mg (without ritonavir) once daily taken with food.

For treatment-experienced patients, the recommended dosage is atazanavir 300 mg with ritonavir 100 mg once daily (all as a single dose with food).

SPECIAL POPULATIONS

RENAL IMPAIRMENT: For patients with renal impairment, including those with severe renal impairment who are not managed with hemodialysis, no dosage adjustment is required for atazanavir. Treatment-naive patients with end-stage renal disease managed with hemodialysis should receive atazanavir 300 mg with ritonavir 100 mg. Atazanavir should not be administered to HIV-treatment–experienced patients with end-stage renal disease managed with hemodialysis.

HEPATIC DYSFUNCTION: Atazanavir should be used with caution in patients with mild-to-moderate hepatic impairment. For patients with Child-Pugh Class B who have not experienced prior virologic failure, a dosage reduction to 300 mg once daily should be considered. Atazanavir should not be used in patients with Child-Pugh Class C. Atazanavir with ritonavir has not been studied in subjects with hepatic impairment and is not recommended.

PEDIATRIC PATIENTS: The recommended daily dosage of atazanavir with ritonavir in patients aged at least 6 years is:

Weight, kg	*Atazanavir*	*Ritonavir*
15 to less than 25	150 mg	80 mg
25 to less than 32	200 mg	100 mg
32 to less than 39	250 mg	100 mg
39 or greater	300 mg	100 mg

For treatment-naive patients aged at least 13 years and at least 39 kg, who are unable to tolerate ritonavir, the recommended dose is atazanavir 400 mg (without ritonavir) once daily with food.

PREGNANCY: Category B.

BREASTFEEDING: It is recommended that HIV-positive mothers not breastfeed their children, to prevent mother-to-child transmission of HIV.

THE ART OF ANTIMICROBIAL THERAPY

Clinical Pearls

1. Atazanavir should always be used in combination with other antiretrovirals.
2. Atazanavir should be taken with food to increase absorption.
3. Atazanavir should be boosted with ritonavir when combined with tenofovir.
4. When atazanavir is boosted with ritonavir, the two medications should be administered at the same time.
5. Avoid proton pump inhibitors or H2 blockers if atazanavir is given unboosted (without ritonavir).
6. Whenever one is initiating atazanavir, make sure to review all medications the patient is receiving to minimize drug interactions.
7. Atazanavir causes an increase in indirect bilirubin by inhibiting glucuronidation.
8. Atazanavir causes nephrolithiasis; patients should be advised to drink adequate water.
9. Rash is not infrequent with atazanavir even though it does not contain a sulfa moiety.

ATOVAQUONE (Mepron)

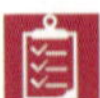

BASIC CHARACTERISTICS

Class: Antimetabolite

Mechanism of Action: Atovaquone is an analogue of ubiquinone. The mechanism of action against *Pneumocystis jiroveci* has not been fully elucidated.

In *Plasmodium* species, the site of action appears to be the cytochrome bc1 complex (complex III). Inhibition of electron transport by atovaquone results in indirect inhibition of these enzymes. The ultimate metabolic effect of such blockade includes inhibition of nucleic acid and ATP synthesis.

Metabolic Route: Atovaquone is excreted unchanged in feces.

FDA FDA-APPROVED INDICATIONS

FDA-Approved Indications: Prevention of *P. jiroveci* pneumonia in patients who are intolerant of trimethoprim plus sulfamethoxazole (TMP-SMX).

Treatment of mild-to-moderate pneumonia caused by *P. jiroveci* in patients who are intolerant of TMP-SMX.

Also Used for: Alternative therapy for toxoplasmosis (in combination with pyrimethamine), babesiosis, malaria therapy, and malaria prophylaxis.

SIDE EFFECTS/TOXICITY

Atovaquone is **contraindicated** for patients who develop or have a history of potentially life-threatening allergic reactions to any of the components of the formulation. Toxic effects include fever, hypersensitivity, rash, insomnia, headache, depression, keratopathy, cough, diarrhea, nausea, pancreatitis, hepatotoxicity, myalgia, renal failure, leukopenia, thrombocytopenia, and methemoglobinemia.

DRUG INTERACTIONS/FOOD INTERACTIONS

Administering atovaquone with food enhances its absorption.

Rifampin lowers atovaquone levels.

DOSING

Prevention of *P. jiroveci* pneumonia: 1500 mg (10 mL) once daily.

Treatment of mild-to-moderate *P. jiroveci* pneumonia: 750 mg (5 mL) administered with meals twice daily for 21 days.

SPECIAL POPULATIONS

RENAL IMPAIRMENT: Unknown.

HEPATIC DYSFUNCTION: Unknown.

PEDIATRICS: Not studied in children.

PREGNANCY: Category C.

BREASTFEEDING: Caution should be exercised when atovaquone is given to breast-feeding mothers.

THE ART OF ANTIMICROBIAL THERAPY

Clinical Pearls

1. Atovaquone is not recommended for treatment of moderate-to-severe *P. jiroveci* pneumonia because of the unreliability of absorption.
2. Atovaquone should be administered with food to increase its absorption.

ATOVAQUONE PLUS PROGUANIL (Malarone)

BASIC CHARACTERISTICS

Class: Antimetabolite

Mechanism of Action: Atovaquone is a selective inhibitor of parasite mitochondrial electron transport. Proguanil hydrochloride primarily exerts its effect by means of the metabolite cycloguanil, a dihydrofolate reductase inhibitor. Inhibition of dihydrofolate reductase in the malaria parasite disrupts deoxythymidylate synthesis.

Atovaquone and cycloguanil are active against the erythrocytic and exoerythrocytic stages of *Plasmodium* species.

Metabolic Route: Atovaquone is excreted unchanged in feces. Proguanil is metabolized by the liver and renally excreted.

FDA FDA-APPROVED INDICATIONS

FDA-Approved Indications: Prophylaxis of *Plasmodium falciparum* malaria and treatment of acute, uncomplicated *P. falciparum* malaria.

SIDE EFFECTS/TOXICITY

Atovaquone plus proguanil is **contraindicated** in:

1. Individuals with known hypersensitivity to atovaquone or proguanil hydrochloride or any component of the formulation. Rare cases of anaphylaxis following treatment with atovaquone plus proguanil have been reported.
2. Prophylaxis of *P. falciparum* malaria in patients with severe renal impairment (creatinine clearance less than 30 mL/min).

Toxicity includes fever, hypersensitivity, rash, angioedema, pruritus, vasculitis, headache, dizziness, insomnia, depression, psychotic events, seizures, cough, keratopathy, stomatitis, hepatotoxicity, anorexia, nausea, vomiting, diarrhea, abdominal pain, pancreatitis, myalgia, renal failure, asthenia, methemoglobinemia, and pancytopenia.

DRUG INTERACTIONS/FOOD INTERACTIONS

Administering atovaquone plus proguanil with food enhances its absorption.

Medications that can decrease the levels of atovaquone are tetracycline, metoclopramide, rifampin, or rifabutin.

Caution should be exercised when one is prescribing atovaquone with indinavir because of the decrease in trough levels of indinavir.

DOSING

Prophylactic treatment with atovaquone plus proguanil should be started 1 or 2 days before entering a malaria-endemic area and should be continued daily during the stay and for 7 days after return. Dosage is 1 atovaquone plus proguanil tablet (adult strength = 250 mg atovaquone and 100 mg proguanil hydrochloride) per day.

Treatment of acute malaria: Four tablets (1 g atovaquone and 400 mg proguanil hydrochloride) as a single dose daily for 3 consecutive days.

SPECIAL POPULATIONS

RENAL IMPAIRMENT: Atovaquone plus proguanil should not be used for malaria prophylaxis in patients with severe renal impairment (creatinine clearance less than 30 mL/min) but may be used with caution for the treatment of malaria if the benefits of the 3-day treatment regimen outweigh the potential risks associated with increased drug exposure. In this case, no dosage adjustment is needed if creatinine clearance is greater than 30 mL/min.

HEPATIC DYSFUNCTION: Atovaquone plus proguanil has not been studied in patients with severe hepatic dysfunction.

PEDIATRICS: Treatment of malaria with atovaquone plus proguanil has not been studied in pediatric patients who weigh less than 5 kg and for treatment for malaria prophylaxis has not been studied in pediatric patients who weigh less than 11 kg.

The dosage for **prophylaxis** of malaria is based upon body weight:

Weight	*Daily Dosage*
11 kg to 20 kg	One pediatric tablet daily (62.5 mg/25 mg)
21 kg to 30 kg	Two pediatric tablets once daily
31 kg to 40 kg	Three pediatric tablets once daily
> 40 kg	One adult tablet daily (250 mg/100 mg)

The dosage for **treatment** of acute malaria is based upon body weight:

Weight	*Regimen*
5 kg to 8 kg	Two pediatric tablets (62.5 mg/25 mg) once daily for 3 days
9 kg to 10 kg	Three pediatric tablets once daily for 3 days
11 kg to 20 kg	One adult tablet daily (250 mg/100 mg) for 3 days
21 kg to 30 kg	Two adult tablets once daily for 3 days
31 kg to 40 kg	Three adult tablets once daily for 3 days
> 40 kg	Four adult tablets once daily for 3 days

Note: Tablets may be crushed and mixed with condensed milk just prior to administration for children who may have difficulty swallowing tablets.

PREGNANCY: Category C.

BREASTFEEDING: Caution should be exercised when atovaquone plus proguanil is given to breastfeeding mothers.

THE ART OF ANTIMICROBIAL THERAPY

Clinical Pearls

1. Atovaquone plus proguanil is not recommended for treatment of severe malaria.
2. Atovaquone plus proguanil should not be used in patients with renal failure.
3. Atovaquone should be administered with food to increase its absorption.
4. Absorption of atovaquone may be reduced in patients with diarrhea or vomiting.
5. Atovaquone plus proguanil may be crushed and mixed with condensed milk just prior to administration for children who may have difficulty swallowing tablets.

AZITHROMYCIN (Zithromax and Zmax)

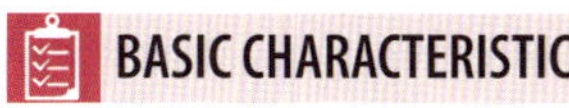

BASIC CHARACTERISTICS

Class: Azalide/macrolide

Mechanism of Action: Binds to the 50S ribosomal subunit of susceptible microorganisms and, thus, interferes with microbial protein synthesis.

Mechanisms of Resistance:

1. Decreased permeability,
2. active efflux,
3. alteration of the 50S ribosomal unit,
4. alteration of the 23S subunit of the 50S ribosomal unit, and
5. enzymatic inactivation of the macrolide.

Metabolic Route: Azithromycin is excreted in the bile.

FDA-APPROVED INDICATIONS

FDA-Approved Indications:

1. **Azithromycin for injection:** community-acquired pneumonia and pelvic inflammatory disease.
2. **Azithromycin 250-mg or 500-mg tablets and solution:** treatment of patients with mild-to-moderate infections caused by susceptible microorganisms in acute bacterial exacerbations of chronic obstructive pulmonary disease, acute bacterial sinusitis, community-acquired pneumonia, pharyngitis/tonsillitis, uncomplicated skin and skin structure infections, urethritis and cervicitis, and genital ulcer disease caused by *Haemophilus ducreyi* (chancroid) in men.
3. **Azithromycin 600-mg tablets:** treatment of serious infections caused by susceptible strains of microorganisms in prophylaxis of disseminated *Mycobacterium avium* complex (MAC), and treatment of disseminated MAC.
4. **Azithromycin 1-g packets:** treatment of sexually transmitted diseases caused by *Chlamydia trachomatis* or *Neisseria gonorrhea.*
5. **Zmax:** treatment of mild-to-moderate infections caused by susceptible microorganisms in acute bacterial sinusitis in adults and community-acquired pneumonia in adults and children aged 6 months and older.

Also Used for: Atypical mycobacteria; with pyrimethamine as alternative for sulfonamide to treat toxoplasmosis.

SIDE EFFECTS/TOXICITY

Contraindicated in patients with known hypersensitivity to azithromycin, erythromycin, or any macrolide or ketolide antibiotic.

Side effects include serious allergic reactions such as anaphylaxis, rash, photosensitivity, angioedema, Stevens-Johnson syndrome and toxic epidermal necrolysis,

Clostridium difficile–associated diarrhea, prolonged cardiac repolarization and QT interval, exacerbation of symptoms of myasthenia gravis and new onset of myasthenic syndrome, nausea, vomiting, diarrhea, abdominal pain, hepatitis, dyspepsia, flatulence, melena, cholestatic jaundice, palpitations, chest pain, candidiasis, vaginitis, nephritis, seizures, hearing loss, dizziness, headache, vertigo, somnolence, thrombocytopenia, and leukopenia.

DRUG INTERACTIONS/FOOD INTERACTIONS

Azithromycin tablets and suspension can be administered with or without food.

The Zmax formulation should be taken on an empty stomach at least 1 hour before or 2 hours after a meal.

Concurrent use of macrolides and **theophylline** has been associated with increases in the serum concentrations of theophylline.

Concomitant administration of azithromycin may potentiate the effects of oral **anticoagulants**. Prothrombin times should be carefully monitored while patients are receiving azithromycin and oral anticoagulants concomitantly.

When azithromycin and these drugs are used concomitantly, careful monitoring of patients is advised:

Digoxin: elevated digoxin levels.

Ergotamine or **dihydroergotamine:** acute ergot toxicity characterized by severe peripheral vasospasm and dysesthesia.

Triazolam: decreased clearance of triazolam, which may increase the pharmacologic effect of triazolam.

Drugs metabolized by the cytochrome P450 system: elevations of serum carbamazepine, cyclosporine, hexobarbital, and phenytoin levels.

DOSING

Azithromycin intravenous (IV) formulation: 500 mg as a single daily dose. For the treatment of severe community-acquired pneumonia, conversion to oral therapy can occur after the second dose and be continued at 500 mg daily. The timing of the switch to oral therapy should be done at the discretion of the physician.

Azithromycin tablets and suspensions in the following strengths: 250-mg and 500-mg tablets; 100 mg/5 mL and 200 mg/5 mL suspensions.

Infection	*Recommended Dosage/Duration of Therapy*
Community-acquired pneumonia (mild severity)	500 mg once daily on day 1, then 250 mg for 4 more days

Infection	*Recommended Dosage/Duration of Therapy*
Pharyngitis/tonsillitis	
Skin/skin structure (uncomplicated)	
Acute bacterial exacerbations of chronic obstructive pulmonary disease	500 mg once daily for 3 days *or* 500 mg once daily on day 1, then 250 mg for 4 more days
Acute bacterial sinusitis	500 mg once daily for 3 days
Genital ulcer disease (chancroid)	One 1-g dose
Nongonoccocal urethritis and cervicitis	One 1-g dose
Gonococcal urethritis and cervicitis	One 2-g dose

Azithromycin 600-mg tablets: Prevention of disseminated MAC infections: 1200 mg taken once weekly.

Treatment of disseminated MAC infections: daily dose of 600 mg, in combination with ethambutol at the recommended daily dosage of 15 mg/kg.

Azithromycin for oral suspension(1-g formulation): The recommended dose for the treatment of nongonococcal urethritis and cervicitis caused by *C. trachomatis* is a single 1-g (1000-mg) packet. The entire contents of the packet should be mixed thoroughly with 2 ounces (approximately 60 mL) of water. The patient should drink the entire contents immediately; then add an additional 2 ounces of water, mix, and drink to ensure complete consumption of dosage. The single-dose packet should not be used to administer doses other than 1000 mg of azithromycin.

Zmax: Zmax should be taken as a single 2-g dose. Zmax provides a full course of antibacterial therapy in a single oral dose. It is recommended that Zmax be taken on an empty stomach (at least 1 hour before or 2 hours after a meal).

SPECIAL POPULATIONS

RENAL IMPAIRMENT: Caution should be used when azithromycin is given to patients with a creatinine clearance of less than 10 mL/min.

HEPATIC DYSFUNCTION: Caution should be used.

PEDIATRIC PATIENTS:

Acute otitis media: Azithromycin for oral suspension 30 mg/kg given as a single dose or 10 mg/kg once daily for 3 days or 10 mg/kg as a single dose on the first day followed by 5 mg/kg/day on days 2 through 5.

Acute bacterial sinusitis: Azithromycin for oral suspension 10 mg/kg once daily for 3 days.

Community-acquired pneumonia: Azithromycin for oral suspension 10 mg/kg as a single dose on the first day followed by 5 mg/kg on days 2 through 5.

Pharyngitis/tonsillitis: Azithromycin for oral suspension 12 mg/kg once daily for 5 days.

For pediatric patients aged 6 months and older, **Zmax** for community-acquired pneumonia should be taken as a single dose of 60 mg/kg body weight; pediatric patients weighing 34 kg or more should receive the adult dosage of 2 g.

The azithromycin 1-g packet is not for pediatric use.

PREGNANCY: Category B

BREASTFEEDING: Caution should be used.

THE ART OF ANTIMICROBIAL THERAPY

Clinical Pearls

1. Multiple formulations of azithromycin are available; caution should be used to administer the appropriate formulation in the correct dosage.
2. When one is treating MAC, azithromycin must be combined with other agents to minimize resistance.
3. Macrolides prolong QT intervals and must be used with caution.
4. Despite successful symptomatic treatment of azithromycin, allergic symptoms have recurred in some patients upon discontinuation of symptomatic therapy, possibly because of the long tissue half-life of azithromycin. This possibility warrants prolonged observation.

BASIC CHARACTERISTICS

Class: Monobactam

Mechanism of Action: Binds penicillin-binding protein (PBP), disrupting cell wall synthesis.

Mechanisms of Resistance:

1. The PBP can be altered, with reduced affinity,
2. production of a β-lactamase resulting in hydrolysis of the β-lactam ring, and
3. decreased ability of the antibiotic to reach the PBP when bacteria increase porins resulting in a decrease of the drug concentration within the cell.

Metabolic Route: Aztreonam is excreted unchanged in the urine.

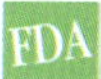

FDA-APPROVED INDICATIONS

FDA-Approved indications: Treatment of the following infections caused by susceptible gram-negative organisms: urinary tract infections, lower respiratory tract infections, septicemia, skin and skin structure infections, intraabdominal infections, and gynecologic infections. Adjunctive therapy to surgery in the management of infections caused by susceptible organisms, including abscesses, infections complicating hollow viscus perforations, cutaneous infections, and infections of serous surfaces.

SIDE EFFECTS/TOXICITY

Side effects include *Clostridium difficile*–associated diarrhea, phlebitis/thrombophlebitis, hypersensitivity, anaphylaxis, fever, rash including toxic epidermal necrolysis and erythema multiforme, seizure, confusion, tinnitus, altered taste, diarrhea, nausea, hepatitis, vomiting, bronchospasm, arrhythmias, hypotension, myalgia, vaginitis, breast tenderness, increased serum creatinine, pancytopenia, neutropenia, eosinophilia, thrombocytopenia, anemia, leukocytosis, thrombocytosis, and prolonged prothrombin time.

DRUG INTERACTIONS/FOOD INTERACTIONS

If an aminoglycoside is used concurrently with aztreonam, renal function should be monitored.

DOSING

Aztreonam may be administered intravenously or by intramuscular injection.

AZTREONAM (Azactam)

Infection	*Dosage*
Urinary tract infections	500 mg or 1 g every 8 to 12 hours
Moderately severe systemic infections	1 g to 2 g every 8 to 12 hours
Severe systemic infections	2 g every 6 to 8 hours
Pseudomonas infections	2 g every 6 to 8 hours

SPECIAL POPULATIONS

RENAL IMPAIRMENT: The dosage of aztreonam should be halved in patients with estimated creatinine clearances between 10 mL/min/1.73 m^2 and 30 mL/min/1.73 m^2 after an initial loading dose of 1 g or 2 g.

In patients with creatinine clearance less than 10 mL/min/1.73 m^2, such as those supported by **hemodialysis**, the usual dose of 500 mg, 1 g, or 2 g should be given **initially**. The **maintenance** dose should be one fourth of the usual initial dose given at the usual fixed interval of 6, 8, or 12 hours.

For serious or life-threatening infections, in addition to the maintenance doses, one eighth of the initial dose should be given after each hemodialysis session.

Continuous Renal Replacement Therapy: administer 50% to 75% of the dose every 8 to 12 hours.

HEPATIC DYSFUNCTION: No dosage adjustment is necessary.

PEDIATRIC PATIENTS: The safety and effectiveness of aztreonam has been established in ages 9 months to 16 years.

Mild-to-moderate infections should be treated with 30 mg/kg every 8 hours.

Moderate-to-severe systemic infections should be treated with 30 mg/kg every 6 to 8 hours.

PREGNANCY: Category B.

BREASTFEEDING: Breastfeeding should be stopped when the patient is receiving aztreonam.

THE ART OF ANTIMICROBIAL THERAPY

Clinical Pearls

1. Although cross-reactivity of aztreonam with other β-lactam antibiotics is rare, this drug should be administered with caution to any patient with a history of hypersensitivity to β-lactams.
2. Aztreonam is similar in structure to ceftazidime and cross-allergies may occur.
3. Aztreonam has no activity against gram-positive organisms.

BASIC CHARACTERISTICS

Class: Nitroimidazole

Mechanism of Action: Data incomplete.

Mechanism of Resistance: Data incomplete.

FDA-APPROVED INDICATIONS

Not FDA-approved, but used for treatment of *Trypanosoma cruzi.*

SIDE EFFECTS/TOXICITY

Side effects include peripheral neuropathy, rash, and granulocytopenia. There is an increased incidence of malignant tumors in patients given benznidazole after cardiac transplantation.

DRUG INTERACTIONS/FOOD INTERACTIONS

Data incomplete.

DOSING

The recommended dose and duration for treatment of all forms of *T cruzi* is 5 mg/kg/day for a total of 60 days.

SPECIAL POPULATIONS

RENAL IMPAIRMENT: Do not administer.

HEPATIC DYSFUNCTION: Do not administer.

PEDIATRIC PATIENTS: Same dosage as adults.

PREGNANCY: Do not administer.

BREASTFEEDING: Do not administer.

THE ART OF ANTIMICROBIAL THERAPY

Clinical Pearls

1. Benznidazole is in stock at the Centers for Disease Control and Prevention, Parasitic Diseases Drug Service (770-488-7775). It may be obtained from a compounding pharmacy through the National Association of Compounding Pharmacies (800-687-7850) or http://www.pccarx.com.
2. Benznidazole is considered the drug of choice for *T. cruzi.*
3. Patients with severe cardiac or gastrointestinal Chagas' disease should not be treated with benznidazole.

BITHIONOL (Bitin)

BASIC CHARACTERISTICS

Class: Chlorinated bisphenol

Mechanism of Action: Unclear; possibly an uncoupler of oxidative phosphorylation.

Metabolic Route: Bithionol is excreted in the urine.

FDA-APPROVED INDICATIONS

Not FDA-approved, but used for treatment of acute and chronic *Fasciola hepatica* and *Paragonimus westermani.*

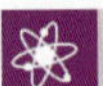

SIDE EFFECTS/TOXICITY

Side effects include nausea, diarrhea, abdominal pain, anorexia, and urticaria.

DRUG INTERACTIONS/FOOD INTERACTIONS

Unknown.

DOSING

The recommended dosage is 30 mg/kg to 50 mg/kg of body weight on alternate days for 10 to 15 doses for the treatment of fascioliasis and paragonimiasis.

SPECIAL POPULATIONS

RENAL IMPAIRMENT: Data incomplete.

HEPATIC DYSFUNCTION: Data incomplete.

PEDIATRIC PATIENTS: 30 mg/kg to 50 mg/kg on alternate days for 10 to 15 doses.

PREGNANCY: Unknown.

BREASTFEEDING: Unknown.

THE ART OF ANTIMICROBIAL THERAPY

Clinical Pearls

1. Bithionol can be obtained from the Centers for Disease Control and Prevention Parasitic Diseases Drug Service (770-488-7775).
2. Treatment with antispasmodics and antihistamines helps reduce side effects.
3. Giving bithionol in two or three divided doses and after meals decreases the incidence of toxicity.

BASIC CHARACTERISTICS

Class: Cyclic polypeptide

Mechanism of Action: Inhibits protein synthesis by binding to the 70S ribosomal unit.

Mechanisms of Resistance: Incompletely understood.

Metabolic Route: Capreomycin is excreted unchanged in the urine.

FDA-APPROVED INDICATIONS

FDA-Approved Indications: Treatment of pulmonary *Mycobacterium tuberculosis* when the primary agents (isoniazid, rifampin, ethambutol, aminosalicylic acid, and streptomycin) have been ineffective or cannot be used because of toxicity or the presence of resistant tubercle bacilli.

SIDE EFFECTS/TOXICITY

> **WARNING:** Use of capreomycin in patients with renal or auditory impairment and use with other non-antituberculosis drugs with similar toxicity must take place only with great caution; use with other parenteral antituberculosis agents with similar toxicity is not recommended.

Contraindicated in patients who are hypersensitive to capreomycin.

Nephrotoxicity and ototoxicity are similar to that with aminoglycosides.

Side effects include hypokalemia, hypomagnesemia, and hypocalcemia.

DRUG INTERACTIONS/FOOD INTERACTIONS

Use with caution when administering neuromuscular blocking agents, other nephrotoxic agents, or ototoxic agents (e.g., polymyxin A sulfate, colistin sulfate, amikacin, gentamicin, tobramycin, vancomycin, kanamycin, and neomycin) because of possible additive effects. Use with great caution in patients with preexisting renal disease or auditory impairment.

DOSING

The recommended dosage is 15 mg/kg/day (maximum 1 g) intravenously or intramuscularly.

Patients aged older than 59 years: 10 mg/kg/day (maximum 750 mg).

After a period of daily administration, capreomycin can be given two or three times per week.

SPECIAL POPULATIONS

RENAL IMPAIRMENT: In patients with creatinine clearance less than 30 mL/min or in dialysis patients: 12 mg/kg to 15 mg/kg two or three times weekly.

HEPATIC DYSFUNCTION: No adjustment necessary.

PEDIATRIC PATIENTS: 15 mg/kg/day to 30 mg/kg/day with a maximum of 1 g daily.

PREGNANCY: Category C

BREASTFEEDING: Use with caution in the breastfeeding mother.

THE ART OF ANTIMICROBIAL THERAPY

Clinical Pearls

1. Capreomycin should never be used alone in the treatment of active tuberculosis.
2. Capreomycin should only be used if resistance to first-line antimycobacterial agents is noted.
3. Serum levels of capreomycin should be monitored, with a goal of peak levels (2 hours after a dose) of 35 μg/mL to 45 μg/mL.
4. Dosage should be based on ideal body weight.
5. May demonstrate cross-resistance with amikacin and kanamycin.
6. Treatment of tuberculosis with capreomycin plus kanamycin or amikacin (double injectable therapy) is not recommended unless the situation is dire and there are no reasonable alternatives.

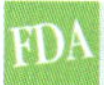 BASIC CHARACTERISTICS

Class: Echinocandin

Mechanism of Action: Inhibits synthesis of 1,3-β-D-glucan, an essential component of fungal cell walls.

Mechanism of Resistance: Data incomplete.

Metabolic Route: Caspofungin is slowly metabolized by hydrolysis and N-acetylation and is eliminated in the feces and urine. It is not metabolized by the cytochrome P450 enzymes.

 FDA-APPROVED INDICATIONS

FDA-Approved Indications: Empirical therapy for presumed fungal infections in febrile, neutropenic patients. Treatment of candidemia and the following *Candida* infections: intraabdominal abscesses, peritonitis, pleural space infections, and esophageal candidiasis. Treatment of invasive aspergillosis in patients who are refractory to or intolerant of other therapies.

 SIDE EFFECTS/TOXICITY

Side effects include fever, chills, anaphylaxis, possible histamine-mediated symptoms, rash, facial swelling, pruritus, sensation of warmth, bronchospasm, pancreatitis, hepatic necrosis, diarrhea, renal failure, seizures, swelling and peripheral edema, hypotension, arrhythmias, thrombocytopenia, hypomagnesemia, hypercalcemia, hyperglycemia, and hypokalemia.

DRUG INTERACTIONS/FOOD INTERACTIONS

Tacrolimus: Standard monitoring of tacrolimus blood concentrations and appropriate tacrolimus dosage adjustments are recommended.

Cyclosporine: Transient increases in liver alanine transaminase (SGPT) and aspartate transaminase (SGOT) have been noted when caspofungin and cyclosporine were coadministered. Monitoring of liver function tests is recommended.

Rifampin: Adult patients on rifampin should receive 70 mg of caspofungin daily.

Nevirapine, efavirenz, carbamazepine, dexamethasone, or **phenytoin:** Increase caspofungin dosage to 70 mg daily.

 DOSING

Empirical therapy, *Candida* infections or *Aspergillus* infections: 70 mg intravenous (IV) loading dose and then 50 mg IV daily.

Esophageal candidiasis: 50 mg IV daily.

SPECIAL POPULATIONS

RENAL IMPAIRMENT: No dosage adjustment is necessary.

HEPATIC IMPAIRMENT: Adult patients with mild hepatic insufficiency (Child-Pugh score 5 to 6) do not need a dosage adjustment.

Adult patients with moderate hepatic insufficiency (Child-Pugh score 7 to 9), caspofungin 35 mg daily is recommended. However, a 70-mg loading dose should still be administered on day 1.

There is no clinical experience in adult patients with severe hepatic insufficiency (Child-Pugh score > 9) and in pediatric patients with any degree of hepatic insufficiency.

PEDIATRIC PATIENTS: For all indications, a single 70-mg/m^2 loading dose (See Mosteller formula for calculating body surface area.) should be administered on day 1, followed by 50 mg/m^2 daily thereafter. The maximum loading dose and the daily maintenance dose should not exceed 70 mg, regardless of the patient's calculated dosage.

When caspofungin is coadministered to pediatric patients with inducers of drug clearance, such as rifampin, efavirenz, nevirapine, phenytoin, dexamethasone, or carbamazepine, a caspofungin dose of 70 mg/m^2 daily (not to exceed 70 mg) should be considered.

PREGNANCY: Category C.

BREASTFEEDING: It is not known if caspofungin is secreted in human milk.

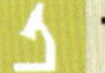

THE ART OF ANTIMICROBIAL THERAPY

Clinical Pearls

1. Echinocandins have activity only against *Candida* species and *Aspergillus* species. They should not be used for any other fungal infections.
2. Caspofungin is active against all pathogenic *Candida* species, including those resistant to fluconazole.

BASIC CHARACTERISTICS

Class: Second-generation cephalosporin

Mechanism of Action: Binds penicillin-binding protein (PBP), disrupting cell wall synthesis.

Mechanisms of Resistance:

1. The PBP can be altered, with reduced affinity,
2. production of a β-lactamase resulting in hydrolysis of the β-lactam ring, and
3. decreased ability of the antibiotic to reach the PBP when bacteria decrease porin production, resulting in a decrease of the drug concentration within the cell.

Metabolic Route: The majority of cefaclor is excreted unchanged in the urine.

FDA-APPROVED INDICATIONS

FDA-Approved Indications: Cefaclor is indicated in the treatment of the following infections when caused by susceptible organisms: otitis media, lower respiratory tract infections, pharyngitis and tonsillitis, urinary tract infections, and skin and skin structure infections.

SIDE EFFECTS/TOXICITY

Cefaclor is **contraindicated** in patients with known allergy to cephalosporins and should be used with caution if hypersensitivity exists to penicillin.

Toxicity includes fever; anaphylaxis; rash including Stevens-Johnson syndrome, erythema multiforme, and toxic epidermal necrolysis; angioedema; flushing; serum sickness–like reactions; encephalopathy; seizures; diarrhea; *Clostridium difficile*–associated diarrhea and pseudomembranous colitis; oral candidiasis; anorexia; nausea; vomiting; stomach cramps; flatulence; hepatitis; renal impairment; genital candidiasis; vaginitis; hemorrhage; prolonged prothrombin time; pancytopenia; hemolytic anemia; and positive Coombs' test.

DRUG INTERACTIONS/FOOD INTERACTIONS

Cefaclor can be taken with or without food.

Probenecid may decrease renal tubular secretion of cephalosporins when used concurrently, resulting in increased and more prolonged cephalosporin blood levels.

Cephalosporins may cause false-positive urine glucose determinations when one is using cupric sulfate solution (Benedict's solution, Clinitest). Tests utilizing glucose oxidase (Tes-Tape, Clinistix) are not affected by cephalosporins.

DOSING

Cefaclor is administered as 250-mg and 500-mg capsules. It can be administered as an oral suspension in the following concentrations: 125 mg/5 mL, 187 mg/5 mL, 250 mg/5 mL, and 375 mg/5 mL.

The usual adult dosage is 250 mg every 8 hours.

For more severe infections (such as pneumonia) or those caused by less-susceptible organisms, doses may be doubled.

SPECIAL POPULATIONS

RENAL IMPAIRMENT: Use with caution, but no dosage adjustment is necessary.

HEPATIC DYSFUNCTION: No dosage adjustment is necessary.

PEDIATRIC PATIENTS: Safety and effectiveness of this product for use in pediatric patients aged younger than 1 month have not been established.

The usual recommended daily dosage for children is 20 mg/kg/day in divided doses every 8 hours.

In more serious infections, otitis media, and infections caused by less-susceptible organisms, 40 mg/kg/day is recommended, with a maximum dosage of 1 g/day.

PREGNANCY: Category B.

BREASTFEEDING: Cefaclor should be used only with caution in breastfeeding mothers.

THE ART OF ANTIMICROBIAL THERAPY

Clinical Pearls

1. Cefaclor is not dose-adjusted for patients with renal impairment.
2. Cross-hypersensitivity among β-lactam antibiotics may occur in up to 10% of patients with a history of penicillin allergy.

BASIC CHARACTERISTICS

Class: First-generation cephalosporin

Mechanism of Action: Binds penicillin-binding protein (PBP), disrupting cell wall synthesis.

Mechanisms of Resistance:

1. The PBP can be altered, with reduced affinity,
2. production of a β-lactamase resulting in hydrolysis of the β-lactam ring, and
3. decreased ability of the antibiotic to reach the PBP when bacteria decrease porin production, resulting in a decrease of the drug concentration within the cell.

Metabolic Route: Cefadroxil is excreted unchanged in the urine.

FDA-APPROVED INDICATIONS

FDA-Approved Indications: Treatment of patients with infection caused by susceptible organisms in urinary tract infections, skin and skin structure infections, and pharyngitis and tonsillitis.

SIDE EFFECTS/TOXICITY

Cefadroxil is **contraindicated** in patients with known allergy to the cephalosporins and should be used with caution if hypersensitivity exists to penicillin.

Toxicity includes fever; anaphylaxis; rash including Stevens-Johnson syndrome, erythema multiforme, and toxic epidermal necrolysis; angioedema; flushing; serum sickness–like reactions; encephalopathy; seizures; diarrhea; *Clostridium difficile*–associated diarrhea and pseudomembranous colitis; oral candidiasis; anorexia; nausea; vomiting; stomach cramps; flatulence; hepatitis; renal impairment; genital candidiasis; vaginitis; hemorrhage; prolonged prothrombin time; pancytopenia; hemolytic anemia; and positive Coombs' test.

DRUG INTERACTIONS/FOOD INTERACTIONS

Cefadroxil may be given with or without food.

Probenecid may decrease renal tubular secretion of cephalosporins when used concurrently, resulting in increased and more prolonged cephalosporin blood levels.

Cephalosporins may cause false-positive urine glucose determinations when one is using cupric sulfate solution (Benedict's solution, Clinitest). Tests utilizing glucose oxidase (Tes-Tape, Clinistix) are not affected by cephalosporins.

CEFADROXIL (Duricef)

DOSING

Cefadroxil is administered as 500-mg or 1-g tablets. It also can be administered as an oral suspension in the following concentrations: 125 mg/5 mL, 250 mg/5 mL, and 500 mg/5 mL.

Urinary tract infections: 1 g or 2 g per day in single (once daily) or divided doses (twice daily).

Skin and skin structure infections: 1 g per day in single (once daily) or divided doses (twice daily).

Pharyngitis and tonsillitis: 1 g per day in single (once daily) or divided doses (twice daily).

SPECIAL POPULATIONS

RENAL IMPAIRMENT: An initial dose of 1 g of cefadroxil should be administered followed by 500 mg at the time intervals listed in the table below:

Renal impairment	*Time intervals*
Creatinine clearance 25 mL/min to 50 mL/min	Every 12 hours
Creatinine clearance 10 mL/min to < 25 mL/min	Every day
Creatinine clearance < 10 mL/min	Every 36 hours
Hemodialysis	500 mg to 1 gram after hemodialysis
Chronic ambulatory peritoneal dialysis	500 mg once daily
Chronic renal replacement therapy	N/A

HEPATIC DYSFUNCTION: No dosage adjustment is necessary.

PEDIATRIC PATIENTS: It is recommended to administer cefadroxil 30 mg/kg/day in divided doses every 12 hours.

PREGNANCY: Category B.

BREASTFEEDING: Cefadroxil should be used with caution in breastfeeding mothers.

THE ART OF ANTIMICROBIAL THERAPY

Clinical Pearls

1. Cefadroxil dosage needs to be adjusted for patients with renal impairment.
2. Cross-allergy with penicillins is less than 10%.

CEFAMANDOLE (Mandol, Mandokef)

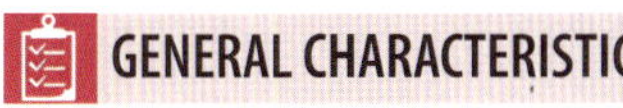

GENERAL CHARACTERISTICS

Class: Second-generation cephalosporin

Mechanism of Action: Binds penicillin-binding protein (PBP), disrupting cell wall synthesis.

Mechanisms of Resistance:

1. The PBP can be altered, with reduced affinity,
2. production of a β-lactamase resulting in hydrolysis of the β-lactam ring, and
3. decreased ability of the antibiotic to reach the PBP when bacteria decrease porin production resulting in a decrease of the drug concentration within the cell.

Metabolic Route: Cefamandole is excreted unchanged in the urine.

FDA-APPROVED INDICATIONS

No longer available in the US; outside the US, used for treatment of lower respiratory infections, urinary tract infections, peritonitis, septicemia, skin and skin structure infections, and bone and joint infections.

Cefamandole preoperatively, intraoperatively, and postoperatively may reduce the incidence of certain postoperative infections.

SIDE EFFECTS/TOXICITY

Cefamandole is **contraindicated** in patients with known allergy to cephalosporins.

Cefamandole should be used with caution if hypersensitivity exists to penicillin.

Toxicity includes phlebitis; fever; anaphylaxis; rash including Stevens-Johnson syndrome, erythema multiforme, and toxic epidermal necrolysis; angioedema; flushing; serum sickness–like reactions; encephalopathy; seizures; diarrhea; *Clostridium difficile*–associated diarrhea and pseudomembranous colitis; oral candidiasis; anorexia; taste perversion; nausea; vomiting; stomach cramps; flatulence; hepatitis; renal impairment; genital candidiasis; vaginitis; hemorrhage; prolonged prothrombin time; pancytopenia; hemolytic anemia, and positive Coombs' test.

DRUG INTERACTIONS/FOOD INTERACTIONS

Concomitant administration of probenecid with cefamandole increases the serum concentration of cefamandole.

Cefamandole inhibits the enzyme acetaldehyde dehydrogenase in laboratory animals. This causes accumulation of acetaldehyde when ethanol is administered concomitantly.

Cephalosporins may cause false-positive urine glucose determinations when one is using cupric sulfate solution (Benedict's solution, Clinitest). Tests utilizing glucose oxidase (Tes-Tape, Clinistix) are not affected by cephalosporins.

CEFAMANDOLE (Mandol, Mandokef)

DOSING

Cefamandole can be administered intravenously (IV) or intramuscularly (IM).

Indication	*Dosage*
Skin and skin structures and uncomplicated pneumonia	500 mg every 6 hours
Uncomplicated urinary tract infections	500 mg every 8 hours
Complicated urinary tract infections	1 g every 8 hours
Severe infections	1 g every 4 to 6 hours
Life-threatening infections with less-susceptible organisms	2 g every 4 hours
Perioperative use	1 g or 2 g IV or IM 30 min to 1 hour before the surgical incision followed by 1 g or 2 g every 6 hours for 24 to 48 hours

SPECIAL POPULATIONS

RENAL IMPAIRMENT:

	For Life-Threatening Infections	*For Less-Severe Infections*
Creatinine clearance 50 mL/min to 80 mL/min	1.5 g every 4 hours or 2 g every 6 hours	0.75 g to 1.5 g every 6 hours
Creatinine clearance 25 mL/min to < 50 mL/min	1.5 g every 6 hours or 2 g every 8 hours	0.75 g to 1.5 g every 8 hours
Creatinine clearance 10 mL/min to < 25 mL/min	1 g every 6 hours or 1.25 g every 8 hours	0.5 g to 1 g every 8 hours
Creatinine clearance 2 mL/min to < 10 mL/min	0.67 g every 8 hours or 1 g every 12 hours	0.5 g to 0.75 g every 12 hours
Creatinine clearance < 2 mL/min	0.5 g every 8 hours or 0.75 g every 12 hours	0.25 g to 0.5 g every 12 hours
Hemodialysis	1 g after dialysis	.5 g after dialysis
Chronic ambulatory peritoneal dialysis	1 g daily	.5 g daily
Continuous renal replacement therapy	1 g every 6 hours	.5 g every 6 hours

HEPATIC DYSFUNCTION: No dosage adjustment is necessary.

PEDIATRIC PATIENTS: 50 mg/kg/day to 100 mg/kg/day in equally divided doses every 4 to 8 hours, which may be increased to a total daily dose of 150 mg/kg (not to exceed the maximum adult dose) for severe infections.

PREGNANCY: Category B.

BREASTFEEDING: The patient should discontinue breastfeeding during treatment.

THE ART OF ANTIMICROBIAL THERAPY

Clinical Pearls

1. The dosage of cefamandole must be adjusted for patients with renal dysfunction.
2. Cross-allergy with penicillins is less than 10%.

GENERAL CHARACTERISTICS

Class: First-generation cephalosporin

Mechanism of Action: Binds penicillin-binding protein (PBP), disrupting cell wall synthesis.

Mechanisms of Resistance:

1. The PBP can be altered, with reduced affinity,
2. production of a β-lactamase resulting in hydrolysis of the β-lactam ring, and
3. decreased ability of the antibiotic to reach the PBP when bacteria decrease porin production resulting in a decrease of the drug concentration within the cell.

Metabolic Route: Cefazolin is excreted unchanged in the urine.

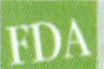

FDA-APPROVED INDICATIONS

FDA-Approved Indications: Treatment of the following infections caused by susceptible organisms: respiratory tract infections, urinary tract infections, skin and skin structure infections, biliary tract infections, bone and joint infections, genital infections, septicemia, endocarditis, and perioperative prophylaxis.

SIDE EFFECTS/TOXICITY

Cefazolin is **contraindicated** in patients with known allergy to cephalosporins and should be used with caution if hypersensitivity exists to penicillin.

Toxicity includes fever; anaphylaxis; rash including Stevens-Johnson syndrome, erythema multiforme, and toxic epidermal necrolysis; angioedema; flushing; serum sickness–like reactions; encephalopathy; seizures; diarrhea; *Clostridium difficile*–associated diarrhea and pseudomembranous colitis; oral candidiasis; anorexia; nausea; vomiting; stomach cramps; flatulence; hepatitis; renal impairment; genital candidiasis; vaginitis; hemorrhage; prolonged prothrombin time; pancytopenia; thrombocytosis; hemolytic anemia; and positive Coombs' test.

DRUG INTERACTIONS/FOOD INTERACTIONS

Probenecid may decrease renal tubular secretion of cephalosporins when used concurrently, resulting in increased and more prolonged cephalosporin blood levels.

Cephalosporins may cause false-positive urine glucose determinations when one is using cupric sulfate solution (Benedict's solution, Clinitest). Tests utilizing glucose oxidase (Tes-Tape, Clinistix) are not affected by cephalosporins.

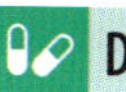

DOSING

USUAL ADULT DOSAGE:

Indication	*Dosage and Frequency*
Moderate-to-severe infections	500 mg to 1 g every 6 to 8 hours
Mild infections (gram-positive)	250 mg to 500 mg every 8 hours
Acute urinary tract infections	1 g every 12 hours
Pneumococcal pneumonia	500 mg every 12 hours
Severe life-threatening infections (e.g., endocarditis or sepsis)	1 g to 1.5 g every 6 hours
Perioperative prophylactic use[a]	1 g 30 min to 1 hour before the start of surgery

[a]For lengthy operations (e.g., 2 hours or more), 500 mg to 1 gram during surgery, *then* 500 mg to 1 gram every 6 to 8 hours for 24 hours postoperatively.

SPECIAL POPULATIONS

RENAL IMPAIRMENT:

	Dosage Adjustment
Creatinine clearance ≥ 55 mL/min	Full dose
Creatinine clearance 35 mL/min to 54 mL/min	Full dose, but at least 8 hours between doses
Creatinine clearance 11 mL/min to 34 mL/min	Half the usual dose every 12 hours
Creatinine clearance ≤ 10 mL/min	Half the usual dose every 18 to 24 hours
Hemodialysis	500 mg to 1 gram after dialysis
Chronic ambulatory peritoneal dialysis	500 mg every 12 hours
Continuous renal replacement therapy	1 g every 12 hours

HEPATIC DYSFUNCTION: No dose adjustment is necessary

PEDIATRIC PATIENTS: Safety and effectiveness for use in premature infants and neonates have not been established.

A total daily dosage of 25 mg/kg to 50 mg/kg divided into three or four equal doses is effective for most mild to moderately severe infections. Total daily dosage may be increased to 100 mg/kg (45 mg/pound) of body weight for severe infections.

RENAL ADJUSTMENT IN CHILDREN:

Creatinine Clearance	*Dosage Adjustment**
40 mL/min to 70 mL/min	60% of the normal daily dosage every 12 hours
20 mL/min to 39 mL/min	25% of the normal daily dosage every 12 hours
<20 mL/min	10% of the normal daily dosage every 24 hours

*All dosage recommendations apply after an initial loading dose.

PREGNANCY: Category B.

BREASTFEEDING: Cefazolin should be used with caution in breastfeeding mothers.

THE ART OF ANTIMICROBIAL THERAPY

Clinical Pearls

1. Dosage of cefazolin must be adjusted in patients with renal impairment.
2. Cross-allergy with penicillins is less than 10% and cefazolin can be used in life-threatening infections with caution if the penicillin allergy is not severe.
3. When one is using cefazolin for surgical prophylaxis, it should be started 30 minutes before incision and continued no longer than 24 hours after surgery.

CEFDINIR (Omnicef)

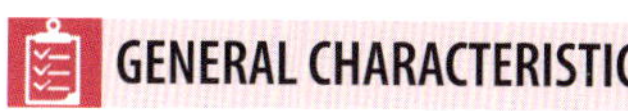

GENERAL CHARACTERISTICS

Class: Third-generation cephalosporin

Mechanism of Action: Binds penicillin-binding protein (PBP), disrupting cell wall synthesis.

Mechanisms of Resistance:

1. The PBP can be altered, with reduced affinity,
2. production of a β-lactamase resulting in hydrolysis of the β-lactam ring, and
3. decreased ability of the antibiotic to reach the PBP when bacteria decrease porin production resulting in a decrease of the drug concentration within the cell.

Metabolic Route: Cefdinir is excreted unchanged in the urine.

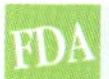

FDA-APPROVED INDICATIONS

FDA-Approved Indications: Treatment of the following infections when caused by susceptible organisms:

Adults: Community-acquired pneumonia, acute exacerbations of chronic bronchitis, acute maxillary sinusitis, pharyngitis and tonsillitis, and uncomplicated skin and skin structure infections.

Pediatrics: Acute bacterial otitis media, pharyngitis and tonsillitis, and uncomplicated skin and skin structure infections.

SIDE EFFECTS/TOXICITY

Cefdinir is **contraindicated** in patients with allergy to cephalosporins. Cefdinir should be used with caution if hypersensitivity exists to penicillins.

Toxicity includes fever; anaphylaxis; rash including Stevens-Johnson syndrome, erythema multiforme, and toxic epidermal necrolysis; angioedema; flushing; serum sickness–like reactions; encephalopathy; seizures; diarrhea; *Clostridium difficile*–associated diarrhea and pseudomembranous colitis; oral candidiasis; anorexia; nausea; vomiting; stomach cramps; flatulence; hepatitis; renal impairment; genital candidiasis; vaginitis; hemorrhage; prolonged prothrombin time; pancytopenia; hemolytic anemia; and positive Coombs' test.

DRUG INTERACTIONS/FOOD INTERACTIONS

Cefdinir can be taken with or without food.

Cefdinir should be taken at least 2 hours before or after an antacid or iron supplement.

Probenecid inhibits the renal excretion of cefdinir.

There have been reports of reddish stools in patients receiving cefdinir.

CEFDINIR (Omnicef)

Cephalosporins may cause false-positive urine glucose determinations when one is using cupric sulfate solution (Benedict's solution, Clinitest). Tests utilizing glucose oxidase (Tes-Tape, Clinistix) are not affected by cephalosporins. False-positive reaction for ketones in the urine may occur with tests using nitroprusside, but not with those using nitroferricyanide.

DOSING

Cefdinir is supplied as 300-mg capsules and a cream-colored powder formulation containing 125 mg/5 mL or 250 mg/5 mL.

The dosages for patients aged older than 13 years:

Infection	*Dosage*	*Duration*
Community-acquired pneumonia	300 mg every 12 hours	10 days
Acute exacerbations of chronic bronchitis	300 mg every 12 hours or 600 mg daily	5 to 10 days
Acute sinusitis	300 mg every 12 hours or 600 mg daily	10 days
Pharyngitis and tonsillitis	300 mg every 12 hours or 600 mg daily	5 to 10 days
Uncomplicated skin and skin structure	300 mg every 12 hours	10 days

SPECIAL POPULATIONS

RENAL IMPAIRMENT:

	Dosage
Creatinine clearance < 30 mg/mL	300 mg once daily
Hemodialysis	300 mg after dialysis
Chronic ambulatory peritoneal dialysis	N/A
Continuous renal replacement therapy	N/A

HEPATIC DYSFUNCTION: No dosage adjustment is necessary.

PEDIATRIC PATIENTS: Safety and efficacy in neonates and infants aged younger than 6 months have not been established.

Infection	*Dosage*	*Duration*
Otitis media	7 mg/kg every 12 hours or 14 mg/kg/day	5 to 10 days

Infection	*Dosage*	*Duration*
Acute maxillary sinusitis	7 mg/kg every 12 hours or 14 mg/kg/day	10 days
Pharyngitis and tonsillitis	7 mg/kg every 12 hours or 14 mg/kg/day	5 to 10 days
Skin and skin structure	7 mg/kg every 12 hours	10 days

For pediatric patients with a creatinine clearance of less than 30 mL/min/1.73 m^2, the dose of cefdinir should be 7 mg/kg (up to 300 mg) given once daily.

PREGNANCY: Category B.

BREASTFEEDING: Cefdinir is not secreted in breastmilk.

THE ART OF ANTIMICROBIAL THERAPY

Clinical Pearls

1. Dosage of cefdinir must be adjusted for patients with renal insufficiency.
2. Cross-allergy with penicillins is less than 10%.

CEFDITOREN PIVOXIL (Spectracef)

GENERAL CHARACTERISTICS

Class: Third-generation cephalosporin

Mechanism of Action: Binds penicillin-binding protein (PBP), disrupting cell wall synthesis.

Mechanisms of Resistance:

1. The PBP can be altered, with reduced affinity,
2. production of a β-lactamase resulting in hydrolysis of the β-lactam ring,
3. decreased ability of the antibiotic to reach the PBP when bacteria decrease porin production resulting in a decrease of the drug concentration within the cell.

Metabolic Route: Cefditoren is excreted unchanged in the urine.

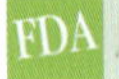

FDA-APPROVED INDICATIONS

FDA-Approved Indications: Treatment of the following infections in adults and adolescents (aged 12 years and older) when caused by susceptible organisms: acute bacterial exacerbation of chronic bronchitis, community-acquired pneumonia, pharyngitis and tonsillitis, and uncomplicated skin and skin-structure infections.

SIDE EFFECTS/TOXICITY

Cefditoren is **contraindicated** in patients with allergy to cephalosporins, in patients with carnitine deficiency, and in patients with milk protein hypersensitivity (not lactose intolerance), because cefditoren contains sodium caseinate, a milk protein.

Cefditoren should be used with caution if hypersensitivity exists to penicillins.

Toxicity includes fever; anaphylaxis; rash including Stevens-Johnson syndrome, erythema multiforme, and toxic epidermal necrolysis; angioedema; flushing; serum sickness–like reactions; encephalopathy; seizures; abnormal dreams; diarrhea; *Clostridium difficile*–associated diarrhea and pseudomembranous colitis; oral candidiasis; anorexia; nausea; vomiting; stomach cramps; flatulence; hepatitis; renal impairment; arthralgia; genital candidiasis; vaginitis; hemorrhage; prolonged prothrombin time; pancytopenia; hemolytic anemia; and positive Coombs' test.

DRUG INTERACTIONS/FOOD INTERACTIONS

Cefditoren should be taken with food.

Probenecid inhibits the renal excretion of cefditoren.

Antacids and H2-receptor antagonists may reduce the absorption of cefditoren.

Cephalosporins may cause false-positive urine glucose determinations when one is using cupric sulfate solution (Benedict's solution, Clinitest). Tests utilizing glucose oxidase (Tes-Tape, Clinistix) are not affected by cephalosporins. False-positive reaction for ketones in the urine may occur with tests using nitroprusside, but not with those using nitroferricyanide.

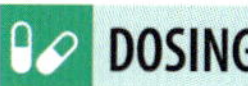

DOSING

Cefditoren is supplied as 200-mg and 400-mg tablets.

Infection	*Dosage*	*Duration*
Community-acquired pneumonia	400 mg every 12 hours	14 days
Acute exacerbations of chronic bronchitis	400 mg every 12 hours	10 days
Pharyngitis	200 mg every 12 hours	10 days
Uncomplicated skin and skin structure	200 mg every 12 hours	10 days

SPECIAL POPULATIONS

RENAL IMPAIRMENT:

	Dosage
Creatinine clearance $\geq$ 30 mL/min	200 mg every 12 hours
Creatinine clearance $<$ 30 mL/min	200 mg daily
Hemodialysis	200 mg daily and 200 mg after hemodialysis
Chronic ambulatory peritoneal dialysis	No data
Continuous renal replacement therapy	No data

HEPATIC DYSFUNCTION: No dosage adjustment is necessary.

PEDIATRIC PATIENTS: Use of cefditoren pivoxil is not recommended for pediatric patients aged younger than 12 years. Dosage in pediatric patients aged 12 years and older should follow adult recommendations.

PREGNANCY: Category B.

BREASTFEEDING: Cefditoren should be used with caution in breastfeeding mothers.

THE ART OF ANTIMICROBIAL THERAPY

Clinical Pearls

1. Cefditoren dosage must be adjusted for patients with renal insufficiency.
2. Cross-allergy with penicillins is less than 10%.
3. It is not recommended that cefditoren be taken with antacids or H2 receptor antagonists.

CEFEPIME (Maxipime)

GENERAL CHARACTERISTICS

Class: Fourth-generation cephalosporin

Mechanism of Action: Binds penicillin-binding protein (PBP), disrupting cell wall synthesis.

Mechanisms of Resistance:

1. The PBP can be altered, with reduced affinity,
2. production of a β-lactamase resulting in hydrolysis of the β-lactam ring, And
3. decreased ability of the antibiotic to reach the PBP when bacteria decrease porin production resulting in a decrease of the drug concentration within the cell.

Metabolic Route: Cefepime is excreted unchanged in the urine.

FDA FDA-APPROVED INDICATIONS

FDA-Approved Indications: Treatment of the following infections when caused by susceptible organisms: pneumonia, empirical therapy for febrile neutropenic patients, uncomplicated and complicated urinary tract infections, uncomplicated skin and skin structure infections, and complicated intraabdominal infections.

SIDE EFFECTS/TOXICITY

Cefepime is **contraindicated** in patients who have shown immediate hypersensitivity reactions to cefepime or cephalosporins, penicillins, or other β-lactam antibiotics. If other forms of hypersensitivity to penicillin exist, cefepime should be used with caution.

Toxicity includes fever; anaphylaxis; rash including Stevens-Johnson syndrome, erythema multiforme, and toxic epidermal necrolysis; angioedema; flushing; serum sickness–like reactions; encephalopathy; seizures; myoclonus; diarrhea; *Clostridium difficile*-associated diarrhea and pseudomembranous colitis; oral candidiasis; anorexia; nausea; vomiting; stomach cramps; flatulence; hepatitis; renal impairment; genital candidiasis; vaginitis; hemorrhage; prolonged prothrombin time; hypercalcemia; hypocalcemia; pancytopenia; hemolytic anemia; and positive Coombs' test.

DRUG INTERACTIONS/FOOD INTERACTIONS

Renal function should be monitored carefully if high doses of aminoglycosides or diuretics are to be administered with cefepime because of the increased potential of nephrotoxicity and ototoxicity of aminoglycoside antibiotics.

Solutions containing dextrose may be contraindicated in patients with known allergy to corn or corn products.

Cephalosporins may cause false-positive urine glucose determinations when one is using cupric sulfate solution (Benedict's solution, Clinitest). Tests utilizing glucose oxidase (Tes-Tape, Clinistix) are not affected by cephalosporins.

DOSING

Type of Infection	*Dosage*	*Duration*
Moderate to severe pneumonia	1g to 2 g every 12 hours	10 days
Febrile neutropenia	2 g every 8 hours	Neutropenia resolution
Urinary tract infection	500 mg to 1 g every 12 hours	7 to 10 days
Severe urinary tract infection	2 g every 12 hours	10 days
Skin and skin structure infection	2 g every 12 hours	10 days
Intraabdominal infection	2 g every 12 hours	7 to 10 days

SPECIAL POPULATIONS

RENAL IMPAIRMENT:

	*Dosages**			
Creatinine clearance > 60 mL/min	500 mg every 12 hours	1 g every 12 hours	2 g every 12 hours	2 g every 8 hours
Creatinine clearance 30 mL/min to 60 mL/min	500 mg once daily	1 g once daily	2 g once daily	2 g every 12 hours
Creatinine clearance 11 mL/min to 29 mL/min	500 mg once daily	500 mg once daily	1 g once daily	2 g once daily
Creatinine clearance < 11 mL/min	250 mg once daily	250 mg once daily	500 mg once daily	1 g once daily
Hemodialysis	1 g on day 1, then 500 mg every 24 hours	1 g on day 1, then 500 mg every 24 hours	1 g on day 1, then 500 mg every 24 hours	1 g every day
Chronic ambulatory peritoneal dialysis	500 mg every 48 hours	1 g every 48 hours	2 g every 48 hours	2 g every 48 hours
Continuous renal replacement therapy	Not recommended			

*Choose the dose that will be used for normal renal function (top row); then select regimen based on creatinine clearance.

HEPATIC DYSFUNCTION: No dosage adjustment is necessary.

PEDIATRIC PATIENTS: Safety and effectiveness in pediatric patients aged younger than 2 months have not been established.

The dosage is 50 mg/kg per dose, administered every 12 hours (50 mg/kg per dose, every 8 hours for febrile neutropenic patients).

PREGNANCY: Category B.

BREASTFEEDING: Cefepime should be used only with caution in breastfeeding mothers.

THE ART OF ANTIMICROBIAL THERAPY

Clinical Pearls

1. Dosage of cefepime is adjusted for patients with renal dysfunction.
2. Cross-allergy with penicillins is less than 10%.
3. Patients with creatinine clearance less than or equal to 60 mL/min must have dosage adjustment to avoid adverse reactions such as encephalopathy, myoclonus, and seizures.
4. Concomitant aminoglycosides increase the potential of nephrotoxicity and ototoxicity.
5. Nephrotoxicity has been reported with concomitant administration of other cephalosporins with potent diuretics such as furosemide.

GENERAL CHARACTERISTICS

Class: Third-generation cephalosporin

Mechanism of Action: Binds penicillin-binding protein (PBP), disrupting cell wall synthesis.

Mechanisms of Resistance:

1. The PBP can be altered, with reduced affinity,
2. production of a β-lactamase resulting in hydrolysis of the β-lactam ring, and
3. decreased ability of the antibiotic to reach the PBP when bacteria decrease porin production resulting in a decrease of the drug concentration within the cell.

Metabolic Route: Cefixime is excreted unchanged in the urine.

FDA-APPROVED INDICATIONS

FDA-Approved Indications: Treatment of the following infections when caused by susceptible organisms: uncomplicated urinary tract infections, otitis media, pharyngitis and tonsillitis, acute bronchitis and acute exacerbations of chronic bronchitis, and uncomplicated gonorrhea.

SIDE EFFECTS/TOXICITY

Cefixime is **contraindicated** in patients with cephalosporin allergy and should be used with caution if hypersensitivity exists to penicillin.

Toxicity includes fever; anaphylaxis; rash including Stevens-Johnson syndrome, erythema multiforme, and toxic epidermal necrolysis; angioedema; flushing; serum sickness–like reactions; encephalopathy; seizures; diarrhea; *Clostridium difficile*–associated diarrhea and pseudomembranous colitis; oral candidiasis; anorexia; nausea; vomiting; stomach cramps; flatulence; hepatitis; renal impairment; genital candidiasis; vaginitis; hemorrhage; prolonged prothrombin time; pancytopenia; hemolytic anemia; and positive Coombs' test.

DRUG INTERACTIONS/FOOD INTERACTIONS

Cefixime can be taken with or without food.

Increased levels of carbamazepine and prothrombin time may be seen when carbamazepine and warfarin are administered with cefixime.

Cephalosporins may cause false-positive urine glucose determinations when one is using cupric sulfate solution (Benedict's solution, Clinitest). Tests utilizing glucose oxidase (Tes-Tape, Clinistix) are not affected by cephalosporins. A false-positive reaction for ketones in the urine may occur with tests using nitroprusside but not with those using nitroferricyanide.

CEFIXIME (Suprax)

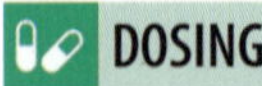

DOSING

Cefixime is available as a 400-mg tablet and an oral suspension of 100 mg/5 mL.

The recommended dosage of the suspension is 400 mg daily.

For the treatment of uncomplicated cervical or urethral gonococcal infections, a single oral dose of 400 mg is recommended.

SPECIAL POPULATIONS

RENAL IMPAIRMENT:

Renal Impairment	*Dosage*
Creatinine clearance 21 mL/min to 60 mL/min or hemodialysis	300 mg daily
Creatinine clearance $\leq$ 20 mL/min, or peritoneal dialysis	200 mg daily
Continuous renal replacement therapy	N/A

HEPATIC DYSFUNCTION: No dosage adjustment is necessary.

PEDIATRIC PATIENTS: Safety and effectiveness of cefixime in children aged younger than 6 months have not been established.

The recommended dose is 8 mg/kg/day of the suspension. This may be administered as a single daily dose or may be given in two divided doses, as 4 mg/kg every 12 hours.

Children weighing more than 50 kg or aged older than 12 years should be treated with the recommended adult dose.

PREGNANCY: Category B.

BREASTFEEDING: Cefixime should be used only with caution in breastfeeding mothers.

THE ART OF ANTIMICROBIAL THERAPY

Clinical Pearls

1. Dosage of cefixime is adjusted for patients with renal dysfunction.
2. Cross-allergy with penicillins is less than 10%.
3. Monitoring is essential when cefixime is coadministered with warfarin and carbamazepine.

CEFOPERAZONE (Cefobid)

GENERAL CHARACTERISTICS

Class: Third-generation cephalosporin

Mechanism of Action: Binds penicillin-binding protein (PBP), disrupting cell wall synthesis.

Mechanisms of Resistance:

1. The PBP can be altered, with reduced affinity,
2. production of a β-lactamase resulting in hydrolysis of the β-lactam ring, and
3. decreased ability of the antibiotic to reach the PBP when bacteria decrease porin production resulting in a decrease of the drug concentration within the cell.

Metabolic Route: Cefoperazone is excreted unchanged in the bile.

FDA-APPROVED INDICATIONS

FDA-Approved Indications: Treatment of patients with infections caused by susceptible strains of organisms in the following conditions: respiratory tract infections, peritonitis and other intraabdominal infections, bacterial septicemia, infections of the skin and skin structures, pelvic inflammatory disease, and urinary tract infections.

SIDE EFFECTS/TOXICITY

Cefoperazone is **contraindicated** in patients who have shown hypersensitivity to the cephalosporin group of antibiotics.

Cefoperazone should be used with caution if hypersensitivity exists to penicillin.

Toxicity includes inflammation at the site of injection; fever; anaphylaxis; rash including Stevens-Johnson syndrome, erythema multiforme, and toxic epidermal necrolysis; angioedema; flushing; serum sickness–like reactions; encephalopathy; seizures; diarrhea; *Clostridium difficile*–associated diarrhea and pseudomembranous colitis; oral candidiasis; anorexia; nausea; vomiting; stomach cramps; flatulence; hepatitis; renal impairment; genital candidiasis; vaginitis; hemorrhage; prolonged prothrombin time; pancytopenia; hemolytic anemia; positive Coombs' test, and a disulfiramlike reaction after alcohol ingestion.

DRUG INTERACTIONS/FOOD INTERACTIONS

Nephrotoxicity has been reported following concomitant administration of cephalosporins with aminoglycoside antibiotics or potent diuretics such as furosemide. Cephalosporins may cause false-positive urine glucose determinations when one is using cupric sulfate solution (Benedict's solution, Clinitest). Tests utilizing glucose oxidase (Tes-Tape, Clinistix) are not affected by cephalosporins.

DOSING

The usual adult daily dosage of cefoperazone is 2 g to 4 g per day administered in equally divided doses every 12 hours. Cefoperazone may be given intramuscularly (with lidocaine) or intravenously.

In severe infections or infections caused by less-sensitive organisms, the total daily dosage and/or frequency may be increased to a total daily dosage of 6 g to 12 g divided into two, three, or four administrations ranging from 1.5 g to 4 g per dose.

SPECIAL POPULATIONS

RENAL IMPAIRMENT: No dosage adjustment is necessary.

HEPATIC DYSFUNCTION OR BILIARY OBSTRUCTION: Daily dosage should not exceed 4 g.

BOTH HEPATIC DYSFUNCTION AND SIGNIFICANT RENAL DISEASE: Daily dosage should not exceed 1 g to 2 g, with monitoring of serum concentrations.

PEDIATRIC PATIENTS: Safety and effectiveness in children have not been established.

PREGNANCY: Category B.

BREASTFEEDING: Cefoperazone should be used with caution in breastfeeding mothers.

THE ART OF ANTIMICROBIAL THERAPY

Clinical Pearls

1. The dosage of cefoperazone is not adjusted for patients with renal dysfunction, but adjustment is necessary for hepatic and/or biliary disease and for combined hepatic and renal dysfunction.
2. Cross-allergy with penicillins is less than 10% and cefoperazone can be used in life-threatening infections with caution if the allergy to penicillin is not severe.
3. Inducible type I β-lactamase resistance has been noted with some organisms (e.g., *Enterobacter* species, *Pseudomonas* species, and *Serratia* species) and can develop during therapy.

 GENERAL CHARACTERISTICS

Class: Third-generation cephalosporin

Mechanism of Action: Binds penicillin-binding protein (PBP), disrupting cell wall synthesis.

Mechanisms of Resistance:

1. The PBP can be altered, with reduced affinity,
2. production of a β-lactamase resulting in hydrolysis of the β-lactam ring, and
3. decreased ability of the antibiotic to reach the PBP when bacteria decrease porin production resulting in a decrease of the drug concentration within the cell.

Metabolic Route: Cefotaxime is predominantly excreted in the urine as unchanged drug and metabolites.

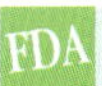 FDA-APPROVED INDICATIONS

FDA-Approved Indications: Treatment of patients with the following serious infections caused by susceptible strains of microorganisms: lower respiratory tract infections, genitourinary infections, gynecologic infections (e.g., pelvic inflammatory disease, endometritis, and pelvic cellulitis), bacteremia/septicemia, skin and skin structure infections, intraabdominal infections, bone and/or joint infections, central nervous system infections (e.g., meningitis and ventriculitis), and prevention of infection perioperatively.

 SIDE EFFECTS/TOXICITY

Cefotaxime is **contraindicated** in patients who have shown hypersensitivity to any cephalosporin and should be used with caution if hypersensitivity exists to penicillin.

Toxicity includes fever; anaphylaxis; rash including Stevens-Johnson syndrome, erythema multiforme, and toxic epidermal necrolysis; angioedema; flushing; serum sickness–like reactions; encephalopathy; seizures; diarrhea; *Clostridium difficile*–associated diarrhea and pseudomembranous colitis; oral candidiasis; anorexia; nausea; vomiting; stomach cramps; flatulence; hepatitis; renal impairment; genital candidiasis; vaginitis; hemorrhage; prolonged prothrombin time; pancytopenia; hemolytic anemia; positive Coombs' test; and potentially life-threatening arrhythmias following rapid (less than 60 seconds) bolus administration via central venous catheter.

 DRUG INTERACTIONS/FOOD INTERACTIONS

Increased nephrotoxicity has been reported following concomitant administration of cephalosporins and aminoglycoside antibiotics.

Cephalosporins may cause false-positive urine glucose determinations when one is using cupric sulfate solution (Benedict's solution, Clinitest). Tests utilizing glucose oxidase (Tes-Tape, Clinistix) are not affected by cephalosporins.

DOSING

Severity or Type of Infection	*Dosage*
Uncomplicated	1 g every 12 hours IM or IV
Moderate to complicated	1 to 2 g every 8 hours IM or IV
Life-threatening	2 g every 4 hours IM or IV
Prevention	1 g 30 to 90 minutes before start of surgery
Gonococcal urethritis or cervicitis	0.5 g IM (single dose)
Rectal gonorrhea in women	0.5 g IM (single dose)
Rectal gonorrhea in men	1 g IM (single dose)

Note: IM = intramuscularly; IV = intravenously.

SPECIAL POPULATIONS

RENAL IMPAIRMENT:

	Dosage
Creatinine clearance 10 mL/min to 50 mL/min	Usual dose every 8 to 12 hours
Creatinine clearance < 10 mL/min	Usual dose once daily
Hemodialysis	1 g after dialysis
Chronic ambulatory peritoneal dialysis	1 g daily
Continuous renal replacement therapy	1 g every 12 hours

HEPATIC DYSFUNCTION: No dosage adjustment is necessary.

PEDIATRIC PATIENTS: For body weights less than 50 kg, the recommended daily dose is 50 mg/kg to 180 mg/kg body weight divided into four to six equal doses. The higher dosages should be used for more severe or serious infections, including meningitis. For body weights 50 kg or more, the usual adult dosage should be used; the maximum daily dosage should not exceed 12 g.

PREGNANCY: Category B.

BREASTFEEDING: Cefotaxime should be used with caution in breastfeeding mothers.

THE ART OF ANTIMICROBIAL THERAPY

Clinical Pearls

1. Dosage of cefotaxime is adjusted for patients with renal impairment.
2. Cross-allergy with penicillins is less than 10% and cefotaxime can be used in life-threatening infections (e.g., meningitis) with caution if the allergy to penicillin is not severe.
3. Cefotaxime may be administered intramuscularly or intravenously.

GENERAL CHARACTERISTICS

Class: Second-generation cephalosporin

Mechanism of Action: Binds penicillin-binding protein (PBP), disrupting cell wall synthesis.

Mechanisms of Resistance:

1. The PBP can be altered, with reduced affinity,
2. production of a β-lactamase resulting in hydrolysis of the β-lactam ring, and
3. decreased ability of the antibiotic to reach the PBP when bacteria decrease porin production resulting in a decrease of the drug concentration within the cell.

Metabolic Route: Cefotetan is predominantly excreted unchanged in the urine.

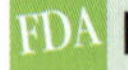

FDA-APPROVED INDICATIONS

FDA-Approved Indications: Treatment of the following infections when caused by susceptible organisms: urinary tract infections, lower respiratory tract infections, skin and skin structure infections, gynecologic infections, intraabdominal infections, and bone and joint infections.

Prophylaxis of surgical procedures that are classified as clean-contaminated or potentially contaminated.

SIDE EFFECTS/TOXICITY

Cefotetan is **contraindicated** in patients with a known allergy to the cephalosporin group of antibiotics and in those individuals who have experienced a cephalosporin-associated hemolytic anemia. Cefotetan should be used with caution if hypersensitivity exists to penicillin.

Toxicity includes fever; anaphylaxis; rash including Stevens-Johnson syndrome, erythema multiforme, and toxic epidermal necrolysis; angioedema; flushing; serum sickness–like reactions; encephalopathy; seizures; diarrhea; *Clostridium difficile*–associated diarrhea and pseudomembranous colitis; oral candidiasis; anorexia; nausea; vomiting; stomach cramps; flatulence; hepatitis; renal impairment; genital candidiasis; vaginitis; hemorrhage; prolonged prothrombin time; pancytopenia; and positive Coombs' test.

There appears to be an increased risk of developing hemolytic anemia on cefotetan relative to other cephalosporins.

DRUG INTERACTIONS/FOOD INTERACTIONS

If cefotetan and an aminoglycoside are used concomitantly, renal function should be carefully monitored, because nephrotoxicity may be potentiated. As with other cephalosporins, high concentrations of cefotetan may produce false increases in the levels of creatinine reported.

Cephalosporins may cause false-positive urine glucose determinations when one is using cupric sulfate solution (Benedict's solution, Clinitest). Tests utilizing glucose oxidase (Tes-Tape, Clinistix) are not affected by cephalosporins.

DOSING

Indication	*Dosage*
Urinary tract infection	500 mg every 12 hours IV or IM or 1 g or 2 g every 24 hours IV or IM or 1 g or 2 g every 12 hours IV or IM
Skin and soft tissue infection	2 g every 24 hours IV or 1 g every 12 hours IV or IM
Severe infections	2 g every 12 hours IV
Life-threatening infections	3 g every 12 hours IV
Prophylaxis	1 g or 2 g 30 to 60 minutes before surgery In patients undergoing cesarean section, the dose should be administered as soon as the umbilical cord is clamped

Note: IV = intravenously; IM = intramuscularly.

SPECIAL POPULATIONS

RENAL IMPAIRMENT: The dosage of cefotetan can be maintained with the interval adjusted as in the table below:

	Dosing Interval
Creatinine clearance > 30 mL/min	Every 12 hours
Creatinine clearance 10 mL/min to 30 mL/min	Every 24 hours
Creatinine clearance < 10 mL/min	Every 48 hours
Hemodialysis	After dialysis only
Chronic ambulatory peritoneal dialysis	Every 24 hours
Continuous renal replacement therapy	750 mg every 12 hours

OR

the dosing interval may remain constant at 12-hour intervals, but the dose reduced to one half for patients with a creatinine clearance of 10 mL/min to 30 mL/min, and one quarter for patients with a creatinine clearance of less than 10 mL/min.

HEPATIC DYSFUNCTION: No dosage adjustment is necessary.

PEDIATRIC PATIENTS: Safety and effectiveness in children have not been established.

PREGNANCY: Category B.

BREASTFEEDING: Cefotetan should be used with caution in breastfeeding mothers.

THE ART OF ANTIMICROBIAL THERAPY

Clinical Pearls

1. Dosage of cefotetan is adjusted for patients with renal dysfunction.
2. Cross-allergy with penicillins is less than 10%.
3. Cefotetan can be given intramuscularly or intravenously.
4. There is an increased risk of hemolytic anemia with cefotetan, relative to other cephalosporins.

CEFOXITIN (Mefoxin)

GENERAL CHARACTERISTICS

Class: Second-generation cephalosporin

Mechanism of Action: Binds penicillin-binding protein (PBP), disrupting cell wall synthesis.

Mechanisms of Resistance:

1. The PBP can be altered, with reduced affinity,
2. production of a β-lactamase resulting in hydrolysis of the β-lactam ring, and
3. decreased ability of the antibiotic to reach the PBP when bacteria decrease porin production resulting in a decrease of the drug concentration within the cell.

Metabolic Route: Cefoxitin is predominantly excreted unchanged in the urine.

FDA-APPROVED INDICATIONS

FDA-Approved Indications: Treatment of serious infections caused by susceptible strains of microorganisms in lower respiratory tract infections, urinary tract infections, intraabdominal infections, gynecologic infections, septicemia, bone and joint infections, and skin and skin structure infections.

Prevention of infection in patients undergoing uncontaminated gastrointestinal surgery, vaginal hysterectomy, abdominal hysterectomy, or cesarean section.

SIDE EFFECTS/TOXICITY

Cefoxitin is **contraindicated** in patients who have shown hypersensitivity to cefoxitin and the cephalosporin group of antibiotics. Cefoxitin should be used with caution if hypersensitivity exists to penicillins.

Toxicity includes fever; anaphylaxis; rash including Stevens-Johnson syndrome, erythema multiforme, and toxic epidermal necrolysis; angioedema; flushing; hypotension; serum sickness–like reactions; encephalopathy; seizures; possible exacerbation of myasthenia gravis; diarrhea; *Clostridium difficile*–associated diarrhea and pseudomembranous colitis; oral candidiasis; anorexia; nausea; vomiting; stomach cramps; flatulence; hepatitis; renal impairment; genital candidiasis; vaginitis; hemorrhage; prolonged prothrombin time; pancytopenia; hemolytic anemia; and positive Coombs' test.

DRUG INTERACTIONS/FOOD INTERACTIONS

Increased nephrotoxicity has been reported following concomitant administration of cephalosporins and aminoglycoside antibiotics.

Cephalosporins may cause false-positive urine glucose determinations when one is using cupric sulfate solution (Benedict's solution, Clinitest). Tests utilizing glucose oxidase (Tes-Tape, Clinistix) are not affected by cephalosporins.

Solutions containing dextrose may be contraindicated in patients with hypersensitivity to corn products.

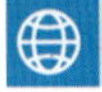 DOSING

Condition	*Dosage*
Uncomplicated infections	1 g every 6 to 8 hours IV
Moderate to severe infections	1 g every 4 hours or 2 g every 6 to 8 hours IV
Prevention	2 g IV 30 to 60 min before incision followed by 2 g IV every 6 hours after first dose for no more than 24 hours

IV = intravenous.

SPECIAL POPULATIONS

RENAL IMPAIRMENT:

	Dosage
Creatinine clearance 30 mL/min to 50 mL/min	1 g to 2 g every 8 to 12 hours
Creatinine clearance 10 mL/min to 29 mL/min	1 g to 2 g every 12 to 24 hours
Creatinine clearance 5 mL/min to 9 mL/min	500 mg to 1 g every 12 to 24 hours
Creatinine clearance < 5 mL/min	500 mg to 1 g every 24 to 48 hours
Hemodialysis	1 g after dialysis
Chronic ambulatory peritoneal dialysis	1 g daily
Continuous renal replacement therapy	1 g to 2 g every 8 to 12 hours

HEPATIC DYSFUNCTION: No dosage adjustment is necessary.

PEDIATRIC PATIENTS: Safety and efficacy in pediatric patients aged younger than 3 months have not been established. In patients aged 3 months and older, the dosage is 80 mg/kg/day to 160 mg/kg/day divided into four to six equal doses. The higher dosages should be used for more severe or serious infections. The total daily dosage should not exceed 12 g.

For surgical infection prevention, 30 mg/kg to 40 mg/kg doses may be given at the times designated above in the dosing section.

PREGNANCY: Category B.

BREASTFEEDING: Cefoxitin should be used with caution in breastfeeding mothers.

THE ART OF ANTIMICROBIAL THERAPY

Clinical Pearls

1. Dosage of cefoxitin is adjusted for patients with renal dysfunction.
2. Cross-allergy with penicillins is less than 10%.
3. Cefoxitin may cause an exacerbation of myasthenia gravis.

CEFPIROME (Cefrom, Keiten, Broact, Cefir)

GENERAL CHARACTERISTICS

Class: Fourth-generation cephalosporin

Mechanism of Action: Binds penicillin binding protein (PBP), disrupting cell wall synthesis.

Mechanisms of Resistance:

1. The PBP can be altered, with reduced affinity,
2. production of a β-lactamase resulting in hydrolysis of the β-lactam ring, and
3. decreased ability of the antibiotic to reach the PBP when bacteria decrease porin production resulting in a decrease of the drug concentration within the cell.

Metabolic Route: Cefpirome is excreted unchanged in the urine.

FDA FDA-APPROVED INDICATIONS

Not FDA approved, but used outside the US for lower respiratory tract infections, complicated upper (pyelonephritis) and lower urinary tract infections, skin and soft tissue infections, bacteremia/septicemia, and infections in neutropenic and immunocompromised patients.

SIDE EFFECTS/TOXICITY

Cefpirome is **contraindicated** in patients who have shown immediate hypersensitivity reactions to cefpirome or cephalosporins, and in patients with porphyria. Caution should be taken in patients with penicillin allergy.

Toxicity includes fever; anaphylaxis; rash including Stevens-Johnson syndrome, erythema multiforme, and toxic epidermal necrolysis; angioedema; flushing; serum sickness–like reactions; encephalopathy; seizures; myoclonus; diarrhea; *Clostridium difficile*–associated diarrhea and pseudomembranous colitis; oral candidiasis; anorexia; nausea; vomiting; stomach cramps; flatulence; hepatitis; renal impairment; genital candidiasis; vaginitis; hemorrhage; prolonged prothrombin time; hypercalcemia; hypocalcemia; pancytopenia; hemolytic anemia; and positive Coombs' test.

DRUG INTERACTIONS/FOOD INTERACTIONS

Renal function should be monitored carefully if high doses of aminoglycosides or diuretics are to be administered with cefpirome because of the increased potential of nephrotoxicity and ototoxicity of aminoglycoside antibiotics.

Cephalosporins may cause false-positive urine glucose determinations when one is using cupric sulfate solution (Benedict's solution, Clinitest). Tests utilizing glucose oxidase (Tes-Tape, Clinistix) are not affected by cephalosporins.

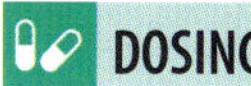

DOSING

Usual adult dosage: 1 g to 2 g intravenously every 12 hours.

SPECIAL POPULATIONS

RENAL IMPAIRMENT:

Renal Impairment	*Dosage*
Creatinine clearance < 50 mL/min	1 g to 2 g loading dose
Then	
Creatinine clearance 20 mL/min to < 50 mL/min	500 mg to 1 g every 12 hours
Creatinine clearance 5 mL/min to < 20 mL/min	500 mg to 1 g every 24 hours
Creatinine clearance < 5, hemodialysis	500 mg to 1 g every 24 hours, then half-dose postdialysis

HEPATIC DYSFUNCTION: No dosage adjustment is necessary.

PEDIATRIC PATIENTS: Cefpirome should not be used in children.

PREGNANCY: Category B.

BREASTFEEDING: Cefpirome should be used only with caution in breastfeeding mothers.

THE ART OF ANTIMICROBIAL THERAPY

Clinical Pearls

1. Cross-allergy with penicillins is less than 10%
2. Patients with creatinine clearance less than or equal to 50 mL/min must have dosage adjustment to avoid adverse reactions such as encephalopathy, myoclonus, and seizures.
3. Concomitant aminoglycosides increase the potential for nephrotoxicity and ototoxicity.
4. Nephrotoxicity has been reported with concomitant administration of other cephalosporins with potent diuretics such as furosemide.

CEFPODOXIME PROXETIL (Vantin)

GENERAL CHARACTERISTICS

Class: Third-generation cephalosporin

Mechanism of Action: Binds penicillin-binding protein (PBP), disrupting cell wall synthesis.

Mechanisms of Resistance:

1. The PBP can be altered, with reduced affinity,
2. production of a β-lactamase resulting in hydrolysis of the β-lactam ring, and
3. decreased ability of the antibiotic to reach the PBP when bacteria decrease porin production resulting in a decrease of the drug concentration within the cell.

Metabolic Route: Cefpodoxime is excreted unchanged in the urine.

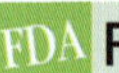

FDA-APPROVED INDICATIONS

FDA-Approved Indications: The following mild-to-moderate infections caused by susceptible strains of microorganisms: acute otitis media, pharyngitis and tonsillitis, community-acquired pneumonia, acute bacterial exacerbation of chronic bronchitis, acute uncomplicated urethral and cervical gonorrhea, acute uncomplicated anorectal infections in women, uncomplicated skin and skin structure infections, acute maxillary sinusitis, and uncomplicated urinary tract infections (cystitis).

SIDE EFFECTS/TOXICITY

Cefpodoxime proxetil is **contraindicated** in patients with a known allergy to cefpodoxime or to the cephalosporin group of antibiotics.

Cefpodoxime should be used with caution if hypersensitivity exists to penicillin.

Toxicity includes fever; anaphylaxis; rash including Stevens-Johnson syndrome, erythema multiforme, and toxic epidermal necrolysis; angioedema; flushing; serum sickness–like reactions; encephalopathy; seizures; hallucination; hyperkinesias; diarrhea; *Clostridium difficile*–associated diarrhea and pseudomembranous colitis; oral candidiasis; anorexia; taste perversion; nausea; vomiting; stomach cramps; flatulence; hepatitis; renal impairment; genital candidiasis; vaginitis; hemorrhage; epistaxis; prolonged prothrombin time; pancytopenia; hemolytic anemia; positive Coombs' test; hyperglycemia; hypoglycemia; hypoalbuminemia; hypoproteinemia; hyperkalemia; and hyponatremia.

DRUG INTERACTIONS/FOOD INTERACTIONS

Oral suspension may be given without regard to food. Tablets should be given with food.

Concomitant administration of high doses of antacids or H2 blockers reduces peak plasma levels of cefpodoxime by 24% to 42%.

Cephalosporins may cause false-positive urine glucose determinations when one is using cupric sulfate solution (Benedict's solution, Clinitest). Tests utilizing glucose oxidase (Tes-Tape, Clinistix) are not affected by cephalosporins.

Probenecid increases levels of cefpodoxime.

Close monitoring of renal function is advised when cefpodoxime proxetil is administered concomitantly with compounds of known nephrotoxic potential.

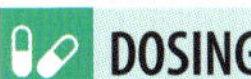

DOSING

Cefpodoxime is available as tablets (100 mg and 200 mg) or suspension (50 mg/5mL or 100 mg/5mL) .

Infection	*Oral Dosage*	*Duration*
Pharyngitis/tonsillitis	100 mg every 12 hours	5 to 10 days
Community-acquired pneumonia	200 mg every 12 hours	14 days
Gonorrhea	400 mg	Single dose
Skin and skin structure	400 mg every 12 hours	7 to 14 days
Acute maxillary sinusitis	200 mg every 12 hours	10 days
Urinary tract	100 mg every 12 hours	7 days

SPECIAL POPULATIONS

RENAL IMPAIRMENT:

Renal Impairment	*Dosage*
Creatinine clearance < 30 mL/min	Usual dose once daily
Hemodialysis	200 mg after dialysis only
Chronic ambulatory peritoneal dialysis	Usual dose once daily
Continuous renal replacement therapy	N/A

HEPATIC DYSFUNCTION: Dosage adjustment is not necessary.

PEDIATRIC PATIENTS: Safety and efficacy in infants aged younger than 2 months have not been established.

Pediatric Infection	*Dosage*	*Duration*
Acute otitis media	5 mg/kg (maximum 200 mg) every 12 hours	5 days
Pharyngitis/tonsillitis	5 mg/kg (maximum 100 mg) every 12 hours	5 to 10 days
Acute maxillary sinusitis	5 mg/kg (maximum 200 mg) every 12 hours	10 days

PREGNANCY: Category B.

BREASTFEEDING: Breastfeeding should be stopped when cefpodoxime is administered.

THE ART OF ANTIMICROBIAL THERAPY

Clinical Pearls

1. Dosage of cefpodoxime is adjusted for patients with renal dysfunction.
2. Cross-allergy with penicillins is less than 10%.
3. Antacids or H2 blockers may decrease serum concentrations of cefpodoxime.

GENERAL CHARACTERISTICS

Class: Second-generation cephalosporin

Mechanism of Action: Binds penicillin-binding protein (PBP), disrupting cell wall synthesis.

Mechanisms of Resistance:

1. The PBP can be altered, with reduced affinity,
2. production of a β-lactamase resulting in hydrolysis of the β-lactam ring, and
3. decreased ability of the antibiotic to reach the PBP when bacteria decrease porin production resulting in a decrease of the drug concentration within the cell.

Metabolic Route: The majority of cefprozil is excreted unchanged in the urine.

FDA-APPROVED INDICATIONS

FDA-Approved Indications: Treatment of patients with the following mild-to-moderate infections caused by susceptible strains of microorganisms: upper respiratory tract infections, otitis media, acute sinusitis, lower respiratory tract infections, secondary bacterial infection of acute bronchitis and acute bacterial exacerbation of chronic bronchitis, complicated and uncomplicated skin and skin structure infections.

SIDE EFFECTS/TOXICITY

Cefprozil is **contraindicated** in patients with known allergy to cephalosporins.

Cefprozil should be used with caution if hypersensitivity exists to penicillin.

Toxicity includes phlebitis; fever; anaphylaxis; rash including Stevens-Johnson syndrome, erythema multiforme, and toxic epidermal necrolysis; angioedema; flushing; serum sickness–like reactions; encephalopathy; seizures; diarrhea; *Clostridium difficile*–associated diarrhea and pseudomembranous colitis; oral candidiasis; anorexia; taste perversion; nausea; vomiting; stomach cramps; flatulence; hepatitis; renal impairment; genital candidiasis; vaginitis; hemorrhage; prolonged prothrombin time; pancytopenia; hemolytic anemia; and positive Coombs' test.

DRUG INTERACTIONS/FOOD INTERACTIONS

Drugs that reduce gastric acidity may result in a lower bioavailability of cefprozil. Cephalosporins may cause false-positive urine glucose determinations when one is using cupric sulfate solution (Benedict's solution, Clinitest). Tests utilizing glucose oxidase (Tes-Tape, Clinistix) are not affected by cephalosporins.

CEFPROZIL AXETIL (Cefzil)

 DOSING

Cefprozil is supplied in 250-mg and 500-mg tablets.

It is also available in a cream-colored suspension 125 mg/5 mL and 250 mg/5 mL.

Infection	*Dosage*	*Duration*
Pharyngitis/tonsillitis	500 mg daily	10 days
Acute sinusitis	250 mg to 500 mg every 12 hours	10 days
Acute bronchitis	500 mg every 12 hours	10 days
Uncomplicated skin and skin structure	250 mg every 12 hours	10 days

SPECIAL POPULATIONS

RENAL IMPAIRMENT:

	Dosage
Creatinine clearance 10 mL/min to 50 mL/min	Reduce dose by 50%
Creatinine clearance < 10 mL/min	Reduce dose by 50% and give once daily
Hemodialysis	Usual dose, but given after dialysis only
Chronic ambulatory peritoneal dialysis	Reduce dose by 50%
Continuous renal replacement therapy	Reduce dose by 50%

HEPATIC DYSFUNCTION: No dosage adjustment is necessary.

PEDIATRIC PATIENTS:

Children Aged 2 to 12 Years

Infection	*Dosage*	*Duration*
Pharyngitis/tonsillitis	7.5 mg/kg every 12 hours	10 days
Uncomplicated skin and skin structure	20 mg/kg daily	10 days

Children Aged 6 Months to 12 Years

Infection	*Dosage*	*Duration*
Otitis media	15 mg/kg every 12 hours	10 days
Sinusitis	7.5 mg/kg to 15 mg/kg every 12 hours	10 days

PREGNANCY: Category B.

BREASTFEEDING: Consideration should be given to discontinuing breastfeeding temporarily during treatment with cefprozil axetil.

THE ART OF ANTIMICROBIAL THERAPY

Clinical Pearls

1. Cefprozil dosage must be adjusted for patients with renal dysfunction.
2. Cross-allergy with penicillins is less than 10%.
3. Phenylketonurics: Cefprozil for oral suspension contains 8.4 mg of phenylalanine per 5 mL (1 teaspoonful) constituted suspension for both the 125 mg/5 mL and 250 mg/5 mL dosage forms.

GENERAL CHARACTERISTICS

Class: Third-generation cephalosporin

Mechanism of Action: Binds penicillin-binding protein (PBP), disrupting cell wall synthesis.

Mechanisms of Resistance:

1. The PBP can be altered, with reduced affinity,
2. production of a β-lactamase resulting in hydrolysis of the β-lactam ring, and
3. decreased ability of the antibiotic to reach the PBP when bacteria decrease porin production resulting in a decrease of the drug concentration within the cell.

Metabolic Route: Ceftazadime is excreted unchanged in the urine.

FDA-APPROVED INDICATIONS

FDA-Approved Indications: Treatment of patients with the following infections caused by susceptible strains of organisms: lower respiratory tract infections; skin and skin structure infections, urinary tract infections, bacterial septicemia, bone and joint infections, gynecologic infections, intraabdominal infections, and central nervous system infections.

SIDE EFFECTS/TOXICITY

Ceftazidime is **contraindicated** in patients who have shown hypersensitivity to ceftazidime or the cephalosporin group of antibiotics.

Ceftazidime should be used with caution if hypersensitivity exists to penicillin.

Toxicity includes inflammation at the site of injection; fever; anaphylaxis; rash including Stevens-Johnson syndrome, erythema multiforme, and toxic epidermal necrolysis; angioedema; flushing; serum sickness–like reactions; encephalopathy; seizures; myoclonus; diarrhea; *Clostridium difficile*–associated diarrhea and pseudomembranous colitis; oral candidiasis; anorexia; nausea; vomiting; stomach cramps; flatulence; hepatitis; renal impairment; genital candidiasis; vaginitis; hemorrhage; prolonged prothrombin time; pancytopenia; hemolytic anemia; and positive Coombs' test.

DRUG INTERACTIONS/FOOD INTERACTIONS

Nephrotoxicity has been reported following concomitant administration of cephalosporins with aminoglycoside antibiotics or potent diuretics such as furosemide. Cephalosporins may cause false-positive urine glucose determinations when one is using cupric sulfate solution (Benedict's solution, Clinitest). Tests utilizing glucose oxidase (Tes-Tape, Clinistix) are not affected by cephalosporins.

DOSING

Infection	*Dosage*
Urinary tract infections	250 mg every 12 hours IV or IM
Bone and joint infections	2 g every 12 hours IV
Complicated urinary tract infections	500 mg every 8 to 12 hours IV or IM
Pneumonia	500 mg to 1 g every 8 hours IV or IM
Skin and skin structure infections	500 mg to 1 g every 8 hours IV or IM
Gynecologic and abdominal infections	2 g every 8 hours IV
Meningitis	2 g every 8 hours IV
Life-threatening infections	2 g every 8 hours IV
Severe *Pseudomonas* lung infections	30 mg/kg to 50 mg/kg up to 6 g/day IV

SPECIAL POPULATIONS

RENAL IMPAIRMENT:

Renal Impairment	*Dose*
Creatinine clearance 31 mL/min to 50 mL/min	1 g every 12 hours
Creatinine clearance 16 mL/min to 30 mL/min	1 g every 24 hours
Creatinine clearance 6 mL/min to 15 mL/min	500 mg every 24 hours
Creatinine clearance $\leq$ 5 mL/min	500 mg every 48 hours
Hemodialysis	1 g after dialysis
Chronic ambulatory peritoneal dialysis	500 mg daily
Continuous renal replacement therapy	1 g every 12 to 24 hours

HEPATIC DYSFUNCTION: No dosage adjustment is necessary.

PEDIATRIC PATIENTS: Neonates aged younger than 1 month: 30 mg/kg every 12 hours. Children aged 1 month to 12 years: 30 mg/kg to 50 mg/kg every 8 hours up to 6 g/day.

PREGNANCY: Category B.

BREASTFEEDING: Ceftazadime should be used with caution in breastfeeding mothers.

THE ART OF ANTIMICROBIAL THERAPY

Clinical Pearls

1. Dosage of ceftazidime is adjusted for patients with renal dysfunction.
2. Cross-allergy with penicillins is less than 10% and ceftazadime can be used in life-threatening infections with caution if the allergy to penicillin is not severe.
3. Inducible type I β-lactamase resistance has been noted with some organisms (e.g., *Enterobacter* species, *Pseudomonas* species, and *Serratia* species) and can develop during therapy.

GENERAL CHARACTERISTICS

Class: Third-generation cephalosporin

Mechanism of Action: Binds penicillin binding protein (PBP), disrupting cell wall synthesis.

Mechanisms of Resistance:

1. The PBP can be altered, with reduced affinity,
2. production of a β-lactamase resulting in hydrolysis of the β-lactam ring, and
3. decreased ability of the antibiotic to reach the PBP when bacteria decrease porin production resulting in a decrease of the drug concentration within the cell.

Metabolic Route: Ceftibuten is excreted predominantly in the urine, with a small amount in the feces.

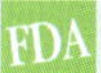

FDA-APPROVED INDICATIONS

FDA-Approved Indications: Treatment of the following infections when caused by susceptible organisms: acute bacterial exacerbations of chronic bronchitis, acute bacterial otitis media, and pharyngitis and tonsillitis.

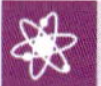

SIDE EFFECTS/TOXICITY

Ceftibuten is **contraindicated** in patients with allergy to cephalosporins. Ceftibuten should be used with caution if hypersensitivity exists to penicillins.

Toxicity includes fever; anaphylaxis; rash including Stevens-Johnson syndrome, erythema multiforme, and toxic epidermal necrolysis; angioedema; flushing; serum sickness–like reactions; encephalopathy; seizures; aphasia; psychosis; stridor; diarrhea; *Clostridium difficile*–associated diarrhea and pseudomembranous colitis; oral candidiasis; anorexia; nausea; vomiting, stomach cramps; flatulence; hepatitis; renal impairment; genital candidiasis; vaginitis; hemorrhage; prolonged prothrombin time; pancytopenia; hemolytic anemia; and positive Coombs' test.

DRUG INTERACTIONS/FOOD INTERACTIONS

Ceftibuten oral suspension must be administered at least 2 hours before or 1 hour after a meal. Probenecid inhibits the renal excretion of ceftibuten. Cephalosporins may cause false-positive urine glucose determinations when one is using cupric sulfate solution (Benedict's solution, Clinitest). Tests utilizing glucose oxidase (Tes-Tape, Clinistix) are not affected by cephalosporins.

CEFTIBUTEN (Cedax)

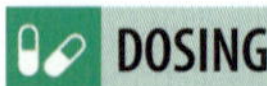

DOSING

Ceftibuten is supplied as a 400-mg capsule and an off-white powder that, when reconstituted, contains 90 mg/5 mL of ceftibuten.

The usual adult dose of ceftibuten is 400 mg daily for 10 days.

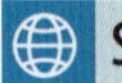

SPECIAL POPULATIONS

RENAL IMPAIRMENT:

	Dosage
Creatinine clearance 30 mL/min to 49 mL/min	4.5 mg/kg or 200 mg daily
Creatinine clearance 5 mL/min to 29 mL/min	2.25 mg/kg or 100 mg daily
Hemodialysis	9 mg/kg or 400 mg after hemodialysis
Chronic ambulatory peritoneal dialysis	N/A
Continuous renal replacement therapy	N/A

HEPATIC DYSFUNCTION: No dosage adjustment is necessary.

PEDIATRIC PATIENTS: 9 mg/kg daily up to 400 mg a day. Safety and efficacy not established in infants aged younger than 6 months.

PREGNANCY: Category B.

BREASTFEEDING: Caution should be used.

THE ART OF ANTIMICROBIAL THERAPY

Clinical Pearls

1. Dosage of ceftibuten must be adjusted for patients with renal insufficiency.
2. Cross-allergy with penicillins is less than 10%.
3. Diabetic patients should be informed that ceftibuten oral suspension contains 1 g sucrose per teaspoon of suspension.

CEFTIZOXIME (Cefizox)

GENERAL CHARACTERISTICS

Class: Third-generation cephalosporin

Mechanism of Action: Binds penicillin-binding protein (PBP), disrupting cell wall synthesis.

Mechanisms of Resistance:

1. The PBP can be altered, with reduced affinity,
2. production of a β-lactamase resulting in hydrolysis of the β-lactam ring, and
3. decreased ability of the antibiotic to reach the PBP when bacteria decrease porin production resulting in a decrease of the drug concentration within the cell.

Metabolic Route: Ceftizoxime is excreted unchanged in the urine.

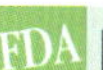

FDA-APPROVED INDICATIONS

FDA-Approved Indications: Treatment of patients with infections caused by susceptible strains of organisms in lower respiratory tract infections, urinary tract infections, gonorrhea including uncomplicated cervical and urethral gonorrhea, pelvic inflammatory disease, intraabdominal infections, septicemia, skin and skin structure infections, bone and joint infections, and meningitis.

SIDE EFFECTS/TOXICITY

Ceftizoxime is **contraindicated** in patients who have shown hypersensitivity to ceftizoxime.

Ceftizoxime should be used with caution if hypersensitivity exists to other cephalosporins or penicillin.

Toxicity includes inflammation at the site of injection; fever; anaphylaxis; rash including Stevens-Johnson syndrome, erythema multiforme, and toxic epidermal necrolysis; angioedema; flushing; serum sickness–like reactions; encephalopathy; seizures; diarrhea; *Clostridium difficile*–associated diarrhea and pseudomembranous colitis; oral candidiasis; anorexia; nausea; vomiting; stomach cramps; flatulence; hepatitis; renal impairment; genital candidiasis; vaginitis; hemorrhage; prolonged prothrombin time; pancytopenia; hemolytic anemia; and positive Coombs' test.

DRUG INTERACTIONS/FOOD INTERACTIONS

Nephrotoxicity has been reported following concomitant administration of cephalosporins with aminoglycoside antibiotics or potent diuretics such as furosemide. Cephalosporins may cause false-positive urine glucose determinations when one is using cupric sulfate solution (Benedict's solution, Clinitest). Tests utilizing glucose oxidase (Tes-Tape, Clinistix) are not affected by cephalosporins.

CEFTIZOXIME (Cefizox)

DOSING

Infection	*Dosage*
Uncomplicated urinary tract infection	500 mg IM or IV every 12 hours
Other infections	1 g IM or IV every 8 to 12 hours
Severe infections	1 g to 2 g IM or IV every 8 to 12 hours
Pelvic inflammatory disease	2 g IV every 8 hours
Life-threatening infections	3 g to 4 g IV every 8 hours
Uncomplicated gonorrhea	1 g IM as 1 dose

Note. IM = intramuscularly; IV = intravenously.

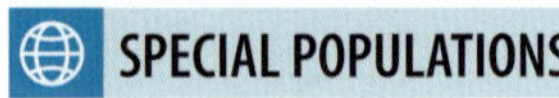

SPECIAL POPULATIONS

RENAL IMPAIRMENT:

	Less Severe Infections	*Severe Infection*
Creatinine clearance 50 mL/min to 79 mL/min	500 mg every 8 hours	750 mg to 1500 mg every 8 hours
Creatinine clearance 5 mL/min to 49 mL/min	250 mg to 500 mg every 12 hours	500 mg to 1000 mg every 12 hours
Creatinine clearance < 5 mL/min	500 mg every 48 hours or 250 mg every 24 hours	500 mg every 24 to 48 hours or 1 g every 48 hours
Hemodialysis	Same as creatinine clearance < 5 mL/min, but after dialysis on dialysis days	
Chronic ambulatory peritoneal dialysis	0.5 g to 1 g every 24 hours	
Continuous renal replacement therapy	250 mg to 500 mg every 12 hours	500 mg to 1000 mg every 12 hours

HEPATIC DYSFUNCTION: No dosage adjustment is necessary.

PEDIATRIC PATIENTS: Aged 6 months and older: 50 mg/kg every 8 hours.

Dosage may be increased to a total daily dose of 200 mg/kg (not to exceed the maximum adult dose for serious infection).

PREGNANCY: Category B.

BREASTFEEDING: Ceftizoxime should be used with caution in breastfeeding mothers.

THE ART OF ANTIMICROBIAL THERAPY

Clinical Pearls

1. Ceftizoxime is dose-adjusted for patients with renal dysfunction.
2. Cross-allergy with penicillins is less than 10% and ceftizoxime can be used in life-threatening infections with caution if the allergy to penicillin is not severe.
3. Because of the serious nature of some urinary tract infections caused by *Pseudomonas aeruginosa* and because many strains of *Pseudomonas* species are only moderately susceptible to ceftizoxime, higher dosage is recommended. Other therapy should be instituted if the response is not prompt.

CEFTRIAXONE (Rocephin)

GENERAL CHARACTERISTICS

Class: Third-generation cephalosporin

Mechanism of Action: Binds penicillin-binding protein (PBP), disrupting cell wall synthesis.

Mechanisms of Resistance:

1. The PBP can be altered, with reduced affinity,
2. production of a β-lactamase resulting in hydrolysis of the β-lactam ring, and
3. decreased ability of the antibiotic to reach the PBP when bacteria decrease porin production resulting in a decrease of the drug concentration within the cell.

Metabolic Route: Approximately 33% of ceftriaxone is excreted in the urine, 67% in the feces.

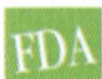

FDA-APPROVED INDICATIONS

FDA-Approved Indications: Treatment of the following syndromes when caused by susceptible organisms: lower respiratory tract infections, acute bacterial otitis media, skin and skin structure infections, urinary tract infections, uncomplicated gonorrhea, pelvic inflammatory disease, bacterial septicemia, bone and joint infections, intraabdominal infections, and meningitis.

Ceftriaxone is also indicated for surgical prophylaxis.

SIDE EFFECTS/TOXICITY

Ceftriaxone is **contraindicated** in patients with cephalosporin allergy and in hyperbilirubinemic neonates.

Ceftriaxone should be used with caution if hypersensitivity exists to penicillin.

Toxicity includes inflammation at the site of injection; fever; anaphylaxis; rash including Stevens-Johnson syndrome, erythema multiforme, and toxic epidermal necrolysis; angioedema; flushing; serum sickness–like reactions; encephalopathy; seizures; myoclonus; diarrhea; *Clostridium difficile*–associated diarrhea and pseudomembranous colitis; oral candidiasis; anorexia; nausea; vomiting; stomach cramps; flatulence; hepatitis; renal impairment; genital candidiasis; vaginitis; hemorrhage; prolonged prothrombin time; pancytopenia; hemolytic anemia; and positive Coombs' test. Crystallization of ceftriaxone salt in the gallbladder may produce gallbladder sludge.

DRUG INTERACTIONS/FOOD INTERACTIONS

Ceftriaxone and intravenous calcium-containing products should not be mixed or coadministered to any patient, even via different sites.

Cephalosporins may cause false-positive urine glucose determinations when one is using cupric sulfate solution (Benedict's solution, Clinitest). Tests utilizing glucose oxidase (Tes-Tape, Clinistix) are not affected by cephalosporins.

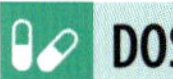

DOSING

Ceftriaxone is given intravenously in doses of 1 g to 2 g daily depending on the type and severity of infection. The total dose may be given once a day or divided equally and given twice a day.

Meningitis: Up to 4 g twice daily.

Gonorrhea: Single dose of 250 mg intramuscularly.

Surgical prophylaxis: 1 g 30 to 60 minutes given preoperatively.

SPECIAL POPULATIONS

RENAL IMPAIRMENT: No dosage adjustment is necessary.

HEPATIC DYSFUNCTION: No dosage adjustment is necessary; however, a dose of 2 g daily should not be exceeded.

PEDIATRIC PATIENTS:

Skin and skin structure infections: 50 mg/kg/day to 75 mg/kg/day (given once a day or in equally divided doses twice a day), not to exceed a daily dose of 2 g.

Acute bacterial otitis media: 50 mg/kg (not to exceed 1 g) as a single intramuscular dose.

Serious miscellaneous infections other than meningitis: 50 mg/kg/day to 75 mg/kg/day, not to exceed 2 g, in divided doses every 12 hours.

Meningitis: Initial dose of 100 mg/kg (not to exceed 4 g), followed by a total daily dose of 100 mg/kg (not to exceed 4 g), administered once daily or in equally divided doses every 12 hours.

Neonates with hyperbilirubinemia should not receive ceftriaxone.

PREGNANCY: Category B.

BREASTFEEDING: Ceftriaxone should be used with caution in breastfeeding mothers.

THE ART OF ANTIMICROBIAL THERAPY

Clinical Pearls

1. Dosage of ceftriaxone is not adjusted for patients with renal impairment.
2. Cross-allergy with penicillins is less than 10% and ceftriaxone can be used in life-threatening infections (e.g., meningitis) with caution if the allergy to penicillin is not severe.

3. Crystallization of ceftriaxone in the gallbladder can occur.
4. Coadministration of ceftriaxone and intravenous calcium products should be avoided.
5. Neonates with hyperbilirubinemia should not receive ceftriaxone.

CEFUROXIME (Zinacef) AND CEFUROXIME AXETIL (Ceftin)

GENERAL CHARACTERISTICS

Class: Second-generation cephalosporin

Mechanism of Action: Binds penicillin binding protein (PBP), disrupting cell wall synthesis.

Mechanisms of Resistance:

1. The PBP can be altered, with reduced affinity,
2. production of a β-lactamase resulting in hydrolysis of the β-lactam ring, and
3. decreased ability of the antibiotic to reach the PBP when bacteria decrease porin production resulting in a decrease of the drug concentration within the cell.

Metabolic Route: Cefuroxime axetil is an ester that is quickly metabolized into the active cefuroxime. Cefuroxime is excreted unchanged in the urine.

FDA FDA-APPROVED INDICATIONS

FDA-Approved Indications:

Cefuroxime tablets are indicated for the treatment of patients with the following mild-to-moderate infections caused by susceptible strains of microorganisms: pharyngitis/tonsillitis, acute bacterial otitis media, acute bacterial maxillary sinusitis, acute bacterial exacerbations of chronic bronchitis and secondary bacterial infections of acute bronchitis, uncomplicated skin and skin structure infections, uncomplicated urinary tract infections, uncomplicated gonorrhea, and early Lyme disease.

Cefuroxime oral suspension is indicated for the treatment of pediatric patients aged 3 months to 12 years with the following mild-to-moderate infections caused by susceptible strains of microorganisms: pharyngitis/tonsillitis, acute bacterial otitis media, and impetigo.

Cefuroxime for injection is indicated for the treatment of patients with the following infections caused by susceptible organisms: lower respiratory tract infections, urinary tract infections, skin and skin structure infections, septicemia, meningitis, gonorrhea, bone and joint infections, and preoperative prophylaxis.

SIDE EFFECTS/TOXICITY

Cefuroxime is **contraindicated** in patients with known allergy to cephalosporins.

Cefuroxime should be used with caution if hypersensitivity exists to penicillin.

Toxicity includes phlebitis; fever; anaphylaxis; rash including Stevens-Johnson syndrome, erythema multiforme, and toxic epidermal necrolysis; angioedema; flushing; serum sickness–like reactions; encephalopathy; seizures; diarrhea; *Clostridium difficile*–associated diarrhea and pseudomembranous colitis; oral candidiasis; anorexia;

taste perversion; nausea; vomiting; stomach cramps; flatulence; hepatitis; renal impairment; genital candidiasis; vaginitis; hemorrhage; prolonged prothrombin time; pancytopenia; hemolytic anemia; and positive Coombs' test.

DRUG INTERACTIONS/FOOD INTERACTIONS

Cefuroxime tablets may be administered with or without food.

Cefuroxime oral suspension must be administered with food.

Concomitant administration of probenecid with cefuroxime axetil tablets increases the serum concentration of cefuroxime axetil.

Drugs that reduce gastric acidity may result in a lower bioavailability of cefuroxime.

Cephalosporins may cause false-positive urine glucose determinations when one is using cupric sulfate solution (Benedict's solution, Clinitest). Tests utilizing glucose oxidase (Tes-Tape, Clinistix) are not affected by cephalosporins.

DOSING

CEFUROXIME TABLETS[a]:

Infection	*Dosage*	*Duration*
Pharyngitis/tonsillitis	250 mg every 12 hours	10 days
Acute maxillary sinusitis	250 mg every 12 hours	10 days
Acute exacerbation of bronchitis	250 mg to 500 mg every 12 hours	10 days
Secondary infections of bronchitis	250 mg to 500 mg every 12 hours	5 to 10 days
Skin and skin structure infections	250 mg to 500 mg every 12 hours	10 days
Urinary tract infections	250 mg every 12 hours	7 to 10 days
Gonorrhea	1 g once	1 dose
Lyme disease	500 mg every 12 hours	20 days

[a]Tablets are available in 250-mg and 500-mg doses. Cefuroxime oral suspension dosages are shown in the "Pediatric Patients" part of the "SPECIAL POPULATIONS" section of this chapter.

CEFUROXIME FOR INJECTION:

Infection	*Dosage*
Uncomplicated urinary tract infections	750 mg or 1.5 g every 8 hours IV or IM
Skin and skin structure infections	750 mg or 1.5 g every 8 hours IV or IM

Infection	*Dosage*
Disseminated gonococcal infections	750 mg or 1.5 g every 8 hours IV or IM
Uncomplicated pneumonia	750 mg or 1.5 g every 8 hours IV or IM
Bone and joint infections	1.5 g every 8 hours IV or IM
Life-threatening infections (e.g., meningitis)	1.5 g every 6 hours IV or IM
Preventive during surgery	1.5 g 30 to 60 min before incision IV or IM, then 750 mg every 8 hours when the procedure is prolonged
Preventive during open-heart surgery	1.5 g at induction, then every 12 hours for a total of 6 g IV or IM

Note: IM = intramuscularly; IV = intravenously.

SPECIAL POPULATIONS

RENAL IMPAIRMENT:

Renal Impairment	*Dosage of Cefuroxime Injection*[a]
Creatinine clearance > 20 mL/min	750 mg to 1.5 g every 8 hours
Creatinine clearance 10 mL/min to 20 mL/min	750 mg every 12 hours
Creatinine clearance < 10 mL/min	750 mg daily
Hemodialysis	750 mg daily, administer after dialysis on dialysis days
Chronic ambulatory peritoneal dialysis	750 mg daily
Continuous renal replacement therapy	1 g every 12 hours

[a]The safety and efficacy of cefuroxime tablet and oral suspension have not been established; renal failure can be expected to prolong the half-life.

HEPATIC DYSFUNCTION: No dosage adjustment is necessary.

PEDIATRIC PATIENTS: The safety and effectiveness of cefuroxime have been established for pediatric patients aged 3 months to 12 years.

Cefuroxime Oral Suspension[a]:

Infection	*Dosage*	*Duration*
Pharyngitis/tonsillitis	10 mg/kg every 12 hours	10 days
Acute otitis media	15 mg/kg every 12 hours	10 days
Acute maxillary sinusitis	15 mg/kg every 12 hours	10 days
Impetigo	15 mg/kg every 12 hours	10 days

[a]Provides the equivalent of 125 mg or 250 mg of cefuroxime per 5 mL.

Cefuroxime for Injection in Pediatric Patients:

Infection	*Dosage*
Mild-to-moderate infections	50 mg/kg/day to 100 mg/kg/day in divided doses every 6 to 8 hours
Severe infections	100 mg/kg/day in divided doses every 6 to 8 hours
Bone and joint infections	150 mg/kg/day in divided doses every 8 hours
Bacterial meningitis	200 mg/kg/day to 240 mg/kg/day in divided doses every 6 to 8 hours

PREGNANCY: Category B.

BREASTFEEDING: Consideration should be given to discontinuing breastfeeding temporarily during treatment with cefuroxime axetil.

THE ART OF ANTIMICROBIAL THERAPY

Clinical Pearls

1. Dosage of cefuroxime must be adjusted for patients with renal impairment.
2. Cross-allergy with penicillins is less than 10% and cefuroxime can be used in life-threatening infections (e.g., meningitis) with caution if the allergy to penicillin is not severe.
3. Cefuroxime tablets and oral suspension are not bioequivalent and are not interchangeable on a milligram-per-milligram basis.
4. Cefuroxime tablets may be administered with or without food. Cefuroxime oral suspension must be administered with food.

GENERAL CHARACTERISTICS

Class: First-generation cephalosporin

Mechanism of Action: Binds penicillin-binding protein (PBP), disrupting cell wall synthesis.

Mechanisms of Resistance:

1. The PBP can be altered, with reduced affinity,
2. production of a β-lactamase resulting in hydrolysis of the β-lactam ring, and
3. decreased ability of the antibiotic to reach the PBP when bacteria decrease porin production resulting in a decrease of the drug concentration within the cell.

Metabolic Route: Cephalexin is excreted unchanged in the urine.

FDA-APPROVED INDICATIONS

FDA-Approved Indications: Treatment of the following infections when caused by susceptible strains of organisms: respiratory tract infections, otitis media, skin and skin structure infections, bone infections, and genitourinary tract infections.

SIDE EFFECTS/TOXICITY

Cephalexin is **contraindicated** in patients with known allergy to the cephalosporin group of antibiotics.

Cephalexin should be used with caution if hypersensitivity exists to penicillin.

Toxicity includes fever, anaphylaxis, rash including Stevens-Johnson syndrome, erythema multiforme, and toxic epidermal necrolysis; angioedema; flushing; hypotension; serum sickness–like reactions; encephalopathy; seizures; diarrhea; *Clostridium difficile*–associated diarrhea and pseudomembranous colitis; oral candidiasis; anorexia; nausea; vomiting; stomach cramps; flatulence; hepatitis; renal impairment; genital candidiasis; vaginitis; hemorrhage; arthritis; prolonged prothrombin time; pancytopenia; hemolytic anemia; and positive Coombs' test.

DRUG INTERACTIONS/FOOD INTERACTIONS

Cephalexin can be administered with or without food.

Probenecid may decrease renal tubular secretion of cephalosporins when used concurrently, resulting in increased and more prolonged cephalosporin blood levels. Cephalosporins may cause false-positive urine glucose determinations when one is using cupric sulfate solution (Benedict's solution, Clinitest). Tests utilizing glucose oxidase (Tes-Tape, Clinistix) are not affected by cephalosporins.

CEPHALEXIN (Keflex)

DOSING

Cephalexin is administered in 250-mg and 500-mg tablets. It can also be administered in a suspension of 125 mg/5 mL or 250 mg/5mL.

The usual adult dosage is 250 mg every 6 hours.

In **streptococcal pharyngitis, skin and skin structure infections,** and **uncomplicated cystitis,** a dosage of 500 mg may be administered every 12 hours.

For **severe infections,** daily doses of cephalexin up to 4 g may be administered.

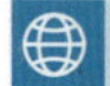

SPECIAL POPULATIONS

RENAL IMPAIRMENT:

	*Dosage**
Creatinine clearance > 50 mL/min	Every 6 hours
Creatinine clearance 10 mL/min to 50 mL/min	Every 8 to 12 hours
Creatinine clearance < 10 mL/min	Every 24 to 48 hours
Supplemental dose after hemodialysis	250 mg to 1 g
Continuous renal replacement therapy	N/A

*Dosage from Dosing section; interval in this table.

HEPATIC DYSFUNCTION: No dosage adjustment is necessary.

PEDIATRIC PATIENTS: The usual recommended daily dosage for pediatric patients is 25 mg/kg to 50 mg/kg in divided doses.

For **streptococcal pharyngitis** in pediatric patients, total daily dose may be divided and administered every 12 hours.

For **severe infections** in pediatric patients, the dosage may be doubled.

In **otitis media** in pediatric patients, 75 mg/kg/day to 100 mg/kg/day in four divided doses is required.

PREGNANCY: Category B.

BREASTFEEDING: Cephalexin should be used with caution in breastfeeding mothers.

THE ART OF ANTIMICROBIAL THERAPY

Clinical Pearls

1. Dosage of cephalexin is adjusted for patients with renal dysfunction.
2. Cross-allergy with penicillins is less than 10%.
3. If more than 4 g of cephalexin are required, parenteral cephalosporins should be used, e.g., cefazolin.

CHLORAMPHENICOL (Chloromycetin)

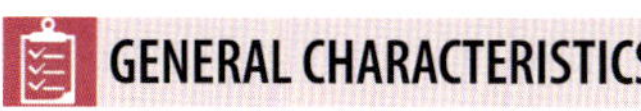

GENERAL CHARACTERISTICS

Class: Antiribosomal antimicrobial

Mechanism of Action: Inhibits bacterial protein synthesis by interfering with the transfer of activated amino acids from soluble RNA to ribsomes.

Mechanisms of Resistance: Data are incomplete.

Metabolic Route: Chloramphenicol is excreted in the urine, predominantly as metabolically inactive metabolites.

FDA-APPROVED INDICATIONS

FDA-Approved Indications: Acute infections caused by *Salmonella typhi.* Serious infections caused by *Salmonella* species; *Haemophilus influenzae,* especially meningeal infections; *Rickettsia,* lymphogranuloma (psittacosis group); various gram-negative bacteria causing bacteremia, meningitis, or other serious gram-negative infections; and other susceptible organisms that have been demonstrated to be resistant to all other appropriate antimicrobial agents.

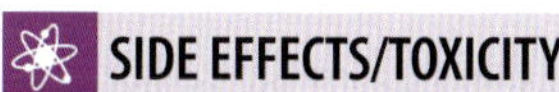

SIDE EFFECTS/TOXICITY

> **WARNING:** Serious and fatal blood dyscrasias (aplastic anemia, hypoplastic anemia, thrombocytopenia, and granulocytopenia) are known to occur after the administration of chloramphenicol. In addition, there have been reports of aplastic anemia attributed to chloramphenicol that later terminated in leukemia. Blood dyscrasias have occurred after both short-term and prolonged therapy with this drug. Chloramphenicol must not be used when less potentially dangerous agents will be effective. *It must not be used in the treatment of trivial infections or where it is not indicated, as in colds, influenza, infections of the throat, or as a prophylactic agent to prevent bacterial infections.*

Chloramphenicol is **contraindicated** in individuals with a history of previous hypersensitivity and/or toxic reaction to it.

Other side effects include hypersensitivity reactions including fever, rash, angioedema, urticaria, and anaphylaxis; toxic reactions including fatalities in the premature baby and neonate ("gray syndrome"); *Clostridium difficile*–associated diarrhea; paroxysmal nocturnal hemoglobinuria; nausea; vomiting; glossitis; stomatitis; diarrhea; enterocolitis; headache; mild depression; mental confusion; delirium; optic neuritis; and peripheral neuritis.

DRUG INTERACTIONS/FOOD INTERACTIONS

Concurrent therapy with other drugs that may cause bone marrow depression should be avoided.

DOSING

Adults should receive 50 mg/kg/day intravenously in divided doses at 6-hour intervals.

SPECIAL POPULATIONS

RENAL IMPAIRMENT: No change.

HEPATIC DYSFUNCTION: No clear recommendations, but dosage should be decreased.

PEDIATRIC PATIENTS: Dosage of 50 mg/kg/day divided into four doses at 6-hour intervals.

In **Neonates:** A total of 25 mg/kg/day in four equal doses at 6-hour intervals.

After the first 2 weeks of life, full-term neonates ordinarily may receive up to a total of 50 mg/kg/day equally divided into four doses at 6-hour intervals.

In young infants and other pediatric patients in whom immature metabolic functions are suspected, a dose of 25 mg/kg/day divided into four equal doses at 6-hour intervals.

PREGNANCY: Category C.

BREASTFEEDING: Mothers should discontinue breastfeeding if chloramphenicol is started.

THE ART OF ANTIMICROBIAL THERAPY

Clinical Pearls

1. Chloramphenicol must be used only in those serious infections for which less potentially dangerous drugs are ineffective or contraindicated.
2. Baseline blood studies should be followed by blood studies every 2 days during therapy. The drug should be discontinued upon appearance of leukopenia, thrombocytopenia, anemia, or any other blood study findings attributable to chloramphenicol.
3. Patients started on intravenous chloramphenicol should be changed to the oral form of another appropriate antibiotic as soon as possible.
4. Repeated courses of chloramphenicol treatment should be avoided if at all possible.

CHLOROQUINE PHOSPHATE (Aralen) AND HYDROXYCHLOROQUINE

GENERAL CHARACTERISTICS

Class: 4-aminoquinolone

Mechanism of Action: Forms toxic complexes with heme molecules, depriving the parasite of hemoglobin.

Mechanism of Resistance: Mutation in transport molecule of digestive vacuole membrane (PfCRT), reducing the amount of drug that accumulates in the digestive vacuoles.

Metabolic Route: Half is excreted in the urine, and the rest is degraded to multiple metabolic products.

FDA-APPROVED INDICATIONS

FDA-Approved Indications:

Chloroquine: Suppressive treatment and treatment of acute attacks of malaria caused by *Plasmodium vivax, Plasmodium malariae, Plasmodium ovale,* and susceptible strains of *Plasmodium falciparum.* Treatment of extraintestinal amebiasis.

Hydroxychloroquine: Suppressive treatment and treatment of acute attacks of malaria caused by *P vivax, P malariae, P ovale,* and susceptible strains of *P falciparum.*

Also used for: Hydroxychloroquine is used in combination with doxycycline to treat Q fever endocarditis.

SIDE EFFECTS/TOXICITY

Side effects include psoriasis; porphyria; hypotension; tachycardia; bradycardia; A-V block or other transient conduction alterations; rash including Stevens-Johnson syndrome and toxic epidermal necrolysis; psychiatric symptoms including anxiety, paranoia, depression, hallucinations and psychosis; nausea; vomiting; diarrhea; hepatitis; seizures; nerve deafness; tinnitus; visual disturbances; myopathy; retinopathy; anemia; leukopenia; and thrombocytopenia.

DRUG INTERACTIONS/FOOD INTERACTIONS

Antacids and kaolin can reduce the absorption of chloroquine; separate by 4 hours.

Concomitant use of cimetidine should be avoided.

An interval of at least 2 hours between intake of ampicillin and chloroquine should be observed.

May increase cyclosporine levels; close monitoring of serum cyclosporine level is recommended.

DOSING

CHLOROQUINE PHOSPHATE

Chloroquine phosphate is calculated as the base. Each 250-mg tablet of chloroquine phosphate is equivalent to 150-mg base and each 500-mg tablet of chloroquine phosphate is equivalent to 300-mg base.

Malaria prophylaxis: 500 mg (300-mg base) on exactly the same day of each week. Prophylactic therapy should begin 2 weeks prior to exposure and be continued for 8 weeks after leaving the endemic area.

Malaria treatment: An initial dose of 1 g (600-mg base) followed by an additional 500 mg (300-mg base) after 6 to 8 hours and a single dose of 500 mg (300-mg base) on each of two consecutive days. This represents a total dose of 2.5 g chloroquine phosphate or 1.5 g base in 3 days.

Extraintestinal amebiasis: 1 g (600-mg base) daily for 2 days, followed by 500 mg (300-mg base) daily for at least 2 to 3 weeks.

HYDROXYCHLOROQUINE

Hydroxychloroquine: One tablet of 200 mg of hydroxychloroquine is equivalent to 155-mg base.

Malaria prophylaxis: *In adults*, 400 mg (310-mg base) on exactly the same day of each week. If circumstances permit, suppressive therapy should begin 2 weeks prior to exposure. The suppressive therapy should be continued for 8 weeks after leaving the endemic area.

Malaria treatment: An initial dose of 800 mg (620-mg base) followed by 400 mg (310-mg base) in 6 to 8 hours and 400 mg (310 mg base) on each of two consecutive days (total 2 g hydroxychloroquine sulfate or 1.55 g base). An alternative method, employing a single dose of 800 mg (620-mg base), has also proved effective.

SPECIAL POPULATIONS

RENAL IMPAIRMENT: There is no adjustment needed.

HEPATIC DYSFUNCTION: Use with caution.

PEDIATRIC PATIENTS:

Chloroquine Phosphate

The weekly **malaria prophylactic** dosage is 5 mg calculated as base, per kg of body weight, but should not exceed the adult dosage regardless of weight.

Malaria treatment: First dose: 10 mg base per kg (but not exceeding a single dose of 600-mg base). Second dose: (6 hours after first dose) 5 mg base per kg (but not exceeding a single dose of 300-mg base). Third dose: (24 hours after first dose) 5 mg base per kg. Fourth dose: (36 hours after first dose) 5 mg base per kg.

Hydroxychloroquine

The weekly **malaria prophylactic** dosage is 5 mg, calculated as base, per kg of body weight, but should not exceed the adult dose regardless of weight.

Malaria treatment: First dose: 10 mg base per kg (but not exceeding a single dose of 620-mg base). Second dose: 5 mg base per kg (but not exceeding a single dose of 310-mg base) 6 hours after first dose. Third dose: 5 mg base per kg 18 hours after second dose. Fourth dose: 5 mg base per kg 24 hours after third dose.

PREGNANCY: Avoid in pregnancy.

BREASTFEEDING: Because of possible severe adverse events in infants, chloroquine or hydroxychloroquine should be given to breastfeeding mothers only if benefit exceeds potential risk.

THE ART OF ANTIMICROBIAL THERAPY

Clinical Pearls

1. *P. falciparum* is usually resistant to chloroquine and hydroxychloroquine in all regions of the world except the Caribbean and the Middle East.
2. Chloroquine and hydroxychloroquine do not eliminate hepatic-phase parasites, and patients with acute *P. vivax* malaria are at high risk of relapse; to avoid relapse, after initial treatment of the acute infection, patients should subsequently be treated with an 8-aminoquinoline derivative (e.g., primaquine).
3. Chloroquine and hydroxychloroquine can induce hemolysis in patients with G6PD deficiency.
4. Caution is urged when chloroquine and hydroxychloroquine is used in patients with history of epilepsy, auditory damage, liver disease, and alcoholism.
5. Because irreversible retinal damage may occur with prolonged or high-dose therapy, ophthalmologic monitoring is advisable.
6. Concomitant use with mefloquine may increase the risk of seizures.
7. Complete blood cell counts should be made periodically if patients are given prolonged therapy.

GENERAL CHARACTERISTICS

Class: Antiviral

Mechanism of Action: Incorporation of cidofovir diphosphate into the growing cytomegalovirus (CMV) viral DNA chain results in reductions in the rate of viral DNA synthesis.

Mechanism of Resistance: Insufficient data.

Metabolic Route: Cidofovir must be administered with probenecid. Cidofovir is cleared unchanged in the urine.

FDA-APPROVED INDICATIONS

FDA-Approved Indications: Treatment of CMV retinitis in patients with acquired immunodeficiency syndrome (AIDS).

Also Used for: Some authorities recommend cidofovir for smallpox and complications of smallpox vaccination (i.e., eczema vaccinatum, progressive vaccinia, and inadvertent inoculation), and for monkeypox. It may also have activity against polyomaviruses and adenovirus.

SIDE EFFECTS/TOXICITY

> **WARNING:** Cidofovir may cause acute renal failure in some cases requiring dialysis. To reduce nephrotoxicity, intravenous prehydration with normal saline and administration of probenecid must be used with each cidofovir infusion. Renal function must be monitored. Initiation of therapy with cidofovir is contraindicated in patients with a serum creatinine greater than 1.5 mg/dL, a calculated creatinine clearance 55 mL/min or less, or a urine protein 100 mg/dL or greater (equivalent to $\geq 2+$ proteinuria). Cidofovir also causes severe neutropenia.

Cidofovir is **contraindicated** in patients with hypersensitivity to cidofovir, in patients receiving other nephrotoxic agents, and in patients with a history of clinically severe hypersensitivity to probenecid or other sulfa-containing medications.

Other toxic effects include proximal tubular cell injury with metabolic acidosis and Fanconi's syndrome; glycosuria; decrease in serum phosphate, uric acid, and bicarbonate; and decreased intraocular pressure with impaired visual acuity, uveitis or iritis, liver dysfunction, and pancreatitis.

DRUG INTERACTIONS/FOOD INTERACTIONS

Probenecid (which is always given with cidofovir) is known to interact with the metabolism or renal tubular excretion of many drugs (e.g., acetaminophen, acyclovir, angiotensin-converting enzyme inhibitors, aminosalicylic acid, barbiturates, benzodiazepines, bumetanide, clofibrate, methotrexate, famotidine, furosemide, nonsteroidal antiinflammatory agents, theophylline, and zidovudine). Concomitant medications should be carefully assessed.

Zidovudine should either be temporarily discontinued or decreased by 50% when coadministered with probenecid on the day of cidofovir infusion.

Nephrotoxic agents: Concomitant administration of cidofovir and agents with nephrotoxic potential is contraindicated.

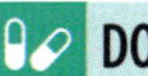

DOSING

Probenecid must be administered orally with each cidofovir dose. Two grams must be administered 3 hours prior to the cidofovir dose and 1 g administered at 2 hours and again at 8 hours after completion of the 1-hour cidofovir infusion (for a total of 4 g).

Ingestion of food prior to each dose of probenecid may reduce drug-related nausea and vomiting.

The recommended induction dose of cidofovir is 5 mg/kg body weight once weekly for 2 consecutive weeks. The recommended maintenance dose of cidofovir is 5 mg/kg administered once every 2 weeks.

SPECIAL POPULATIONS

RENAL IMPAIRMENT: The maintenance dose of cidofovir must be reduced from 5 mg/kg to 3 mg/kg for an increase in serum creatinine of 0.3 mg/dL to 0.4 mg/dL above baseline. Cidofovir therapy must be discontinued for an increase in serum creatinine of 0.5 mg/dL or more above baseline or development of 3+ or more proteinuria.

Cidofovir is contraindicated in patients with a serum creatinine concentration greater than 1.5 mg/dL, a calculated creatinine clearance 55 mL/min or less, or a urine protein 100 mg/dL or more (equivalent to 2+ or more proteinuria).

HEPATIC DYSFUNCTION: No adjustment is needed.

PEDIATRIC PATIENTS: Cidofovir has not been studied in children.

PREGNANCY: Category C.

BREASTFEEDING: The use of cidofovir is not recommended for breastfeeding mothers.

THE ART OF ANTIMICROBIAL THERAPY

Clinical Pearls

1. To minimize potential nephrotoxicity, probenecid and intravenous saline prehydration must be administered with each cidofovir infusion. Patients should be

warned of potential adverse events caused by probenecid (e.g., headache, nausea, vomiting, and hypersensitivity reactions, including rash, fever, chills, and anaphylaxis).

2. Cidofovir is contraindicated in patients with creatinine greater than 1.5 mg/dL, those with creatinine clearance less than or equal to 55 mL/min, or those with a urine protein greater than or equal to 100 mg/dL.
3. Cidofovir should not be administered with other nephrotoxic agents.
4. Patients should be monitored for neutropenia.

CIPROFLOXACIN (Cipro and Cipro XR)

GENERAL CHARACTERISTICS

Class: Fluoroquinolone

Mechanism of Action: Inhibits bacterial topoisomerase IV and DNA gyrase.

Mechanisms of Resistance: Mutations in DNA gyrase and/or topoisomerase IV, or through altered efflux.

Metabolic Route: Ciprofloxacin is predominantly excreted in the urine.

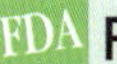

FDA APPROVED INDICATIONS

FDA-Approved Indications: Ciprofloxacin is indicated for the treatment of the following serious infections caused by susceptible strains of microorganisms: urinary tract infections, acute uncomplicated cystitis in females, chronic bacterial prostatitis, lower respiratory tract infections, acute sinusitis, skin and skin structure infections, bone and joint infections, complicated intraabdominal infections, infectious diarrhea, typhoid fever (enteric fever), uncomplicated cervical and urethral gonorrhea, and inhalational anthrax prophylaxis.

Also used for: Ciprofloxacin is also used for treatment of *Mycobacterium tuberculosis* and nontuberculous mycobacteria, inhalational and cutaneous anthrax, plague, tularemia, and traveler's diarrhea.

Cipro XR is indicated only for the treatment of urinary tract infections, including uncomplicated urinary tract infections (acute cystitis), complicated urinary tract infections, and acute uncomplicated pyelonephritis, caused by susceptible microorganisms.

SIDE EFFECTS/TOXICITY

> **WARNING:** Fluoroquinolones, including ciprofloxacin tablets, are associated with an increased risk of tendonitis and tendon rupture in all ages. This risk is further increased in patients aged older than 60 years, in patients taking corticosteroids, and in patients with kidney, heart, or lung transplants.

Ciprofloxacin is contraindicated in persons with a history of hypersensitivity associated with the use of ciprofloxacin or any quinolone.

Side effects: hypersensitivity; angioedema; headache; seizures; increased intracranial pressure; psychosis; tremors; agitation; lightheadedness; confusion; hallucinations; paranoia; depression; nightmares; insomnia; suicidal thoughts or acts; tendon ruptures of the shoulder, hand, or Achilles' tendon; photosensitivity; prolongation of the QT interval and arrhythmia; rare cases of torsades de pointes; renal failure; peripheral neuropathy; *Clostridium difficile*–associated diarrhea; nausea; vomiting; elevations in alanine transaminase (SGPT) and aspartate transaminase (SGOT); blurred vision; and pancytopenia.

DRUG INTERACTIONS/FOOD INTERACTIONS

1. Ciprofloxacin absorption may be decreased by antacids containing calcium, magnesium, or aluminum; sucralfate; divalent or trivalent cations such as iron; or multivitamins containing zinc. Ciprofloxacin should be taken 2 hours before or 6 hours after these products.
2. Concomitant administration with tizanidine is contraindicated.
3. Cimetidine results in significant increases in half-life of some quinolones.
4. Ciprofloxacin inhibits cytochrome P450 enzyme activity. This may result in a prolonged half-life for some drugs that are also metabolized by this system such as caffeine, cyclosporine, theophylline/methylxanthines, and warfarin when coadministered with quinolones.
5. The concomitant administration of a nonsteroidal antiinflammatory drug with a quinolone may increase the risk of central nervous system stimulation and seizures.
6. The concomitant use of probenecid decreases renal tubular secretion.
7. Disturbances of blood glucose, including hyperglycemia and hypoglycemia, may be seen in patients treated concurrently with antidiabetic agents.
8. Ciprofloxacin may produce false-positive urine screening results for opiates.

DOSING

Cipro

Ciprofloxacin is available as 250-mg, 500-mg, and 750-mg tablets, as a suspension that is 5% (250 mg/5 mL) and 10% (500 mg/5 mL), and in an intravenous (IV) formulation.

Usual adult dosage: 500 mg to 750 mg orally twice daily or 400 mg IV every 8 to 12 hours.

Usual duration: 7 to 14 days

Exceptions: Urinary tract infection: 250 mg every 12 hours for 3 days (uncomplicated) or 250 mg every 12 hours for 7 to 14 days (mild-to-moderate).

Traveler's diarrhea: 750 mg for one dose 1(mild), or 500 mg twice a day for 3 days (severe).

Duration for chronic prostatitis and bone or joint infections: more than 4 weeks.

Duration for anthrax: 60 days.

Cipro XR

Cipro XR is supplied as 500-mg and 1000-mg extended-release capsules.

Indication	*Dosage*	*Usual Duration*
Uncomplicated urinary tract infection (acute cystitis)	500 mg every 24 hours	3 days

Indication	*Dosage*	*Usual Duration*
Complicated urinary tract infection	1000 mg every 24 hours	7 to 14 days
Acute uncomplicated pyelonephritis	1000 mg every 24 hours	7 to 14 days

SPECIAL POPULATIONS

RENAL IMPAIRMENT:

Ciprofloxacin Oral Tablet or Suspension:

	Dosage
Creatinine clearance > 50 mL/min	Usual dosage
Creatinine clearance 30 mL/min to 50 mL/min	250 mg to 500 mg every 12 hours
Creatinine clearance 5 mL/min to 29 mL/min	250 mg to 500 mg every 18 hours
Hemodialysis	250 mg to 500 mg every 24 hours (after dialysis)
Chronic ambulatory peritoneal dialysis	250 mg every 8 hours
Continuous renal replacement therapy	250 mg to 500 mg every 12 hours

Cipro XR:

	Dosage
Creatinine clearance < 30 mL/min	500 mg daily
Hemodialysis	500 mg daily; administer after dialysis on dialysis days
Chronic ambulatory peritoneal dialysis	500 mg daily
Continuous renal replacement therapy	N/A

HEPATIC DYSFUNCTION: A maximum dosage of 400 mg of ciprofloxacin per day should not be exceeded.

PEDIATRIC PATIENTS: Safety and efficacy in pediatric patients aged younger than 18 years have not yet been established. However, it is approved as an alternative agent for complicated urinary tract infections and pyelonephritis and prophylaxis for inhaled anthrax.

Infection	*Route of Administration*	*Dosage*	*Total Duration*
Complicated urinary tract infection or pyelonephritis	Intravenous	6 mg/kg to 10 mg/kg every 8 hours	
	Oral	10 mg/kg to 20 mg/kg every 12 hours	10 to 21 days

CIPROFLOXACIN (Cipro and Cipro XR)

Infection	*Route of Administration*	*Dosage*	*Total Duration*
Inhalational anthrax (postexposure, cutaneous)	Intravenous	10 mg/kg every 12 hours	
	Oral	15 mg/kg every 12 hours	60 days

PREGNANCY: Category C.

BREASTFEEDING: Ciprofloxacin should not be administered to breastfeeding mothers.

THE ART OF ANTIMICROBIAL THERAPY

Clinical Pearls

1. Ciprofloxacin should be given at least 2 hours before cations or 6 hours after.
2. Cipro XR and Cipro are not interchangeable.
3. The oral Cipro and IV Cipro doses are not the same. For every 250 mg oral, the equivalent is 200 mg intravenously.
4. All fluoroquinolones can cause tendon rupture, especially in patients aged older than 60 years.
5. All fluoroquinolones can prolong QT intervals and caution should be used when they are given with other medications that affect QT intervals.
6. All fluoroquinolones can cause phototoxicity.
7. All fluoroquinolones can lower seizure threshold and cause other central nervous system side effects.
8. Ciprofloxacin should be avoided if possible in children, pregnant women, and breastfeeding mothers because of concern for cartilage developmental problems.
9. Ciprofloxacin has activity against mycobacteria; therefore, ciprofloxacin monotherapy (e.g., for pneumonia) should be avoided if mycobacterial infection is possible.
10. Treatment of gonorrhea with fluoroquinolones should be undertaken with caution because of rising resistance.

CLARITHROMYCIN (Biaxin and Biaxin XL)

GENERAL CHARACTERISTICS

Class: Macrolide

Mechanism of Action: Binds to the 50S ribosomal subunit of susceptible microorganisms and, thus, interferes with microbial protein synthesis.

Mechanisms of Resistance:

1. Decreased permeability,
2. active efflux,
3. alteration of the 50S ribosomal unit,
4. alteration of the 23S subunit of the 50S ribosomal unit, and
5. enzymatic inactivation of the macrolide.

Metabolic Route: About 30% of clarithromycin is excreted in the urine with the remainder excreted in the bile.

FDA FDA-APPROVED INDICATIONS

FDA-Approved Indications:

1. **Clarithromycin (tablets and oral suspension):** susceptible organisms causing pharyngitis/tonsillitis (adults and children); acute maxillary sinusitis (adults and children); acute bacterial exacerbation of chronic bronchitis (adults); community-acquired pneumonia (adults and children); uncomplicated skin and skin structure infections (adults and children); acute otitis media (children); disseminated infection caused by *Mycobacterium avium* or *Mycobacterium intracellulare* (adults and children); in combination with amoxicillin and lansoprazole or omeprazole delayed-release capsules, as triple therapy, treatment of patients with *Helicobacter pylori* infection and duodenal ulcer disease; in combination with omeprazole or ranitidine bismuth citrate tablets, treatment of patients with an active duodenal ulcer associated with *H pylori* infection; prevention of disseminated *M avium* complex (MAC) disease in patients with advanced HIV infection.
2. **Clarithromycin extended release (XL):** Acute maxillary sinusitis (adults), acute bacterial exacerbation of chronic bronchitis (adults), and community-acquired pneumonia (adults).

SIDE EFFECTS/TOXICITY

Contraindicated in patients with known hypersensitivity to clarithromycin, erythromycin, or any macrolide or ketolide antibiotic.

Side effects include: Serious allergic reactions, including rash, photosensitivity, anaphylaxis, angioedema, Stevens-Johnson syndrome and toxic epidermal necrolysis, *Clostridium difficile*–associated diarrhea, tooth discoloration, nausea, vomiting, diarrhea, abdominal pain, pancreatitis, hepatitis, cholestatic jaundice, dyspepsia, flatulence, melena, prolonged cardiac repolarization and QT interval, palpitations, chest pain, exacerbation of symptoms of myasthenia gravis and new onset of myasthenic syndrome, genital candidiasis, vaginitis, nephritis, dizziness, headache, vertigo, somnolence, fatigue, seizure, deafness, thrombocytopenia, and leukopenia.

DRUG INTERACTIONS/FOOD INTERACTIONS

Clarithromycin can be administered with or without food.

Clarithromycin extended-release tablets should be taken with food.

Clarithromycin and other macrolides are known to inhibit enzymes, particularly CYP3A; therefore, coadministration of clarithromycin and a drug primarily metabolized by CYP3A may be associated with elevations in concentrations of the latter. As a result:

1. It is **contraindicated** to use clarithromycin with terfenadine, oral midazolam, triazolam, alprazolam, ergotamine, dihydroergotamine, cisapride, pimozide, or astemizole.
2. Clarithromycin should be **used with caution** with theophylline, oral anticoagulants, digoxin, verapamil, zidovudine, colchicine, sildenafil, tadalafil, vardenafil, tolterodine, intravenous midazolam, itraconazole, HMG-CoA reductase inhibitors (e.g., lovastatin and simvastatin), cyclosporine, carbamazepine, tacrolimus, alfentanil, disopyramide, rifabutin, quinidine, methylprednisolone, cilostazol, bromocriptine, vinblastine, hexobarbital, phenytoin, and valproate.
3. If one is giving clarithromycin with **ritonavir** to patients with renal impairment, the following dosage adjustments should be considered. For patients with creatinine clearance 30 mL/min to 60 mL/min, the dosage of clarithromycin should be reduced by 50%. For patients with creatinine clearance less than 30 mL/min, the dosage of clarithromycin should be decreased by 75%.
4. When one is giving clarithromycin with **atazanavir** to patients with moderate renal impairment (creatinine clearance 30 mL/min to 60 mL/min), the dosage of clarithromycin should be decreased by 50%. For patients with creatinine clearance less than 30 mL/min, the dosage of clarithromycin should be decreased by 75%.
5. Doses of clarithromycin greater than 1000 mg per day should not be coadministered with protease inhibitors.
6. There have been reports of torsades de pointes occurring with concurrent use of clarithromycin and **quinidine** or **disopyramide**; if given, electrocardiogram and serum levels of these drugs should be monitored.
7. Clarithromycin in combination with **ranitidine bismuth citrate** therapy is not recommended in patients with creatinine clearance less than 25 mL/min. Clarithromycin in combination with ranitidine bismuth citrate should not be used in patients with a history of acute porphyria.

DOSING

Clarithromycin is administered in 250-mg and 500-mg tablets; and as granules in 2 concentrations: 125 mg/5 mL and 250 mg/5mL.

Clarithromycin extended release (XL) is administered in 500-mg tablets.

CLARITHROMYCIN DOSAGES:

Infection	*Tablets or suspension*		*Extended Release*	
	Dosage, Every 12 hours	*Duration, days*	*Dosage, Every 24 hours*	*Duration, days*
Pharyngitis/tonsillitis	250 mg	10	NA	NA
Acute maxillary sinusitis	500 mg	14	2 500-mg tablets	14
Acute exacerbation of chronic bronchitis	500 mg	7 to 14	2 500-mg tablets	7
Community-acquired pneumonia	250 mg	7	2 500-mg tablets	7
Uncomplicated skin and skin structure	250 mg	7 to 14	NA	NA

***For H pylori* eradication to reduce the risk of duodenal ulcer recurrence:**

1. Triple therapy (clarithromycin with lansoprazole and amoxicillin): The recommended adult dosage is 500 mg clarithromycin, 30 mg lansoprazole, and 1 g amoxicillin, all given twice daily (every 12 hours) for 10 or 14 days.
2. Triple therapy (clarithromycin with omeprazole and amoxicillin): The recommended adult dosage is 500 mg clarithromycin, 20 mg omeprazole, and 1 g amoxicillin, all given twice daily (every 12 hours) for 10 days. In patients with an ulcer present at the time of initiation of therapy, an additional 18 days of omeprazole 20 mg once daily is recommended for ulcer healing and symptom relief.
3. Dual therapy (clarithromycin with omeprazole): The recommended adult dosage is 500 mg clarithromycin given three times daily (every 8 hours) and 40 mg omeprazole given once daily (every morning) for 14 days. An additional 14 days of omeprazole 20 mg once daily is recommended for ulcer healing and symptom relief.
4. Dual therapy (clarithromycin with ranitidine bismuth citrate): The recommended adult dosage is 500 mg clarithromycin given twice daily (every 12 hours) or three times daily (every 8 hours) and 400 mg ranitidine bismuth citrate given twice daily (every 12 hours) for 14 to 28 days.

The recommended dosage of clarithromycin for the prevention of disseminated *M avium* disease (MAC) is 500 mg twice daily.

The recommended dose of clarithromycin for the treatment of disseminated MAC is 500 mg twice daily in combination with other medications.

SPECIAL POPULATIONS

RENAL IMPAIRMENT:

	Clarithromycin Dosage
Creatinine clearance < 30 mL/min	500 mg once daily
Hemodialysis	Give dose after dialysis
Chronic ambulatory peritoneal dialysis and continuous renal replacement therapy	N/A

HEPATIC DYSFUNCTION: No adjustment is necessary.

PEDIATRIC PATIENTS: Safety and effectiveness of clarithromycin in pediatric patients aged younger than 6 months have not been established.

The usual recommended daily dosage is 15 mg/kg/day divided every 12 hours for 10 days.

The recommended dosage of clarithromycin for the prevention of disseminated MAC is 7.5 mg/kg twice daily up to 500 mg twice daily.

For treatment of MAC, the recommended dosage is 7.5 mg/kg twice daily up to 500 mg twice daily. The safety of clarithromycin has not been studied in MAC patients aged younger than 20 months.

PREGNANCY: Category C

BREASTFEEDING: Clarithromycin should be used with caution in breastfeeding mothers.

THE ART OF ANTIMICROBIAL THERAPY

Clinical Pearls

1. When one is treating MAC, clarithromycin must be combined with other agents to minimize resistance.
2. Macrolides prolong QT intervals and must be used with caution.
3. Clarithromycin should not be used in pregnant women unless there is no alternative.

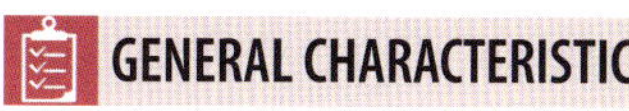

CLINDAMYCIN (Cleocin)

GENERAL CHARACTERISTICS

Class: Lincosamide

Mechanism of Action: Inhibits bacterial protein synthesis by binding to the 50S subunit of the ribosome.

Mechanisms of Resistance:

1. Alteration of the 50S ribosomal protein by an amino acid substitution,
2. alteration in the 23S ribosomal RNA subunit by methylation (MLS gene), and
3. nucleotidylation of the hydroxyl group of clindamycin.

Metabolic Route: Clindamycin is metabolized and excreted in the urine and feces.

FDA-APPROVED INDICATIONS

FDA-Approved Indications: Clindamycin capsules and granules for suspension are indicated in the treatment of serious infections caused by susceptible anaerobic bacteria, streptococci, pneumococci, and staphylococci.

Clindamycin for injection is indicated in the treatment of the following serious infections caused by susceptible organisms: lower respiratory tract infections including pneumonia, empyema, and lung abscess; skin and skin structure infections; gynecologic infections including endometritis, nongonococcal tubo-ovarian abscess, pelvic cellulitis, and postsurgical vaginal cuff infection; intraabdominal infections including peritonitis and intraabdominal abscess caused by susceptible anaerobic organisms; septicemia; and bone and joint infections.

Also Used for: Clindamycin in combination with primaquine has been used to treat *Pneumocystis jiroveci* pneumonia (PCP).

Clindamycin in combination with pyrimethamine has been used to treat *Toxoplasma gondii* infections in HIV-infected patients.

Clindamycin in combination with primaquine has been used to treat *Plasmodium falciparum* malaria.

Clindamycin in combination with quinine has been used to treat babesiosis.

SIDE EFFECTS/TOXICITY

Contraindicated in individuals with a history of hypersensitivity to preparations containing clindamycin or lincomycin.

Side effects include *Clostridium difficile*–associated diarrhea, esophagitis, abdominal pain, nausea, vomiting, diarrhea, morbilliform and vesiculobullous rash, urticaria, erythema multiforme, Stevens-Johnson syndrome, pruritus, vaginitis, abnormal liver function tests, neutropenia, eosinophilia, polyarthritis, and neuromuscular blockade.

DRUG INTERACTIONS/FOOD INTERACTIONS

Clindamycin capsules and granules can be taken without regard to food.

Use with caution in patients receiving musculoskeletal blocking agents.

Antagonism has been demonstrated between clindamycin and erythromycin in vitro.

DOSING

Clindamycin is supplied as 75-mg, 150-mg, and 300-mg capsules.

Clindamycin flavored granules for oral solution is supplied in a concentration of 75 mg/5 mL.

Clindamycin can also be administered intravenously.

CLINDAMYCIN CAPSULES

Serious infections: 150 mg to 300 mg every 6 hours.

More severe infections: 300 mg to 450 mg every 6 hours.

CLINDAMYCIN FOR INJECTION

Serious infections: 600 mg/day to 1200 mg/day in two, three, or four equal doses.

More severe infections: 1200 mg/day to 2700 mg/day in two, three, or four equal doses.

In life-threatening situations, doses of as much as 4800 mg/day have been given intravenously.

SPECIAL POPULATIONS

RENAL IMPAIRMENT: No dosage adjustment is necessary.

HEPATIC DYSFUNCTION: No dosage adjustment is necessary.

PEDIATRIC PATIENTS:

Clindamycin Capsules or IV:

Serious infections: 8 mg/kg/day to 16 mg/kg/day divided into three or four equal doses.

More severe infections: 16 mg/kg/day to 20 mg/kg/day divided into three or four equal doses.

Clindamycin Granules:

Serious infections: 8 mg/kg/day to 12 mg/kg/day divided into three or four equal doses.

Severe infections: 13 mg/kg/day to 16 mg/kg/day divided into three or four equal doses.

More severe infections: 17 mg/kg/day to 25 mg/kg/day divided into three or four equal doses.

In pediatric patients weighing 10 kg or less, 37.5 mg three times a day should be considered the minimum recommended dose.

PREGNANCY: Category B.

BREASTFEEDING: Clindamycin should be used with caution in breastfeeding mothers.

THE ART OF ANTIMICROBIAL THERAPY

Clinical Pearls

1. To avoid the possibility of esophageal irritation, clindamycin capsules should be taken with a full glass of water.
2. Clindamycin in combination with other agents has been effective in treating PCP, toxoplasmosis, and *P. falciparum* malaria.
3. When one is treating staphylococcal infections, be sure to assess for inducible resistance (D-Test) to clindamycin in organisms demonstrating erythromycin resistance and clindamycin susceptibility.
4. The 75-mg and 150-mg capsules contain tartrazine, which may cause allergic reactions (including bronchospasm). Tartrazine allergy is frequently seen in patients who also have aspirin hypersensitivity.

CLOFAZIMINE (Lamprene)

GENERAL CHARACTERISTICS

Class: Iminophenazine

Mechanisms of Action: Inhibits mycobacterial growth and binds preferentially to mycobacterial DNA.

Mechanism of Resistance: Incompletely understood.

Metabolic Route: Clofazimine is partially metabolized with more than 50% excreted unchanged in feces.

FDA-APPROVED INDICATIONS

FDA-Approved Indications: Second-line treatment of lepromatous leprosy, including dapsone-resistant lepromatous leprosy; initial treatment of multibacillary leprosy, in combination with one or more other antileprosy agents; and treatment of lepromatous leprosy complicated by erythema nodosum leprosum reactions.

Also Used for: Resistant *Mycobacterium tuberculosis* infection, in combination with other antituberculosis agents.

SIDE EFFECTS/TOXICITY

Side effects include rash, photosensitivity, splenic infarction, bowel obstruction, hepatitis, jaundice, gastrointestinal bleeding, eosinophilic enteritis, retinopathy, and pink or red to brownish-black discoloration of the skin, cornea, conjunctiva, and body fluids.

DRUG INTERACTIONS/FOOD INTERACTIONS

Most patients tolerate clofazimine better when it is taken with food, and absorption is improved.

DOSING

Clofazimine is supplied in 50-mg and 100-mg tablets. The usual adult dosage is 200 mg daily for 2 months followed by 100 mg daily.

SPECIAL POPULATIONS

RENAL IMPAIRMENT: No dosage adjustment is necessary.

HEPATIC DYSFUNCTION: Use with caution.

PEDIATRICS: The accepted dose is 1 mg/kg/day but data are limited.

PREGNANCY: Category C.

BREASTFEEDING: Use of clofazimine is not recommended in breastfeeding mothers.

THE ART OF ANTIMICROBIAL THERAPY

Clinical Pearls

1. Clofazimine should never be used alone in the treatment of active mycobacterial infections.
2. Food increases the levels of clofazimine.
3. Although clofazimine demonstrates in vitro activity against *Mycobacterium avium* complex (MAC), disseminated MAC has shown increased mortality when treated with clofazimine, and clofazimine is not recommended for this indication.

COLISTIMETHATE SODIUM (Coly-Mycin)

GENERAL CHARACTERISTICS

Class: Cell membrane–altering antibiotic

Mechanism of Action: Colistimethate sodium is a surface-active agent that penetrates into and disrupts the bacterial cell membrane.

Mechanism of Resistance: Data incomplete.

Metabolic Route: Colistimethate is excreted in the urine.

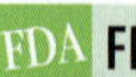

FDA-APPROVED INDICATIONS

FDA-Approved Indications: Treatment of acute or chronic infections caused by sensitive strains of gram-negative bacilli.

SIDE EFFECTS/TOXICITY

Side effects include **nephrotoxicity and transient neurological disturbances** including circumoral paresthesia or numbness, tingling of the extremities, generalized pruritus, vertigo, dizziness, and slurring of speech. **Also seen**: Gastrointestinal upset, generalized itching, urticaria, rash, fever, respiratory arrest (after intramuscular administration), and *Clostridium difficile*–associated diarrhea.

DRUG INTERACTIONS/FOOD INTERACTIONS

Aminoglycosides, curariform muscle relaxants, ether, succinylcholine, gallamine, decamethonium, sodium citrate, and polymyxin interfere with nerve transmission at the neuromuscular junction and should not be given concomitantly with colistin except with the greatest caution.

Cephalothin may enhance the nephrotoxicity.

DOSING

Colistimethate should be given in two to four divided doses of 2.5 mg/kg every 6–12 hours to 5 mg/kg every 6–12 hours for patients with normal renal function, depending on the severity of the infection.

In obese individuals, dosage should be based on ideal body weight.

SPECIAL POPULATIONS

RENAL IMPAIRMENT:

	Dosage
Creatinine clearance 40 mL/min to 60 mL/min	2.5 mg/kg every 12 hours
Creatinine clearance 10 mL/min to 39 mL/min	2.5 mg/kg every 24 hours

	Dosage
Creatinine clearance < 10 mL/min	1.5 mg/kg every 36 hours
After hemodialysis or peritoneal diaysis	1.5 mg/kg every 36 hours; no extra dose
Continuous renal replacement therapy	2.5 mg/kg every 24 hours

HEPATIC DYSFUNCTION: No dosage adjustment is necessary.

PEDIATRIC PATIENTS: As for adults. Close clinical monitoring of pediatric patients is recommended.

PREGNANCY: Category C

BREASTFEEDING: Caution should be used when one is administering colistimethate to a breastfeeding mother.

THE ART OF ANTIMICROBIAL THERAPY

Clinical Pearls

1. Colistimethate is not indicated for infections caused by *Proteus* or *Neisseria.*
2. Overdosage can result in renal insufficiency, muscle weakness, and apnea.
3. Avoid the administration of nephrotoxic agents or neuromuscular blocking agents when one is administering colistimethate.

GENERAL CHARACTERISTICS

Class: Analogue of D-alanine

Mechanisms of Action: Inhibits cell wall synthesis in gram-positive and gram-negative bacteria and in *Mycobacterium tuberculosis.*

Mechanism of Resistance: Incompletely understood.

Metabolic Route: About two thirds of cycloserine is excreted in the urine and the other third is metabolized to unknown substances.

FDA-APPROVED INDICATIONS

FDA-Approved Indications: Treatment of active pulmonary and extrapulmonary tuberculosis when the causative organisms are susceptible to this drug and when treatment with the primary medications has proved inadequate; and treatment of urinary tract infections caused by susceptible strains of gram-positive and gram-negative bacteria, but cycloserine should be considered only when conventional therapy has failed.

SIDE EFFECTS/TOXICITY

Contraindicated in patients with hypersensitivity to cycloserine, epilepsy, depression, severe anxiety, psychosis, or excessive use of alcohol.

Side effects include central nervous system toxicity, including inability to concentrate and lethargy, headache, tremor, vertigo, paresis, dysarthria, seizure, depression, psychosis, and suicidal ideation; peripheral neuropathy; allergic dermatitis; lichenoid eruptions; Stevens-Johnson syndrome; elevated serum transaminases; congestive heart failure; vitamin B12 and/or folic acid deficiency; megaloblastic anemia; and sideroblastic anemia.

DRUG INTERACTIONS/FOOD INTERACTIONS

Absorption modestly decreased by food; avoid large, fatty meals.

Concurrent administration of ethionamide has been reported to potentiate neurotoxic side effects.

Alcohol and cycloserine are incompatible because alcohol increases risk of epileptic episodes.

Concurrent administration of isoniazid may result in increased incidence of central nervous system effects, such as dizziness or drowsiness.

DOSING

Usually 10 mg/kg/day to 15 mg/kg/day: 250 mg orally twice a day; can increase to 250 mg orally three times a day or 250 mg orally each morning and 500 mg orally each night if peak levels are kept below 35 μg/mL.

SPECIAL POPULATIONS

RENAL IMPAIRMENT: The manufacturer contraindicates the use of cycloserine in severe renal insufficiency; if it must be used, for patients with creatinine clearance less than 30 mL/min or on hemodialysis, give 250 mg once daily, or a 500-mg dose three times per week; monitor levels.

HEPATIC DYSFUNCTION: No dosage adjustment necessary.

PEDIATRIC PATIENTS: Safety and effectiveness in pediatric patients have not been established. If it must be used: 10 mg/kg/day to 20 mg/kg/day in divided doses every 12 hours (daily maximum 1 g).

PREGNANCY: Category C

BREASTFEEDING: Cycloserine may be used in breastfeeding mothers; however, infant should be given B6.

THE ART OF ANTIMICROBIAL THERAPY

Clinical Pearls

1. Cycloserine should never be used alone in the treatment of active tuberculosis.
2. Cycloserine should only be used if resistance to first-line antimycobacterial agents is noted.
3. Cycloserine may cause increased neurotoxic side effects when administered with ethionamide.
4. Even though cycloserine has activity against usual bacteria, it is not routinely used to treat nonmycobacterial infection.
5. A patient should not consume alcohol while on cycloserine.
6. Neuropsychiatric side effects usually occur at serum levels greater than 35 μg/mL; serum levels of cycloserine should be monitored, with a goal of peak levels (2 hours after a dose) of 20 μg/mL to 35 μg/mL.
7. Hematologic, renal, and hepatic function should be monitored.
8. Some patients tolerate cycloserine best if treatment is begun with a small dose that is gradually increased over a few days to a week (ramping).
9. All patients should receive vitamin B6 while taking cycloserine. Adults need 100 mg to 300 mg (or 50 mg per 250 mg of cycloserine) and children should receive a dose proportionate to their weight.

BASIC CHARACTERISTICS

Class: Sulfone

Mechanism of Action: Inhibits bacterial dihydropteroate synthase.

Mechanisms of Resistance:

1. Overproduction of PABA para-aminobenzoic acid,
2. production of drug-resistant dihydropteroate synthase, and
3. decrease in cell permeability of dapsone.

Metabolic Route: Dapsone is excreted in the urine.

FDA-APPROVED INDICATIONS

FDA-Approved Indications: Dermatitis herpetiformis and leprosy (all forms).

Also Used for: Alternative prophylaxis for *Pneumocystis jiroveci,* alternate treatment of *P. jiroveci* pneumonia (with trimethoprim), and alternative prophylaxis for toxoplasmosis (with pyrimethamine and leucovorin).

SIDE EFFECTS/TOXICITY

Side effects/toxicities include hemolysis, (especially in those with G6PD deficiency), peripheral neuropathy, nausea, vomiting, abdominal pain, pancreatitis, vertigo, blurred vision, tinnitus, insomnia, fever, headache, psychosis, phototoxicity, pulmonary eosinophilia, tachycardia, albuminuria, nephrotic syndrome, hypoalbuminemia, renal papillary necrosis, male infertility, drug-induced lupus erythematosus, cutaneous reactions, hepatitis, cholestatic jaundice, agranulocytosis, aplastic anemia, and methemoglobinemia.

DRUG INTERACTIONS/FOOD INTERACTIONS

Dapsone can be taken with or without food.

Rifampin lowers dapsone levels but (in leprosy) no adjustment is necessary.

Folic acid antagonists such as pyrimethamine may increase the likelihood of hematologic reactions.

DOSING

PCP prophylaxis: 100 mg daily.

PCP treatment: 100 mg daily (plus trimethoprim 15 mg/kg/day).

Toxoplasmosis prophylaxis: 50 mg daily (plus pyrimethamine 50 mg weekly and leucovorin 25 mg weekly).

For leprosy: In bacteriologically negative **tuberculoid** and indeterminate disease, the recommendation is the coadministration of dapsone 100 mg daily with 6 months of rifampin 600 mg daily. Then dapsone should be continued for an additional 3 years for tuberculoid and indeterminate patients and for 5 years for borderline-tuberculoid patients.

In **lepromatous** and borderline-lepromatous patients, the recommendation is the coadministration of dapsone 100 mg daily with 2 years of rifampin 600 mg daily. Dapsone 100 mg daily is continued for 3 to 10 years until all signs of clinical activity are controlled with skin scrapings and biopsies negative for 1 year. Dapsone should then be continued for an additional 10 years for borderline patients and for life for lepromatous patients.

SPECIAL POPULATIONS

RENAL IMPAIRMENT: No dosage adjustment is necessary.

HEPATIC DYSFUNCTION: No dosage adjustment is necessary.

PEDIATRIC PATIENTS:

- PCP prophylaxis: 2 mg/kg (maximum 100 mg).
- Toxoplasma prophylaxis: 2 mg/kg with pyrimethamine 1 mg/kg daily, plus leucovorin 5 mg every 3 days.

PREGNANCY: Category C.

BREASTFEEDING: Do not administer dapsone to breastfeeding mothers.

THE ART OF ANTIMICROBIAL THERAPY

Clinical Pearls

1. Dapsone should be used in combination with one or more antileprosy drugs when one is treating leprosy.
2. Dapsone should not be used in patients who are G6PD-deficient.

DAPTOMYCIN (Cubicin)

BASIC CHARACTERISTICS

Class: Cyclic lipopeptide

Mechanism of Action: Binds to bacterial membranes and causes a rapid depolarization of membrane potential resulting in bacterial cell death.

Mechanisms of Resistance: Not fully understood; however, increasing minimum inhibitory concentrations (MICs) in *Staphylococcus aureus* have been reported while patients were receiving daptomycin.

Metabolic Route: Daptomycin is excreted unchanged in the urine.

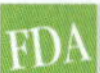

FDA-APPROVED INDICATIONS

FDA-Approved Indications: Complicated skin and skin structure infections caused by susceptible gram-positive organisms, and *S. aureus* bloodstream infections (bacteremia), including those in patients with right-sided infective endocarditis.

SIDE EFFECTS/TOXICITY

Side effects/toxicities include anaphylaxis, rash, rhabdomyolysis, arrhythmias, blurred vision, oral and vaginal candidiasis, gram-negative infections, *Clostridium difficile*–associated diarrhea, abnormal liver function tests, elevated CPK (daptomycin should be discontinued in symptomatic patients with CPK elevation greater than 1000 U/L, or in patients without reported symptoms who have elevations in CPK greater than 2000 U/L), peripheral neuropathy, thrombocytopenia and eosinophilic pneumonia.

DRUG INTERACTIONS/FOOD INTERACTIONS

Caution is warranted when daptomycin is coadministered with tobramycin.

Daptomycin can cause a false prolongation of prothrombin time (PT) and elevation of international normalized ratio (INR); it is recommended that the PT/INR be repeated with blood drawn just before the next dose of daptomycin. If still elevated, PT should be evaluated with an alternative method if possible, and other causes of prolonged PT should be sought.

Consideration should be given to temporarily suspending use of HMG-CoA reductase inhibitors.

DOSING

Complicated skin and skin structure infections: 4 mg/kg IV daily for 7 to 14 days.

***S. aureus* bloodstream infections:** 6 mg/kg IV daily for 2 to 6 weeks.

SPECIAL POPULATIONS

RENAL IMPAIRMENT: The same dosage is administered to those with a creatinine clearance less than 30 mL/min but it is given every 48 hours. This includes those on hemodialysis, chronic ambulatory peritoneal dialysis, and continuous renal replacement therapy.

HEPATIC DYSFUNCTION: No dosage adjustment is necessary.

PEDIATRIC PATIENTS: Safety and efficacy in patients aged younger than 18 years have not been established.

PREGNANCY: Category B.

BREASTFEEDING: Daptomycin should be used with caution in breastfeeding mothers.

THE ART OF ANTIMICROBIAL THERAPY

Clinical Pearls

1. Daptomycin dosage should be adjusted in patients with renal impairment.
2. CPK should be monitored while the patient is receiving daptomycin.
3. Daptomycin may cause false elevation of PT/INR results.
4. Increased MIC in *S. aureus* may develop while a patient is on daptomycin therapy.
5. Daptomycin should not be used to treat pneumonia in view of the high failure rate.

BASIC CHARACTERISTICS

Class: Protease inhibitor

Mechanism of Action: Reversibly binds the active site of the enzyme protease. Inhibition of protease prevents cleavage of the *gag* and *gag-pol* polyprotein resulting in the production of immature, noninfectious virus.

Mechanism of Resistance: Development of mutations on the enzyme protease causes a conformational change that prevents darunavir from binding the active site, allowing protease activity to continue. There are many protease mutations identified for darunavir, of which five are required to inhibit its activity.

Metabolic Route: Darunavir is metabolized in the liver and excreted in the feces.

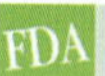

FDA-APPROVED INDICATIONS

FDA-Approved Indications: Treatment of HIV-1 in combinations with other antiretroviral agents.

SIDE EFFECTS/TOXICITY

Side effects/toxicities include new-onset diabetes mellitus; exacerbation of preexisting diabetes mellitus; hyperglycemia; increased bleeding, including spontaneous skin hematomas and hemarthrosis in patients with hemophilia type A or B; redistribution or accumulation of body fat including central obesity, dorsocervical fat enlargement (buffalo hump), peripheral wasting, facial wasting, and breast enlargement; cushingoid appearance; immune reconstitution syndrome; hepatitis; rash; QTc prolongation; torsades de pointes; abdominal pain; headache; anorexia; dyspepsia; epigastric pain; hepatitis; mouth ulceration; pancreatitis; vomiting; anemia; leukopenia; thrombocytopenia; increases in alkaline phosphatase, amylase, creatine phosphokinase, lactic dehydrogenase, SGOT, SGPT, and gamma glutamyl transpeptidase; hyperlipemia; hyperuricemia; hyperglycemia; hypoglycemia; and dehydration.

DRUG INTERACTIONS/FOOD INTERACTIONS

Darunavir should be taken with a meal.

Drugs that **should not be coadministered** with darunavir include amiodarone, quinidine, rifampin, ergot derivatives, Saint-John's-wort, HMG-CoA reductase inhibitors, simvastatin or lovastatin, pimozide, proton pump inhibitors, benzodiazepines, voriconazole, phenobarbital, phenytoin, carbamazepine, lopinavir, or saquinavir.

Darunavir is an inhibitor of the CYP3A enzyme; coadministration of darunavir and drugs primarily metabolized by CYP3A may result in increased plasma concentrations of the other drug that could increase or prolong its therapeutic and adverse effects.

Darunavir is metabolized by CYP3A; coadministration of darunavir and drugs that induce CYP3A may decrease darunavir plasma concentrations and reduce its therapeutic effect. Coadministration of darunavir and drugs that inhibit CYP3A may increase darunavir plasma concentrations. Because of these metabolic effects, potential drug interactions that may require dosage change or clinical/laboratory monitoring are listed in the following table:

Medication	*Adjustment or Action*
Itraconzole	Do not exceed 200 mg of itraconazole
Ketoconazole	Do not exceed 200 mg of ketoconazole
Clarithromycin	Reduce clarithromycin dosage in patients with renal impairment
Rifabutin	Decrease rifabutin to 150 mg every other day
Hormonal contraceptives	Use alternative or additional method
Atorvastatin	Use lowest possible dosage with close monitoring
Pravastatin	Use lowest possible dosage with close monitoring
Methadone	Monitor; may require higher methadone dosage
Sildenafil	25 mg every 48 hours
Tadalafil	5 mg; no more than 10 mg in 72 hours
Vardenafil	2.5 mg in 24 hours
Paroxetine, sertraline	Monitor for antidepressant response
Tenofovir	Monitor for tenofovir toxicity
Maraviroc	Maraviroc dosage should be 150 mg twice daily
Cyclosporine, tacrolimus, sirolimus	Monitor levels of immunosuppressants

DOSING

Darunavir is supplied in 75-mg, 150-mg, 300-mg, 400-mg, and 600-mg tablets. Darunavir **must** be taken with ritonavir to achieve adequate levels. The recommended dosage of darunavir in antiretroviral therapy–naïve patients is 800 mg (two 400-mg tablets) taken with ritonavir 100 mg once daily and with food. The type of food does not affect exposure to darunavir.

For treatment-experienced patients, the recommended dosage of darunavir tablets is 600 mg taken with ritonavir 100 mg twice daily and with food.

SPECIAL POPULATIONS

RENAL IMPAIRMENT: There is no adjustment needed.

HEPATIC DYSFUNCTION: No dosage adjustment is required in patients with mild or moderate hepatic impairment. Darunavir is not recommended for use in patients with severe hepatic impairment.

PEDIATRIC PATIENTS: Darunavir is approved for pediatric patients aged 6 years and older. Once daily dosing is not recommended.

- **Body weight 20 kg to 30 kg:** darunavir 375 mg plus ritonavir 50 mg twice daily
- **Body weight >30 kg to 40 kg:** darunavir 450 mg plus ritonavir 60 mg twice daily
- **Body weight greater than 40 kg:** darunavir 600 mg plus ritonavir 100 mg twice daily

The safety and efficacy of darunavir plus ritonavir in pediatric patients aged 3 years to less than 6 years have not been established. Do not use darunavir plus ritonavir in patients aged younger than 3 years.

PREGNANCY: Category C.

BREASTFEEDING: It is recommended that HIV-positive mothers not breastfeed their children to decrease mother-to-child transmission of HIV.

THE ART OF ANTIMICROBIAL THERAPY

Clinical Pearls

1. Darunavir should always be used in combination with other antiretrovirals.
2. Darunavir must be administered with ritonavir to achieve adequate levels.
3. Darunavir should be taken with food to increase absorption.
4. Darunavir has a sulfa moiety; use caution when using it in patients with sulfa allergies.
5. When one is assessing for resistance to darunavir, a phenotype assay may be helpful.
6. Whenever initiating darunavir, one should make sure to review all medications the patient is receiving, to minimize drug interactions.

BASIC CHARACTERISTICS

Class: Nonnucleoside reverse transcriptase inhibitor

Mechanism of Action: Inhibits reverse transcriptase activity by binding the enzyme.

Mechanism of Resistance: Changes in the structure of reverse transcriptase lead to the inability of delavirdine to bind the enzyme and allow transcription to continue. The most frequent resistance mutations include K103N and Y181C.

Metabolic Route: Delavirdine is metabolized by the cytochrome P450 system to several inactive metabolites.

FDA-APPROVED INDICATION

FDA-Approved Indication: Treatment of HIV-1 in combinations with other antiretroviral agents.

SIDE EFFECTS/TOXICITY

Side effects/toxicities include immune reconstitution; redistribution or accumulation of body fat including central obesity, dorsocervical fat enlargement (buffalo hump), peripheral wasting, facial wasting, and breast enlargement; cushingoid appearance; severe rash; abdominal pain; abnormal cardiac rate and rhythm; diarrhea; hyperglycemia; hypertriglyceridemia; increased AST; increased GGT; increased lipase; increased serum alkaline phosphatase; hemolytic anemia; and rhabdomyolysis.

DRUG INTERACTIONS/FOOD INTERACTIONS

Food has no significant effect on delavirdine.

Delavirdine should not be administered concurrently with astemizole, cisapride, midazolam, pimozide, terfenadine, triazolam, ergot derivatives, Saint-John's-wort, etravirine, phenobarbitol, phenytoin, carbamazepine, rifabutin, rifampin, fosamprenavir, lovastatin, or simvastatin.

Delavirdine causes hepatic enzyme inhibition of CYP3A4; coadministration of delavirdine with drugs primarily metabolized by CYP3A4 isozymes may result in altered plasma concentrations of the coadministered drug. Drugs that induce CYP3A4 activity would be expected to increase the clearance of delavirdine resulting in lowered plasma concentrations. Because of these metabolic activities, the following drug interactions warrant consideration of dosage adjustment and monitoring of clinical effects and serum levels of affected drugs:

DELAVIRDINE (Rescriptor)

Medication	*Adjustment or Action*
Atorvastatin	Use lowest possible dosage and monitor for toxicity
Clarithromycin	Consider alternative agent
Methadone	Monitor for methadone toxicity
Voriconazole	Monitor for delavirdine toxicity
Oral contraceptives	Levels of contraceptive may increase
Sildenafil	25 mg every 48 hours
Vardenafil	2.5 mg; no more than 2.5 mg in 24 hours
Tadalafil	5 mg; no more than 10 mg in 72 hours
Warfarin	Monitor INR closely
Quinidine	Monitor for quinidine toxicity
Indinavir	Indinavir 600 mg three times a day
Maraviroc	Maraviroc 150 mg twice a day

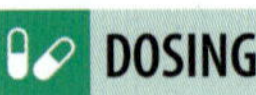

DOSING

Delavirdine is delivered in 100-mg or 200-mg tablets. The recommended dosage is 400 mg three times daily. The 100-mg tablets may be dispersed in water prior to consumption. The 200-mg tablets should be taken as intact tablets because they are not readily dispersed in water. Patients with achlorhydria should take delavirdine with an acidic beverage (e.g., orange or cranberry juice). Patients taking both delavirdine and antacids should be advised to take them at least 1 hour apart.

SPECIAL POPULATIONS

RENAL IMPAIRMENT: There is no dosage adjustment needed.

HEPATIC DYSFUNCTION: Caution should be exercised when one is administering delavirdine to patients with impaired hepatic function.

PEDIATRIC PATIENTS: Safety and effectiveness have not been established in individuals aged younger than 16 years.

PREGNANCY: Category C.

BREASTFEEDING: It is recommended that HIV-positive mothers not breastfeed their children to decrease mother-to-child transmission of HIV.

THE ART OF ANTIMICROBIAL THERAPY

Clinical Pearls

1. Delavirdine should always be used in combination with other antiretrovirals.
2. Delavirdine 100-mg tablets can be dissolved in water. The 200-mg tablets cannot.
3. Delavirdine should be given with a pH-lowering agent such as a cola beverage.
4. Whenever initiating delavirdine, one should make sure to review all medications the patient is receiving, to limit drug interactions.

 BASIC CHARACTERISTICS

Class: Semisynthetic penicillin

Mechanism of Action: Binds penicillin-binding protein (PBP), disrupting cell wall synthesis.

Mechanisms of Resistance:

1. The PBP can be altered, with reduced affinity,
2. production of a β-lactamase resulting in hydrolysis of the β-lactam ring, and
3. decreased ability of the antibiotic to reach the PBP when bacteria decrease porin production, resulting in reduced drug concentration within the cell.

Metabolic Route: Dicloxacillin is excreted as unchanged drug in the urine.

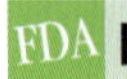 FDA-APPROVED INDICATIONS

FDA-Approved Indications: Treatment of infections caused by susceptible penicillinase-producing staphylococci.

 SIDE EFFECTS/TOXICITY

A history of allergic reaction to any of the penicillins is a **contraindication.**

Side effects/toxicities include *Clostridium difficile*– associated diarrhea; interstitial nephritis including rash, fever, eosinophilia, hematuria, proteinuria, and renal insufficiency; esophageal ulceration; thrombophlebitis; hypersensitivity reactions including rash, erythema multiforme, and Stevens-Johnson syndrome; hepatitis; nausea; vomiting; diarrhea; stomatitis; black or hairy tongue; hyperactivity; seizures; anemia; thrombocytopenia; neutropenia; and eosinophilia.

DRUG INTERACTIONS/FOOD INTERACTIONS

Dicloxacillin is best absorbed when taken on an empty stomach, and should be administered at least 1 hour before or 2 hours after meals. Chloramphenicol, macrolides, sulfonamides, and tetracyclines may interfere with the bactericidal effects of penicillins.

When dicloxacillin and warfarin are used concomitantly, the prothrombin time should be closely monitored.

High urine concentrations of dicloxacillin may result in false-positive reactions when one is testing for the presence of glucose in urine by using Clinitest. It is recommended that glucose tests based on enzymatic glucose oxidase reactions (such as Clinistix) be used instead.

DOSING

Dicloxacillin is supplied as 250-mg and 500-mg capsules.

Mild to moderate infections: 125 mg every 6 hours

Severe infections: 250 mg every 6 hours

SPECIAL POPULATIONS

RENAL IMPAIRMENT: No dosage adjustment is necessary.

HEPATIC DYSFUNCTION: No dosage adjustment is necessary.

COMBINED RENAL AND HEPATIC INSUFFICIENCY: Measurement of dicloxacillin serum levels should be performed and dosage should be adjusted accordingly.

PEDIATRIC PATIENTS: Dicloxacillin should be avoided in the neonate.

- **Mild to moderate infections:** 12.5 mg/kg every 6 hours
- **Severe infections:** 25 mg/kg every 6 hours

PREGNANCY: Category B.

BREASTFEEDING: Dicloxacillin should be used only with caution in breastfeeding mothers.

THE ART OF ANTIMICROBIAL THERAPY

Clinical Pearls

1. Dosage of dicloxacillin does not need to be adjusted for patients with renal impairment.
2. Dicloxacillin should be used with caution in patients with both renal and hepatic insufficiency.
3. Dicloxacillin should be taken with at least 4 fluid ounces (120 mL) of water and should not be taken in the supine position or immediately before going to bed.
4. Dicloxacillin should be taken on an empty stomach.

DIDANOSINE (Videx EC)

BASIC CHARACTERISTICS

Class: Nucleoside reverse transcriptase inhibitor.

Mechanism of Action: Converted by cellular enzymes to its active drug, dideoxyadenosine triphosphate, an analogue of adenosine triphosphate. The dideoxyadenosine triphosphate competes with the naturally occurring nucleotide for incorporation in newly forming HIV DNA. Because dideoxyadenosine triphosphate does not have a terminal hydroxyl group, it halts transcription and replication of the virus.

Mechanism of Resistance: Changes in the structure of HIV reverse transcriptase lead to preferred incorporation of adenosine triphosphate and decreased incorporation of dideoxyadenosine triphosphate, which allows transcription of DNA to continue. Resistance mutations include L74V and K65R.

Metabolic Route: Approximately 20% of didanosine is excreted in the urine unchanged; the remainder is excreted similarly to endogenous purines.

FDA FDA-APPROVED INDICATIONS

FDA-Approved Indications: Treatment of HIV infection in combination with other antiretrovirals.

SIDE EFFECTS/TOXICITY

> **WARNING:** Fatal and nonfatal **pancreatitis** have occurred during therapy with didanosine. Didanosine should be suspended in patients with suspected pancreatitis and discontinued in patients with confirmed pancreatitis. **Lactic acidosis** and hepatomegaly with steatosis have been reported with nucleoside analogues, including didanosine. This is magnified when didanosine is used in combination with stavudine and, therefore, they should not be used together. If this syndrome occurs, the drug should be discontinued.

Other side effects/toxicities: Immune reconstitution inflammatory syndrome; fat redistribution including central obesity and dorsocervical fat enlargement, peripheral wasting, facial wasting, and breast enlargement; peripheral neuropathy; hepatotoxicity and hepatic failure; retinal changes; and optic neuritis.

DRUG INTERACTIONS/FOOD INTERACTIONS

Didanosine must be taken without food.

Didanosine should not be administered with stavudine because of increased risk of lactic acidosis and peripheral neuropathy.

Coadministration with allopurinol or ribavirin is not recommended.

Coadministration with drugs that may cause pancreatic toxicity or neuropathy may increase risk of their respective adverse reactions.

Didanosine should be used with caution when given with tenofovir because the combination decreased CD4 counts. If used together, the dosage of didanosine should be decreased to 250 mg daily.

DOSING

Didanosine is administered in 125-mg, 200-mg, 250-mg, and 400-mg tablets or in a powder that can be placed in solution. The recommended adult dosage is 400 mg daily for those who weigh more than or equal to 60 kg. For those who weigh from 25 kg to 59.9 kg, the dosage should be reduced to 250 mg daily. For those who weigh from 20 kg to 24.9 kg, 200 mg daily should be given.

SPECIAL POPULATIONS

RENAL IMPAIRMENT:

Dosage Adjustment:

CrCl Measurement	*≥ 60 kg*	*< 60 kg*
≥ 60	400 mg once daily	250 mg once daily
30 to 59	200 mg once daily	125 mg once daily
10 to 29	125 mg once daily	125 mg once daily
< 10	125 mg once daily	Not recommended

Note: CrCl = Creatinine Clearance.

HEPATIC DYSFUNCTION: No dosage adjustment is necessary.

PEDIATRIC PATIENTS: Didanosine is approved for use in children that weigh at least 20 kg. The dosing is the same as that for adults.

PREGNANCY: Category B.

BREASTFEEDING: It is recommended that HIV-positive mothers not breastfeed their children to decrease mother-to-child transmission of HIV.

THE ART OF ANTIMICROBIAL THERAPY

Clinical Pearls

1. Didanosine should be used in combination with other antiretroviral agents.
2. Didanosine should not be used with either stavudine or ribavirin because of increased risk of lactic acidosis.
3. Didanosine and tenofovir combination should be avoided if possible.
4. Periodic eye examinations should be considered in patients taking didanosine.

DIETHYLCARBAMAZINE (Hetrazan)

BASIC CHARACTERISTICS

Class: Piperazine derivative

Mechanisms of Action (incompletely understood):

1. Free radicals, from platelet-mediated release of antigen from microfilariae result in death of the organisim.
2. alteration of prostaglandin metabolism, leading to immobilization of microfilariae, and
3. inhibition of microtubule polymerization.

Metabolic Route: Diethylcarbamazine is excreted in the urine, 50% in unchanged form.

FDA-APPROVED INDICATIONS

Not FDA-approved, but used for treatment of *Wuchereria bancrofti*, *Brugia malayi*, *Brugia timori*, and *Loa loa*.

SIDE EFFECTS/TOXICITY

Side effects/toxicities include anorexia, nausea, vomiting, headache, and somnolence. The Mazzotti reaction (fever, tachypnea, tachycardia, and hypotension) is seen predominantly in individuals with onchocerciasis; milder forms of the Mazzotti reaction may also be seen in patients with bancroftian filariasis and *Loiasis*. May also see local inflammatory reaction at site of dying worms or microfilariae (e.g., pain, abscess formation, adenitis and lymphangitis). In loiasis, encephalitis may develop if level of parasitemia is high.

DRUG INTERACTIONS/FOOD INTERACTIONS

Efficacy may be reduced by corticosteroids. Synergism is seen with albendazole or ivermectin.

DOSING

Diethylcarbamazine is administered in 50-mg tablets.

- **Bancroftian filariasis:** 6 mg/kg/day, divided into three doses for 12 days or 6 mg/kg/day for 12 days plus albendazole or ivermectin
- **Loaiasis:** 8 mg/kg/day to 10 mg/kg/day divided into three doses for 21 days
- **Prophylaxis of *Loa loa*:** 300 mg weekly

SPECIAL POPULATIONS

RENAL IMPAIRMENT: One should decrease the dosage in patients with renal insufficiency.

HEPATIC DYSFUNCTION: Data incomplete.

PEDIATRIC PATIENTS: Same dosage as adults.

PREGNANCY: Contraindicated.

BREASTFEEDING: Do not administer DEC to breastfeeding mothers.

THE ART OF ANTIMICROBIAL THERAPY

Clinical Pearls

1. Diethylcarbamazine can be obtained from the Centers for Disease Control and Prevention's Parasitic Diseases Drug Service: 770–488–7775.
2. Diethylcarbamazine is not used for onchocerciasis because of the Mazzotti reaction and the risk of increased ocular side effects including blindness. Before one treats a patient with DEC for lymphatic filariasis or *Loiasis*, co-infection with *Onchocerca* should be excluded.
3. Corticosteroids may ameliorate the Mazzotti reaction but may also reduce the efficacy of DEC.
4. In individuals with high-level *Loa loa* infection, pretreatment apheresis may decrease the likelihood of encephalitis.
5. If DEC is given as a single large daily dose it should be administered at night to minimize adverse effects.

DILOXANIDE FUROATE (Furamide)

BASIC CHARACTERISTICS

Class: Dichloroacetamide derivative

Mechanism of Action: Interferes with protein synthesis.

Metabolic Route: More than 50% of diloxanide furoate is excreted in the urine with about 10% in the feces.

FDA-APPROVED INDICATIONS

Not FDA-approved, but used for treatment of *Entamoeba histolytica*—used as monotherapy for asymptomatic cyst passers; given with other amoebicides to treat invasive or extraintestinal amoebiasis.

SIDE EFFECTS/TOXICITY

Side effects/toxicities include anorexia, nausea, flatulence, abdominal cramps and diarrhea, and urticaria.

DRUG INTERACTIONS/FOOD INTERACTIONS

Unknown.

DOSING

500 mg three times a day for 10 days.

SPECIAL POPULATIONS

RENAL IMPAIRMENT: Unknown.

HEPATIC DYSFUNCTION: Unknown.

PEDIATRIC PATIENTS: 20 mg/kg daily in three divided doses for 10 days. The maximum dosage for children is 1.5 g a day.

PREGNANCY: Defer treatment until after the first trimester of pregnancy.

BREASTFEEDING: Unknown.

THE ART OF ANTIMICROBIAL THERAPY

Clinical Pearls

Diloxanide furoate is not available commercially in the United States. It may be obtained from a compounding pharmacy through the National Association of Compounding Pharmacies (800-687-7850) or http://www.pccarx.com.

DORIPENEM (Doribax)

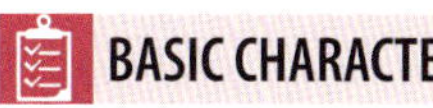

BASIC CHARACTERISTICS

Class: Carbapenem

Mechanism of Action: Binds penicillin-binding protein (PBP), disrupting cell wall synthesis.

Mechanisms of Resistance:

1. The PBP can be altered, with reduced affinity,
2. production of a β-lactamase resulting in hydrolysis of the β-lactam ring,
3. decreased ability of the antibiotic to reach the PBP when bacteria decrease porins, resulting in a decrease of the drug concentration within the cell, and
4. increased expression of efflux pump components.

Metabolic Route: Doripenem is excreted in the urine.

FDA-APPROVED INDICATIONS

FDA-Approved Indications: Treatment of serious infections caused by susceptible strains of microorganisms in complicated intraabdominal infections and complicated urinary tract infections, including pyelonephritis.

SIDE EFFECTS/TOXICITY

Doripenem is **contraindicated** in patients with known hypersensitivity to any component of this product or to other drugs in the same class or in patients who have demonstrated anaphylactic reactions to β-lactams. Before initiation of therapy with doripenem, careful inquiry should be made concerning previous hypersensitivity reactions to carbapenems, penicillins, cephalosporins, other β-lactams, and other allergens, because of the increased possibility of hypersensitivity.

Side effects/toxicities include seizures; phlebitis; fever; anaphylaxis; rash including Stevens-Johnson syndrome, erythema multiforme, and toxic epidermal necrolysis; angioedema; hypotension; encephalopathy; hearing loss; diarrhea; *Clostridium difficile*–associated diarrhea and pseudomembranous colitis; oral candidiasis; glossitis; anorexia; nausea; vomiting; stomach cramps; hepatitis; renal impairment; pyuria; hematuria; genital pruritis; dyspnea; polyarthralgia; prolonged prothrombin time; pancytopenia; positive Coombs' test; increased ALT (SGPT), AST (SGOT), alkaline phosphatase, bilirubin, and LDH; decreased serum sodium; and increased potassium and chloride.

DRUG INTERACTIONS/FOOD INTERACTIONS

Doripenem may reduce serum valproic acid concentrations; levels should be monitored. It is not recommended that probenecid be given with doripenem.

DORIPENEM (Doribax)

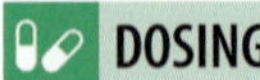

DOSING

The recommended dosage of doripenem is 500 mg every 8 hours by intravenous infusion.

SPECIAL POPULATIONS

RENAL IMPAIRMENT:

CrCl Measurement/Hemodialysis	*Dosage*
30 mL/min to 50 mL/min	250 mg every 8 hours
10 mL/min to < 30 mL/min	250 mg every 12 hours
< 10 mL/min	No information
After hemodialysis or peritoneal dialysis	No information
Continuous renal replacement therapy	No information

Note: CrCl = Creatinine Clearance.

HEPATIC DYSFUNCTION: No dosage adjustment is necessary.

PEDIATRIC PATIENTS: Safety and effectiveness in pediatric patients have not been established.

PREGNANCY: Category B.

BREASTFEEDING: Doripenem should be used with caution in breastfeeding mothers.

THE ART OF ANTIMICROBIAL THERAPY

Clinical Pearls

1. Dosage of doripenem must be adjusted for patients with renal impairment.
2. Cross-allergy with penicillins is less than 10%.
3. Doripenem is active against many organisms that carry extended-spectrum β-lactamases.
4. Among the carbapenems, doripenem has the most potent gram-negative activity and may be active against organisms that are resistant to other carbapenems.

DOXYCYCLINE (Vibramycin) and DOXYCYCLINE DELAYED-RELEASE (Doryx)

 BASIC CHARACTERISTICS

Class: Tetracycline

Mechanism of Action: Reversibly binds the 30s ribosomal subunit preventing the addition of new amino acids into the growing peptide chain.

Mechanisms of Resistance: Decreased entry into the cell or increased excretion of the drug. Rarely the tetracyclines are inactivated.

Metabolic Route: Doxycycline and doxycycline delayed-release are concentrated by the liver in the bile, and excreted in the urine and feces at high concentrations and in a biologically active form.

 FDA-APPROVED INDICATIONS

FDA-Approved Indications: Treatment of the following serious infections caused by susceptible strains of microorganisms: respiratory and genitourinary tract infections, Rocky Mountain spotted fever, typhus fever and the typhus group, Q fever, rickettsialpox and tick fevers caused by *Rickettsiae, Mycoplasma pneumoniae*, lymphogranuloma venereum, psittacosis, trachoma, inclusion conjunctivitis, chlamydial genital and rectal infection, nongonococcal urethritis, relapsing fever, chancroid, plague, tularemia, cholera, *Campylobacter fetus* infections, brucellosis, bartonellosis, granuloma inguinale, gonorrhea, syphilis, yaws, listeriosis, anthrax, actinomycosis, Vincent's infection, intestinal amebiasis, *Clostridium* infections, prophylaxis of malaria, and severe acne.

Also Used for: Treatment of malaria, anaplasmosis, ehrlichiosis, borreliosis including Lyme disease, rapidly growing mycobacteria, community-acquired methacillin-resistant *Staphylococcus aureus*, and *Mycobacterium marinum*.

 SIDE EFFECTS/TOXICITY

Doxycycline is **contraindicated** in persons who have shown hypersensitivity to any of the tetracyclines.

Tetracyclines should not be used during pregnancy or up to the age of 8 years unless absolutely necessary and no reasonable alternative exists.

Side effects/toxicities include hypersensitivity reactions including rash, anaphylaxis, urticaria, angioneurotic edema, serum sickness, photosensitivity, pericarditis, exacerbation of systemic lupus erythematosus, nausea, vomiting, diarrhea, glossitis, esophagitis, hepatotoxicity, pseudomembranous colitis, bulging fontanels in infants and benign intracranial hypertension in adults, vertigo, pseudotumor cerebri, tinnitus and decreased hearing, dose-related rise in blood urea nitrogen, hemolytic anemia, thrombocytopenia, neutropenia, and eosinophilia.

DRUG INTERACTIONS/FOOD INTERACTIONS

Although absorption of tetracycline is impaired by bismuth subsalicylate, antacids, and iron-containing preparations, doxycycline may be given with food or milk.

Concurrent use of tetracycline may render oral contraceptives less effective.

Patients who are on anticoagulant therapy may require downward adjustment of their anticoagulant dosage.

It is advisable to avoid giving tetracycline-class drugs in conjunction with penicillin.

The concurrent use of tetracycline and methoxyflurane has been reported to result in fatal renal toxicity.

DOSING

Doxycycline

Doxycycline is supplied as 50-mg and 100-mg capsules, and a syrup containing 50 mg/5 mL. It is also administered intravenously; however, oral therapy should be instituted as soon as possible. If intravenous therapy is given over prolonged periods of time, thrombophlebitis may result.

Usual dosage of doxycycline: 200 mg on the first day of treatment (administered as 100 mg every 12 hours) followed by a maintenance dosage of 100 mg per day. The maintenance dosage may be administered as a single dose or as 50 mg every 12 hours.

In the management of **more severe infections**, 100 mg every 12 hours is recommended.

Gonococcal infections, chlamydial genitourinary or rectal infection, nongonococcal urethritis: 100 mg twice daily for 7 days

Syphilis: early – 100 mg twice daily for 2 weeks; syphilis of more than 1 year's duration – 100 mg twice daily for 4 weeks.

Gonococcal or chlamydial epididymo-orchitis: 100 mg twice daily for 10 days.

Malaria prophylaxis: 100 mg daily; children aged older than 8 years – 2 mg/kg once daily up to the adult dosage. Prophylaxis is begun 1 to 2 days before travel to the malarious area and continued during travel and for 4 weeks after leaving the malarious area.

Anthrax (treatment and prophylaxis)**:** 100 mg twice daily for 60 days; children weighing less than 45 kg – 2.2 mg/kg twice daily for 60 days. Children weighing 45 kg or more receive the adult dosage.

Doxycycline Delayed-Release Capsules

Doxycycline delayed-release capsules are administered in 75-mg and 100-mg capsules. They are dosed similarly to regular doxycycline; however, they may also be administered by carefully opening the capsules and sprinkling the capsule contents on a spoonful of applesauce. The applesauce should be swallowed immediately without chewing and followed with a cool 8-ounce glass of water to ensure complete swallowing of the capsule contents.

SPECIAL POPULATIONS

RENAL IMPAIRMENT: No dosage adjustment is necessary.

HEPATIC DYSFUNCTION: No dosage adjustment is necessary.

PEDIATRIC PATIENTS: **For children aged older than 8 years:** The recommended dosage schedule for children weighing 100 pounds or less is 2 mg/lb of body weight divided into two doses on the first day of treatment, followed by 1 mg/lb of body weight given as a single daily dose or divided into two doses, on subsequent days. For more severe infections up to 2 mg/lb of body weight may be used. For children who weigh more than 100 pounds the usual adult dosage should be used.

PREGNANCY: Category D.

BREASTFEEDING: Do not administer doxycycline to breastfeeding mothers.

THE ART OF ANTIMICROBIAL THERAPY

Clinical Pearls

1. To reduce the risk of esophageal irritation and ulceration, doxycycline should be taken with adequate amounts of fluid and should not be taken immediately before going to bed.
2. Doxycycline can cause fetal harm when administered to a pregnant woman.
3. The use of drugs of the tetracycline class during tooth development (last half of pregnancy, infancy, and childhood to the age of 8 years) may cause permanent discoloration of the teeth (yellow-gray-brown).
4. The Oracea brand of doxycycline is indicated only for the treatment of inflammatory lesions (papules and pustules) of rosacea in adult patients. It has not been evaluated in the treatment of infections and should not be substituted for the doxycycline preparations discussed previously.
5. The absorption of doxycycline is NOT markedly influenced by simultaneous ingestion of food or milk.

EFAVIRENZ (Sustiva)

Note: Also available combined with tenofovir and emtricitabine as Atripla; *see* tenofovir plus emtricitabine plus efavirenz)

BASIC CHARACTERISTICS

Class: Nonnucleoside reverse transcriptase inhibitor

Mechanism of Action: Inhibits reverse transcriptase activity by binding the enzyme.

Mechanism of Resistance: Changes in the structure of reverse transcriptase lead to the inability of efavirenz to bind the enzyme and allow transcription to continue. The most frequent resistance mutations include K103N and Y181C.

Metabolic Route: Efavirenz is metabolized by the cytochrome P450 system to hydroxylated metabolites with subsequent glucuronidation.

FDA-APPROVED INDICATION

FDA-Approved Indication: Treatment of HIV-1 in combinations with other antiretroviral agents.

SIDE EFFECTS/TOXICITY

Side effects/toxicities include serious psychiatric toxicity, including severe depression, suicidal ideation, nonfatal suicide attempts, aggressive behavior, paranoid reactions, manic reactions, insomnia, impaired concentration, somnolence, dizziness, abnormal dreams, and hallucinations. Other side effects/toxicities include rash, elevated liver enzymes, convulsions, elevated cholesterol, fat redistribution, immune reconstitution syndrome, nausea and vomiting, headache, and fatigue.

DRUG INTERACTIONS/FOOD INTERACTIONS

Efavirenz should be taken on an empty stomach at bedtime to decrease central nervous system side effects.

Efavirenz should not be administered concurrently with astemizole, bepridil, cisapride, midazolam, pimozide, triazolam, ergot derivatives, Saint-John's-wort, or etravirine.

Efavirenz causes hepatic enzyme induction of CYP3A4; coadministration of efavirenz with drugs primarily metabolized by 2C9, 2C19, and 3A4 isozymes may result in altered plasma concentrations of the coadministered drug. Drugs that induce CYP3A4 activity would be expected to increase the clearance of efavirenz resulting in lowered plasma concentrations. Because of these metabolic activities, the following drug interactions warrant consideration of dosage adjustment and monitoring of clinical effects and serum levels of affected drugs:

Medication	*Adjustment or Action*
Voriconazole	Increase voriconazole to 400 mg twice daily and decrease efavirenz to 300 mg daily
Clarithromycin	Consider alternative agent to clarithromycin
Rifabutin	Increase rifabutin to 450 to 600 mg daily or 600 mg three times per week
Rifampin	Consider increasing efavirenz to 800 mg/day
Hormonal contraceptives	Use alternative or additional method
Phenobarbitol, phenytoin, or carbamazepine	Monitor anticonvulsant level; consider alternative
Methadone	Opiate withdrawal common, titrate methadone
Warfarin	Monitor INR closely
Fosamprenavir	Fosamprenavir 1400 mg plus ritonavir 300 mg daily or usual twice daily dosage
Darunavir	Monitor levels with normal dosing
Indinavir	Indinavir 800 mg twice daily plus ritonavir 100 mg twice daily
Maraviroc	Increase maraviroc to 600 mg twice daily

DOSING

Efavirenz is administered in 50-mg, 200-mg, and 600-mg tablets.

The recommended dosage of efavirenz is 600 mg orally, once daily, in combination with other antiretrovirals.

SPECIAL POPULATIONS

RENAL IMPAIRMENT: There is no dosage adjustment needed.

HEPATIC DYSFUNCTION: In patients with known or suspected history of hepatitis B or C infection and in patients treated with other medications associated with liver toxicity, monitoring of liver enzymes is recommended.

PEDIATRIC PATIENTS: Should only be administered to children aged older than 3 years as follows:

Weight, kg	*Dose, mg/day*
10 to < 15	200
15 to < 20	250
20 to < 25	300
25 to < 32.5	350
32.5 to < 40	400
≥40	600

PREGNANCY: Category D.

BREASTFEEDING: It is recommended that HIV-positive mothers not breastfeed their children, to decrease mother-to-child transmission of HIV.

THE ART OF ANTIMICROBIAL THERAPY

Clinical Pearls

1. Efavirenz should always be used in combination with other antiretrovirals.
2. Efavirenz should be dosed at bedtime to decrease the central nervous system adverse events.
3. If efavirenz is given without food, less is absorbed and side effects can be decreased.
4. Efavirenz has a very long half life. If a patient is stopping an antiretroviral regimen, to decrease development of resistance the other medications should be continued for at least another 48 hours.
5. Women receiving efavirenz should use two methods of birth control.
6. Whenever initiating efavirenz, one should make sure to review all medications the patient is receiving, to limit drug interactions.

EFLORNITHINE (Ornidyl)

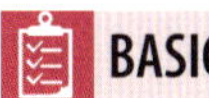

BASIC CHARACTERISTICS

Class: Fluorinated analogue of ornithine

Mechanism of Action: Inhibits of ornithine decarboxylase resulting in a decrease in spermidine and trypanothione.

Metabolic Route: Eflornithine is excreted unchanged in the urine.

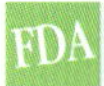

FDA-APPROVED INDICATION

Not FDA-approved, but used for treatment of *Trypanosoma brucei gambiense* trypanosomiasis. However, because of shortage, the World Health Organization recommends using eflornithine only in relapsing cases of late-stage *Trypanosoma brucei gambiense* trypanosomiasis.

SIDE EFFECTS/TOXICITY

Side effects/toxicities include anemia, leukopenia, thrombocytopenia, seizures, diarrhea, hearing loss, and alopecia.

DRUG INTERACTIONS/FOOD INTERACTIONS

Data incomplete.

DOSING

New cases of late-stage Gambian trypanosomiasis: 100 mg/kg every 6 hours IV for 14 days.

Relapse: same dosage for 7 days.

SPECIAL POPULATIONS

RENAL IMPAIRMENT: The dosage should be reduced in patients with renal insufficiency.

HEPATIC DYSFUNCTION: No dosage adjustment is necessary.

PEDIATRIC PATIENTS: Children aged younger than 12 years should receive 125 mg/kg every 6 hours IV for 14 days. Older children should receive 100 mg/kg every 6 hours for 14 days.

PREGNANCY: Eflornithine may induce abortion.

BREASTFEEDING: Unknown.

THE ART OF ANTIMICROBIAL THERAPY

Clinical Pearls

1. Patients treated with eflornithine should be followed for 2 years, with a lumbar puncture every 6 months.
2. Eflornithine monotherapy should not be used to treat *Trypanosoma brucei rhodesiense* trypanosomiasis because it is much less active.
3. Eflornithine and melarsoprol may be synergistic for the treatment of old world trypanosomiasis.
4. Eflornithine is a licensed drug, but the only source in the United States is the Centers for Disease Control and Prevention, Parasitic Diseases Drug Service: 770-488-7775.

EMTRICITABINE (Emtriva)

Note: Also available combined with tenofovir in Truvada (*see* tenofovir plus emtricitabine) and with both tenofovir and efavirenz in Atripla (*see* tenofovir plus emtricitabine plus efavirenz)

BASIC CHARACTERISTICS

Class: Nucleoside reverse transcriptase inhibitor.

Mechanism of Action: Converted by cellular enzymes to its active drug, emtricitabine triphosphate, an analogue of cytosine triphosphate. The emtricitabine triphosphate competes with the naturally occurring nucleotides for incorporation in newly forming HIV DNA. Because emtricitabine triphosphate does not have a terminal hydroxyl group, it halts transcription and replication of the virus.

Mechanism of Resistance: Changes in the structure of HIV reverse transcriptase lead to preferred incorporation of cytosine triphosphate and decreased incorporation of emtricitabine triphosphate, which allows transcription of DNA to continue. Resistance mutations include M184V.

Metabolic Route: Emtricitabine is mainly excreted unchanged in the urine.

FDA-APPROVED INDICATIONS

FDA-Approved Indications: Emtricitabine is approved to be used in combination with other antiretrovirals for the treatment of HIV infection.

Also used for: Emtricitabine has activity against hepatitis B (HBV).

SIDE EFFECTS/TOXICITY

> **WARNING: Severe acute exacerbations of hepatitis B** have been reported in patients who have discontinued emtricitabine. Hepatic function should be monitored closely with both clinical and laboratory follow-up for at least several months in patients who are co-infected with HIV-1 and HBV and discontinue emtricitabine. If appropriate, initiation of anti–hepatitis B therapy may be warranted. **Lactic acidosis** and hepatomegaly with steatosis have been reported with nucleoside analogues, including emtricitabine. If this syndrome occurs, the drug should be discontinued.

Other side effects/toxicities: Immune reconstitution inflammatory syndrome, fat redistribution including central obesity and dorsocervical fat enlargement, peripheral wasting, facial wasting, breast enlargement, headache, diarrhea, nausea, fatigue, dizziness, depression, insomnia, abnormal dreams, rash, abdominal pain, asthenia, increased cough, and rhinitis. Skin hyperpigmentation is common in pediatric patients.

DRUG INTERACTIONS/FOOD INTERACTIONS

Emtricitabine can be taken with or without food and is unaffected by pH.

Emtricitabine should not be administered with any medication that contains lamivudine because they are both cytosine analogues and may be antagonistic.

Emtricitabine should not be administered with other medications containing emtricitabine (i.e., Truvada or Atripla).

DOSING

Emtricitabine is administered in a 200-mg tablet or in a clear orange liquid, which contains 10 mg/mL of emtricitabine. The recommended adult dosage is 200 mg daily.

SPECIAL POPULATIONS

RENAL IMPAIRMENT: Dosage adjustment is necessary as follows:

For creatinine clearance:

- 30 mL/min to 49 mL/min: 200 mg every 48 hours
- 15 mL/min to 29 mL/min: 200 mg every 72 hours
- < 15 mL/min or hemodialysis: 200 mg every 96 hours

HEPATIC DYSFUNCTION: No dosage adjustment is necessary.

PEDIATRIC PATIENTS: The approved dosage is 6 mg/kg up to a maximum of 240 mg oral solution or a 200-mg capsule daily.

PREGNANCY: Category B.

BREASTFEEDING: It is recommended that HIV-positive mothers not breastfeed their children, to decrease mother-to-child transmission of HIV.

THE ART OF ANTIMICROBIAL THERAPY

Clinical Pearls

1. Emtricitabine should be used in combination with other antiretroviral agents.
2. Emtricitabine is present in three different medications: Emtriva, Truvada, and Atripla.
3. Patients with HIV-1 should be tested for HBV before initiating antiretroviral therapy with emtricitabine.

BASIC CHARACTERISTICS

Class: Fusion inhibitor

Mechanism of Action: Interferes with the entry of HIV-1 into cells by inhibiting fusion of viral and cellular membranes.

Mechanism of Resistance: Resistant isolates have shown mutations that resulted in amino acid substitutions at the enfuvirtide binding HR1 domain positions 36 to 38 of the HIV-1 envelope glycoprotein gp41.

Metabolic Route: Enfuvirtide undergoes catabolism to its constituent amino acids, with subsequent recycling of the amino acids in the body pool.

FDA-APPROVED INDICATIONS

FDA-Approved Indications: Treatment of HIV-1 in combinations with other antiretroviral agents in treatment-experienced patients with evidence of HIV-1 replication despite ongoing antiretroviral therapy.

SIDE EFFECTS/TOXICITY

Side effects/toxicities include hypersensitivity reactions including rash and fever, nausea, vomiting, chills, rigors, hypotension, elevated serum liver transaminases; injection site reactions that include pain and discomfort, induration, erythema, nodules and cysts, pruritus, and ecchymosis; immune reconstitution syndrome; bacterial pneumonia; primary immune complex reaction; respiratory distress; glomerulonephritis; and Guillain-Barré syndrome. There is a theoretical risk that enfuvirtide use may lead to the production of anti-enfuvirtide antibodies that cross-react with HIV gp41. This could result in a false-positive HIV test with an enzyme-linked immunosorbent assay (ELISA).

DRUG INTERACTIONS/FOOD INTERACTIONS

There are no drug interactions.

DOSING

The recommended dosage of enfuvirtide is 90 mg (1 mL) twice daily injected subcutaneously into the back of the upper arm, anterior thigh, or abdomen. Each injection should be given at a site different from the preceding injection site.

SPECIAL POPULATIONS

RENAL IMPAIRMENT: There is no dosage adjustment needed.

HEPATIC DYSFUNCTION: There is no dosage adjustment needed.

PEDIATRIC PATIENTS: Enfuvirtide should not be used in children aged younger than 6 years. In those aged 6 through 16 years, the recommended dosage of enfuvirtide is 2 mg/kg twice daily up to a maximum dosage of 90 mg twice daily injected subcutaneously.

PREGNANCY: Category B.

BREASTFEEDING: It is recommended that HIV-positive mothers not breastfeed their children, to decrease mother-to-child transmission of HIV.

THE ART OF ANTIMICROBIAL THERAPY

Clinical Pearls

1. Enfuvirtide should always be used in combination with other antiretrovirals.
2. Enfuvirtide must be administered within 24 hours of reconstitution.
3. Injection site reactions may be decreased if the enfuvirtide is at room temperature or warmer.
4. Enfuvirtide should only be administered subcutaneously in the anterior thigh, abdomen, or back of the upper arms to ensure good absorption.

 BASIC CHARACTERISTICS

Class: Nucleoside reverse transcriptase inhibitor.

Mechanism of Action: Entecavir is a guanosine nucleoside analogue that is phosphorylated to the active triphosphate form. It competes with guanosine triphosphate to inhibit all three activities of the HBV polymerase (reverse transcriptase):

1. base priming,
2. reverse transcription of the negative strand from the pregenomic messenger RNA, and
3. synthesis of the positive strand of HBV DNA.

Mechanism of Resistance: Lamivudine-resistant HBV caries 8- to 30-fold reduction in entecavir susceptibility. The mutations rtM204I/V with or without rtL180M in HBV polymerase lead to decreased incorporation of entecavir.

Metabolic Route: Entecavir is excreted unchanged in the urine.

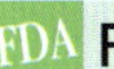 FDA-APPROVED INDICATIONS

FDA-Approved Indications: Treatment of chronic HBV infection in adults with evidence of active viral replication and either evidence of persistent elevations in serum aminotransferases (ALT or AST) or histologically active disease.

 SIDE EFFECTS/TOXICITY

> **WARNING: Lactic acidosis and severe hepatomegaly** with steatosis, including fatal cases, have been reported with the use of nucleoside analogues. **Severe acute exacerbations of hepatitis B** have been reported in patients who have discontinued anti–hepatitis B therapy, including entecavir.

Entecavir is not recommended for patients co-infected with HIV and HBV who are not also receiving highly active antiretroviral therapy (HAART), because of the potential for the development of resistance to HIV nucleoside reverse transcriptase inhibitors. Before initiation of entecavir therapy, HIV antibody testing should be offered to all patients.

Other side effects/toxicities include headache, fatigue, rash, dizziness, and nausea.

 DRUG INTERACTIONS/FOOD INTERACTIONS

Entecavir should be administered at least 2 hours after a meal and 2 hours before the next meal.

There are no significant drug interactions.

ENTECAVIR (Baraclude)

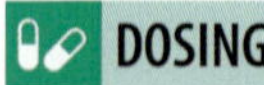

DOSING

Entecavir is supplied in 0.5-mg and 1-mg tablets and an orange-flavored, clear, colorless to pale yellow aqueous solution containing 0.05 mg/mL. The recommended dosage in nucleoside-treatment–naïve adults and adolescents aged 16 years and older is 0.5 mg once daily. The recommended dosage in those who are receiving lamivudine or have virus resistant to either lamivudine or telbivudine is 1 mg once daily.

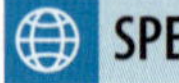

SPECIAL POPULATIONS

RENAL IMPAIRMENT:

CrCl Measurement/ Hemodialysis	*Nucleoside-Treatment Naïve Dosage*	*Lamivudine-Resistant Dosage*
≥ 50 mL/min	0.5 mg once daily	1 mg once daily
30 mL/min to < 50 mL/min	0.25 mg once daily or 0.5 mg every 48 hours	0.5 mg once daily or 1 mg every 48 hours
10 mL/min to < 30 mL/min	0.15 mg once daily or 0.5 mg every 72 hours	0.3 mg once daily or 1 mg every 72 hours
<10 mL/min, hemodialysis, or peritoneal dialysis	0.05 mg once daily or 0.5 mg every 7 days	0.1 mg once daily or 1 mg every 7 days

Note: CrCl = Creatinine Clearance.

HEPATIC DYSFUNCTION: No dosage adjustment.

PEDIATRIC PATIENTS: Safety and effectiveness of entecavir in patients aged younger than 16 years have not been established.

PREGNANCY: Category C.

BREASTFEEDING: It is not recommended to administer entecavir to breastfeeding mothers.

THE ART OF ANTIMICROBIAL THERAPY

Clinical Pearls

1. Lamivudine resistance leads to decreased susceptibility to entecavir.
2. Resistance mutations are similar for entecavir and telbivudine.
3. Before initiation of entecavir therapy, HIV testing should be offered to all patients.
4. Do not initiate entecavir in HIV co-infected patients unless they are on HAART; M184V mutations on HIV reverse transcriptase have been reported.

ERTAPENEM (Invanz)

BASIC CHARACTERISTICS

Class: Carbapenem

Mechanism of Action: Binds penicillin binding protein (PBP), disrupting cell wall synthesis.

Mechanisms of Resistance:

1. The PBP can be altered, with reduced affinity,
2. production of a β-lactamase resulting in hydrolysis of the β-lactam ring,
3. decreased ability of the antibiotic to reach the PBP when bacteria decrease porin production, resulting in a decrease of the drug concentration within the cell, and
4. increased expression of efflux pump components.

Metabolic Route: Ertapenem is excreted in the urine.

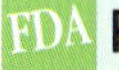

FDA-APPROVED INDICATIONS

FDA-Approved Indications: Treatment of serious infections caused by susceptible strains of microorganisms in the following conditions: complicated intraabdominal infections; complicated skin and skin structure infections, including diabetic foot infections without osteomyelitis; community-acquired pneumonia; complicated urinary tract infections including pyelonephritis with or without concurrent bacteremia; acute pelvic infections including postpartum endomyometritis, septic abortion, and post-surgical gynecologic infections; and prophylaxis of surgical site infection following elective colorectal surgery.

SIDE EFFECTS/TOXICITY

Ertapenem is **contraindicated** in patients with known hypersensitivity to any component of this product or to other drugs in the same class or in patients who have demonstrated anaphylactic reactions to β-lactams. Before initiation of therapy with ertapenem, careful inquiry should be made concerning previous hypersensitivity reactions to penicillins, cephalosporins, other β-lactams, and other allergens, because of the increased possibility of hypersensitivity.

Side effects/toxicities include phlebitis; fever; anaphylaxis; rash including Stevens-Johnson syndrome, erythema multiforme, and toxic epidermal necrolysis; angioedema; hypotension; encephalopathy; seizures; hearing loss; diarrhea; *Clostridium difficile*–associated diarrhea and pseudomembranous colitis; oral candidiasis; glossitis; anorexia; nausea; vomiting; stomach cramps; hepatitis; renal impairment; pyuria; hematuria; genital pruritis; dyspnea; polyarthralgia; prolonged prothrombin time; pancytopenia; positive Coombs' test; increased ALT (SGPT), AST (SGOT), alkaline phosphatase, bilirubin, and LDH; decreased serum sodium; and increased potassium and chloride.

 DRUG INTERACTIONS/FOOD INTERACTIONS

Ertapenem may reduce serum valproic acid concentrations; levels should be monitored. It is not recommended that probenecid be given with ertapenem.

 DOSING

The dosage of ertapenem in patients aged 13 years and older is 1 g given once a day by intravenous infusion or intramuscular injection.

Type of Infection	*Dosage (Patients ≥ 13 Years)*	*Duration*
Complicated skin and skin structure infection	1 g daily	7 to 14 days
Community-acquired pneumonia	1 g daily	10 to 14 days
Complicated urinary tract infection	1 g daily	10 to 14 days
Acute pelvic infections	1 g daily	3 to 10 days
Surgical prophylaxis	1 g	Given 60 minutes before incision

 SPECIAL POPULATIONS

RENAL IMPAIRMENT:

- **Creatinine clearance < 30 mL/min:** 500 mg daily
- **After hemodialysis:** if dose was received less than 6 hours before hemodialysis, give supplemental dose of 150 mg
- **Continuous renal replacement therapy or peritoneal dialysis:** unknown

HEPATIC DYSFUNCTION: No dosage adjustment is necessary.

PEDIATRIC PATIENTS:

Type of Infection	*Dosage (Patients < 13 Years)*	*Duration*
Complicated skin and skin structure infections	15 mg/kg every 12 hours	7 to 14 days
Community-acquired pneumonia	15 mg/kg every 12 hours	10 to 14 days
Complicated urinary tract infection	15 mg/kg every 12 hours	10 to 14 days
Acute pelvic infections	15 mg/kg every 12 hours	3 to 10 days

PREGNANCY: Category B.

BREASTFEEDING: Ertapenem should be used with caution in breastfeeding mothers.

THE ART OF ANTIMICROBIAL THERAPY

Clinical Pearls

1. Dosage of ertapanem must be adjusted for patients with renal impairment.
2. Cross-allergy with penicillins is less than10%.
3. Unlike other carbapenems, ertapenem is not active against *Pseudomonas* species and other highly resistant gram-negative rods.
4. Ertapenem is active against extended-spectrum β-lactamase–producing gram-negative enteric rods.
5. Ertapanem is associated with seizure risk predominantly in patients with central nervous system disease or renal impairment.

Note: Including (1) erythromycin ethylsuccinate tablets, suspension, and delayed-release formulation; (2) erythromycin lactobionate for injection; (3) erythromycin stearate (base); (4) erythromycin estolate; and (5) erythromycin coated pellets and delayed-release pellets.

BASIC CHARACTERISTICS

Class: Macrolide

Mechanism of Action: Binds to the 50S ribosomal subunit of susceptible microorganisms and, thus, interferes with microbial protein synthesis.

Mechanisms of Resistance:

1. Decreased permeability,
2. active efflux,
3. alteration of the 50S ribosomal unit,
4. alteration of the 23S subunit of the 50S ribosomal unit, and
5. enzymatic inactivation of the macrolide.

Metabolic Route: Erythromycin is excreted in the bile.

FDA FDA-APPROVED INDICATIONS

FDA-Approved Indications: All formulations of erythromycin have the following indications; any exceptions are noted: Treatment of the following infections caused by susceptible strains of the designated organisms: upper and lower respiratory tract infections; *Mycoplasma* infection; listeriosis; pertussis; skin and skin structure infections; diphtheria; erythrasma caused by *Corynebacterium minutissimum;* intestinal amebiasis caused by *Entamoeba histolytica* (oral erythromycins only); *Chlamydia trachomatis* conjunctivitis of the newborn, pneumonia of infancy, and urogenital infections during pregnancy; alternative to penicillin for gonococcal pelvic inflammatory disease and syphilis; alternative to tetracyclines for uncomplicated urethral, endocervical, or rectal infections in adults caused by *C. trachomatis*, nongonococcal urethritis caused by *Ureaplasma urealyticum;* Legionnaires' disease; and alternative to penicillin for prevention of rheumatic fever.

SIDE EFFECTS/TOXICITY

Contraindicated in patients with known hypersensitivity to this antibiotic.

Side effects/toxicities include allergic reactions, rash, nausea, vomiting, abdominal pain, diarrhea, anorexia, elevations of liver enzymes, jaundice, pancreatitis, pseudomembranous colitis, rhabdomyolysis, exacerbation of symptoms of myasthenia gravis and new onset of symptoms of myasthenic syndrome, infantile hypertrophic pyloric stenosis, QT prolongation and ventricular arrhythmias, convulsions, and reversible hearing loss.

DRUG INTERACTIONS/FOOD INTERACTIONS

Erythromycin tablets and suspension can be administered with or without food.

Erythromycin is a substrate and inhibitor of the P450 enzyme system (CYP3A). Erythromycin is **contraindicated** in patients taking terfenadine, astemizole, pimozide, or cisapride.

Erythromycin should be used with **caution**, with monitoring of serum concentrations when possible, with the following medications: theophylline, oral anticoagulants, digoxin, verapamil, carbamazapine, sildenafil, midazolam, triazolam, HMG-CoA reductase inhibitors (e.g., lovastatin and simvastatin), ergotamine, cyclosporine, tacrolimus, alfentanil, disopyramide, rifabutin, quinidine, methylprednisolone, cilostazol, vinblastine, and bromocriptine.

Erythromycin interacts with other drugs not metabolized by the CYP3A system, including hexobarbital, phenytoin, and valproate.

DOSING

There are multiple formulations of erythromycin.

Oral (erythromycin ethylsuccinate): usual dosage is 400 mg every 6 hours; delayed-release formulations can be given in 6-hour, 8-hour, and 12-hour intervals with a total of 1000 mg in the day; for severe infections, the dosage can be increased to 4 g in a 24-hour period.

For adult dosage calculation, use a ratio of 400 mg of erythromycin as the ethylsuccinate to 250 mg of erythromycin stearate (base) or estolate.

Intravenous (erythromycin lactobionate): 15 mg/kg/day to 20 mg/kg/day, in divided doses every 6 hours. Higher dosages, up to 4 g/day, may be given for severe infections.

SPECIAL POPULATIONS

RENAL IMPAIRMENT: For creatinine clearance less than 10 mL/min, administer half the usual daily dose.

HEPATIC DYSFUNCTION: Caution should be used.

PEDIATRIC PATIENTS: In mild-to-moderate infections, the usual dosage of erythromycin ethylsuccinate for children is 30 mg/kg/day to 50 mg/kg/day in equally divided doses every 6 hours. For more severe infections this dosage may be doubled. If twice-a-day dosage is desired, one half of the total daily dose may be given every 12 hours. Doses may also be given three times daily by administering one third of the total daily dose every 8 hours.

PREGNANCY: Category B.

BREASTFEEDING: Caution should be used.

 THE ART OF ANTIMICROBIAL THERAPY

Clinical Pearls

1. Multiple formulations of erythromycin are available; caution should be used as the dosage regimens differ.
2. Macrolides prolong QT intervals and must be used with caution.

ETHAMBUTOL HYDROCHLORIDE (Myambutol)

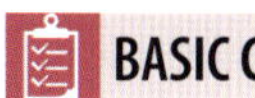 BASIC CHARACTERISTICS

Class: N-substituted ethylenediamine

Mechanism of Action: Inhibits arabinosyl transferase enzymes involved in biosynthesis of mycobacterial cell wall.

Mechanism of Resistance: Point mutations in the arabinosyl transferase enzyme.

Metabolic Route: Approximately 50% of ethambutol is excreted in the urine, 25% is metabolized by the liver, and 25% is excreted in the feces unchanged.

FDA FDA-APPROVED INDICATIONS

FDA-Approved Indications: Treatment of *Mycobacterium tuberculosis* in combination with other antimycobacterial agents.

Also Used for: Treatment of non-tuberculous mycobacterial infection, including *Mycobacterium avium intracellulare* complex, *Mycobacterium kansasii, Mycobacterium bovis,* and infection caused by Bacillus Calmette-Guerin.

 SIDE EFFECTS/TOXICITY

Side effects/toxicities include optic neuritis, peripheral neuropathy, rash, thrombocytopenia, anaphylaxis, dermatitis, arthralgias, fever, and elevations of serum uric acid with precipitation of acute gout.

DRUG INTERACTIONS/FOOD INTERACTIONS

Antacids may reduce absorption and should be separated from ethambutol administration by 2 hours.

 DOSING

Note: Dose should never be divided, but should be given a single dose.

Dosage is 15 mg/kg/day to 25 mg/kg/day in one daily dose. If the larger dose is initiated, reduce it to 15 mg/kg/day after 60 days. Maximum daily dose: 1600 mg.

Twice-weekly dosage:

- 40 kg to 55 kg: 2000 mg
- 56 kg to 75 kg: 2800 mg
- 76 kg to 90 kg: 4000 mg (maximum)

Thrice-weekly dosage:

- 40 kg to 55kg: 1200 mg
- 56 kg to 75 kg: 2000 mg
- 76 kg to 90 kg: 2400 mg (maximum)

SPECIAL POPULATIONS

RENAL IMPAIRMENT: Renal failure (creatinine clearance < 30) or hemodialysis: 15 mg/kg to 25 mg/kg three times weekly; monitor assays in patients with renal failure (usual levels 2 μg/mL to 5μg/mL).

HEPATIC DYSFUNCTION: No dosage adjustment necessary.

PEDIATRIC PATIENTS: 15 mg/kg/day to 20 mg/kg/day in one daily dose; maximum 1000 mg. Twice-weekly dosage: 50 mg/kg; maximum 2500 mg.

PREGNANCY: Category C.

BREASTFEEDING: It is safe to administer to breastfeeding mothers.

THE ART OF ANTIMICROBIAL THERAPY

Clinical Pearls

1. Ethambutol should always be used in combination with other antimycobacterial agents.
2. All patients receiving ethambutol should have evaluation of visual acuity and color vision at initiation of therapy and at least monthly during therapy.
3. Because the visual toxicity is dose-related, serum levels should be assayed in patients with renal impairment.
4. Visual toxicity is less common with intermittent therapy (e.g., twice- or thrice-weekly administration).
5. Visual toxicity is uncommon at the lower dosage of 15 mg/kg/day.

BASIC CHARACTERISTICS

Class: Derivative of isonicotinic acid

Mechanism of Action: Blocks mycolic acid synthesis.

Mechanisms of Resistance: Incompletely understood.

Metabolic Route: Ethionamide metabolism is presumed to occur in the liver and six metabolites have been isolated.

FDA-APPROVED INDICATIONS

FDA-Approved Indications: Treatment of active tuberculosis in patients with *Mycobacterium tuberculosis* that is resistant to isoniazid or rifampin, or when there is intolerance on the part of the patient to other antituberculosis drugs.

SIDE EFFECTS/TOXICITY

Contraindicated in patients with severe hepatic impairment and in patients who are hypersensitive to the drug.

Side effects/toxicities include hepatitis, hypoglycemia, hypothyroidism, nausea, vomiting, diarrhea, abdominal pain, excessive salivation, metallic taste, stomatitis, anorexia, weight loss, headache, psychotic disturbances, rash, photosensitivity, thrombocytopenia, gynecomastia, impotence, peripheral neuritis, optic neuritis, diplopia, blurred vision, and a pellagralike syndrome.

DRUG INTERACTIONS/FOOD INTERACTIONS

Ethionamide tablets may be administered without regard to the timing of meals.

Ethionamide has been found to raise serum concentrations of isoniazid.

Convulsions have been reported when ethionamide is administered with cycloserine. Excessive ethanol ingestion should be avoided because a psychotic reaction has been reported.

DOSING

Ethionamide is supplied as 250-mg tablets. The usual adult dosage is 15 mg/kg/day to 20 mg/kg/day frequently divided (maximum dosage 1 g per day); usually 500 mg to 750 mg per day in two divided doses or a single daily dose.

A single daily dose can sometimes be given at bedtime or with the main meal.

SPECIAL POPULATIONS

RENAL IMPAIRMENT: No dosage adjustment is necessary.

HEPATIC DYSFUNCTION: Contraindicated in patients with severe hepatic dysfunction.

PEDIATRIC PATIENTS: Should not be used in patients aged younger than 12 years except when the organisms are definitely resistant to primary therapy and systemic dissemination of the disease, or other life-threatening complications of tuberculosis, are judged to be imminent. Dosage is 15 mg/kg/day to 20 mg/kg/day usually divided into two or three doses (maximum dosage 1 g per day).

PREGNANCY: Category C.

BREASTFEEDING: Administer only if the benefits outweigh the risks. If given, treat infant with B6.

THE ART OF ANTIMICROBIAL THERAPY

Clinical Pearls

1. Ethionamide should never be used alone in the treatment of active tuberculosis.
2. Ethionamide should only be used if resistance or intolerance of the first-line antituberculosis medications occurs.
3. Ethionamide may cause increased side effects when used with cycloserine.
4. Pyridoxine should be given to all patients receiving ethionamide to prevent or relieve neurotoxic effects. Adults need 100 mg (more if also taking cycloserine) and children should receive a dose proportionate to their weight.
5. Alcohol should be avoided in patients receiving ethionamide.
6. Monitor thyroid-stimulating hormone and liver function tests.
7. Cross-resistance may occur with isoniazid and thiacetazone.
8. Ethionamide should be taken with food to minimize gastrointestinal distress.
9. Some patients tolerate ethionamide best if it is begun with a small dose that is gradually increased over a few days to a week (ramping).

ETRAVIRINE (Intelence)

BASIC CHARACTERISTICS

Class: Nonnucleoside reverse transcriptase inhibitor (NNRTI)

Mechanism of Action: Inhibits reverse transcriptase activity by binding the enzyme.

Mechanism of Resistance: Changes in the structure of reverse transcriptase lead to the inability of etravirine to bind the enzyme and allow transcription to continue. The most frequent resistance mutations that lead to resistance to other NNRTIs do not affect etravirine.

Metabolic Route: Etravirine is metabolized by the cytochrome P450 system and is excreted in both urine and feces.

FDA-APPROVED INDICATIONS

FDA-Approved Indication: Treatment of HIV-1 in combination with other antiretroviral agents.

SIDE EFFECTS/TOXICITY

Side effects/toxicities include hypersensitivity with fever, general malaise, fatigue, muscle or joint aches, blisters, oral lesions, conjunctivitis, facial edema, hepatitis, eosinophilia, Stevens-Johnson syndrome, and erythema multiforme; elevated liver enzymes; elevated cholesterol; fat redistribution; and immune reconstitution syndrome.

DRUG INTERACTIONS/FOOD INTERACTIONS

Etravirine must be administered with food.

Etravirine should not be administered concurrently with astemizole, bepridil, cisapride, midazolam, pimozide, triazolam, ergot derivatives, Saint-John's-wort, rifampin, phenobarbitol, phenytoin, carbamazepine, efavirenz, fosamprenavir, atazanavir, indinavir, nevirapine, full-dose ritonavir, or tipranavir.

Etravirine causes hepatic enzyme induction of CYP3A4; coadministration of etravirine with drugs primarily metabolized by 2C9, 2C19, and 3A4 isozymes may result in altered plasma concentrations of the coadministered drug. Drugs that induce CYP3A4 activity would be expected to increase the clearance of etravirine resulting in lowered plasma concentrations. Because of these metabolic activities, the following drug interactions warrant consideration of dosage adjustment and monitoring of clinical effects and serum levels of affected drugs:

Medication	*Adjustment or Action*
Itraconazole, ketoconazole, voriconazole	Monitor azole levels
Clarithromycin	Consider alternative agent

Medication	*Adjustment or Action*
Rifabutin	Normal dosage unless etravirine is combined with ritonavir, then consider an alternative to etravirine
Methadone	Monitor for methadone withdrawal
Warfarin	Monitor INR closely
Dexamethasone	Use with caution
Diazepam	Decrease diazepam as needed
Cyclosporine, sirolimus, tacrolimus	Monitor immunosuppressant levels
Atorvastatin, fluvastatin, simvastatin, lovastatin	Dosage adjustment of the HMG-CoA may be necessary
Antiarrhythmics	Use with caution

DOSING

Etravirine is administered in 100-mg tablets. The recommended oral dosage of etravirine is two 100-mg tablets taken twice daily. Etravirine tablets may be dispersed in a glass of water.

SPECIAL POPULATIONS

RENAL IMPAIRMENT: There is no dosage adjustment needed.

HEPATIC DYSFUNCTION: In patients with known or suspected hepatitis and in patients treated with other medications associated with liver toxicity, monitoring of liver enzymes is recommended.

PEDIATRIC PATIENTS: Not studied in pediatric populations.

PREGNANCY: Category B.

BREASTFEEDING: It is recommended that HIV-positive mothers not breastfeed their children, to decrease mother-to-child transmission of HIV.

THE ART OF ANTIMICROBIAL THERAPY

Clinical Pearls

1. Etravirine should always be used in combination with other antiretrovirals.
2. Etravirine should be dosed with food.
3. Etravirine can be dissolved in water to create a slurry.
4. Whenever initiating etravirine, one should make sure to review all medications the patient is receiving, to limit drug interactions.

5. Etravirine has a higher barrier to resistance than do the other NNRTIs.
6. The only protease inhibitors that can be coadministered with etravirine are darunavir, lopinavir, or saquinavir.
7. Etravirine is not recommended for naïve antiretroviral therapy.
8. Etravirine should not be used alone with 2 NRTIs; it is recommended to be used in the salvage setting with at least one other class in addition to the NRTIs.

BASIC CHARACTERISTICS

Class: Nucleoside analogue

Mechanism of Action: Famciclovir is the prodrug of penciclovir. Penciclovir is a guanine analogue. After hydrolysis, it is phosphorylated by thymidine kinase to the active triphosphate form. Penciclovir triphosphate stops replication of herpes viral DNA. This is accomplished in three ways:

1. competitive inhibition of viral DNA polymerase,
2. incorporation into and termination of the growing viral DNA chain, and
3. inactivation of the viral DNA polymerase. The greater antiviral activity of acyclovir against herpes simplex virus (HSV) compared with varicella zoster virus (VZV) is because of its more efficient phosphorylation by the viral thymidine kinase.

Mechanism of Resistance: Resistance of HSV and VZV to penciclovir can result from qualitative or quantitative changes in the viral thymidine kinase or DNA polymerase.

Metabolic Route: After oral administration, famciclovir is deacetylated and hydrolyzed to penciclovir. Penciclovir is excreted in the urine.

FDA FDA-APPROVED INDICATIONS

FDA-Approved Indications: Treatment of herpes zoster, suppression of recurrent genital herpes in immunocompetent patients, and the treatment of recurrent mucocutaneous herpes simplex infections in HIV-infected patients.

SIDE EFFECTS/TOXICITY

Side effects/toxicities include headache, parasthesia, migraine, confusion, hallucinations, nausea, vomiting, diarrhea, flatulence, abdominal pain, fatigue, pruritus, rash, and dysmenorrhea.

DRUG INTERACTIONS/FOOD INTERACTIONS

Famciclovir can be administered orally with or without food.

Concurrent use with probenecid or other drugs significantly eliminated by active renal tubular secretion may result in increased plasma concentrations of penciclovir.

DOSING

Famciclovir is supplied in 125-mg, 250-mg, and 500-mg tablets.

Herpes zoster: 500 mg every 8 hours for 7 days

Suppression of recurrent genital herpes: 250 mg twice daily for up to 1 year

Recurrent orolabial or genital herpes simplex in HIV-infected individuals: 500 mg twice daily for 7 days

SPECIAL POPULATIONS

RENAL IMPAIRMENT:

Indication	*CrCl 40 mL/min to 59 mL/min*	*CrCl 20 mL/min to 39 mL/min*	*CrCl < 20 mL/min*	*Hemodialysis*
Herpes zoster	500 mg every 12 hours	500 mg every 24 hours	250 mg every 24 hours	250 mg post-hemodialysis
Suppression of genital herpes	250 mg every 12 hours	125 mg every 12 hours	125 mg every 24 hours	125 mg post-hemodialysis
Treatment of recurrent orolabial and genital herpes in HIV	500 mg every 12 hours	500 mg every 24 hours	250 mg every 24 hours	250 mg post-hemodialysis

Note: CrCl = Creatinine Clearance.

HEPATIC DYSFUNCTION: No dosage adjustment is needed.

PEDIATRIC PATIENTS: Famciclovir has not been studied in patients aged younger than 18 years. Use acyclovir.

PREGNANCY: Category B.

BREASTFEEDING: It may be administered with caution to breastfeeding mothers.

THE ART OF ANTIMICROBIAL THERAPY

Clinical Pearls

1. Famciclovir is effective against HSV and VZV. It has no activity against the other herpesviruses.
2. Famciclovir is not recommended for children; acyclovir is recommended in this age group.

FLUCONAZOLE (Diflucan)

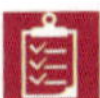 BASIC CHARACTERISTICS

Class: Triazole

Mechanism of Action: Inhibition of lanosterol 14-α-demethylase, which is involved in the synthesis of ergosterol, an essential component of fungal cell membranes.

Mechanisms of Resistance:

1. Point mutations in the gene (*ERG11*) encoding for the target enzyme lead to an altered target with decreased affinity for azoles,
2. overexpression of *ERG11* results in the production of high concentrations of the target enzyme, creating the need for higher intracellular drug concentrations to inhibit all of the enzyme molecules in the cell, and
3. active efflux of fluconazole out of the cell through the activation of two types of multidrug efflux transporters.

Metabolic Route: Fluconazole can be administered orally or intravenously. It can be taken with or without food. It is metabolized by the liver; however, up to 22% can be excreted unchanged in the urine.

FDA FDA-APPROVED INDICATIONS

FDA-Approved Indications: Vaginal candidiasis, oropharyngeal and esophageal candidiasis, *Candida* urinary tract infections, peritonitis, candidemia, disseminated candidiasis, candida pneumonia, cryptococcal meningitis, and prophylaxis of candidiasis in patients undergoing bone marrow transplantation who receive cytotoxic chemotherapy or radiation therapy.

Also used for: *Coccidioides immitis* infections including meningitis.

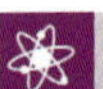 SIDE EFFECTS/TOXICITY

Fluconazole is **contraindicated** in patients who have shown hypersensitivity to fluconazole or to any of its excipients.

Side effects/toxicities include hepatic toxicity, anaphylaxis, exfoliative skin disorder, prolongation of the QT interval and torsades de pointes, nausea, vomiting, abdominal pain, leukopenia, thrombocytopenia, hypercholesterolemia, hypertriglyceridemia, hypokalemia, and taste perversion.

DRUG INTERACTIONS/FOOD INTERACTIONS

Fluconazole can be taken with or without food.

Fluconazole is an inhibitor of the cytochrome P450-CYP3A4; caution should be used when one is using fluconazole with other drugs that are metabolized by P450-CYP3A4, as the serum levels of the coadministered drugs may be elevated. The following list comprises significant drug interactions:

Medication	*Adjustment or Action*
Astemizole	Monitor for astemizole toxicity
Benzodiazepines (short-acting)	Monitor for benzodiazepine toxicity and consider decreasing the benzodiazepine dosage
Cisapride	Contraindicated
Cyclosporine	Monitor for elevated cyclosporine concentration
Oral hypoglycemics	Monitor for hypoglycemia
Phenytoin	Monitor for phenytoin toxicity
Rifabutin	Monitor for rifabutin toxicity
Rifampin	Monitor for decreased fluconazole effect
Tacrolimus	Monitor for toxicity
Terfenadine	The combined use of fluconazole at doses of 400 mg/day or greater with terfenadine is contraindicated. The coadministration of fluconazole at dosages lower than 400 mg/day with terfenadine should be carefully monitored for QTc prolongation and dysrhythmias.
Theophylline	Monitor for theophylline toxicity
Warfarin	Monitor for increased warfarin effect

DOSING

Vaginal candidiasis: 150 mg as a single oral dose.

Note: The following regimens utilize the same dosage, either oral or intravenous:

Oropharyngeal candidiasis: 200 mg on the first day, followed by 100 mg once daily for 2 weeks.

Esophageal candidiasis: 200 mg on the first day, followed by 100 mg once daily; dosages up to 400 mg/day may be used for a minimum of 3 weeks and for at least 2 weeks following resolution of symptoms.

Systemic *Candida* infections: 800 mg on the first day followed by 400 mg daily; duration of therapy has not been determined.

Urinary tract infections and peritonitis: 50 mg to 200 mg may be used daily.

Cryptococcal meningitis: 400 mg on the first day, followed by 200 mg once daily. A dosage of 400 mg once daily may be used based on medical judgment of the patient's response to therapy for 10 to 12 weeks after the cerebrospinal fluid becomes culture-negative. The recommended dosage for suppression of relapse of cryptococcal meningitis in patients with AIDS is 200 mg once daily.

Prophylaxis in patients undergoing bone marrow transplantation: 400 mg, once daily. Patients who are anticipated to have severe granulocytopenia should start fluconazole prophylaxis several days before the anticipated onset of neutropenia, and continue for 7 days after the neutrophil count rises above 1000 cells per mm^3.

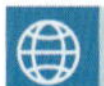

SPECIAL POPULATIONS

RENAL IMPAIRMENT: There is no need to adjust single-dose therapy for vaginal candidiasis because of impaired renal function. For multiple dose regimens:

CrCl Measurement/Hemodialysis	*Dosage*
≥ 50 mL/min	Full dose
< 50 mL/min	Half dose
Hemodialysis	Full dose after each dialysis
Continuous renal replacement therapy	400 mg to 800 mg every 24 hours

Note: CrCl = Creatinine Clearance.

HEPATIC IMPAIRMENT: Caution should be used when used in patients with hepatic impairment. Liver function tests should be monitored.

PEDIATRIC PATIENTS: Efficacy of fluconazole has not been established in infants aged younger than 6 months. For children aged 6 months and older, 3 mg/kg is equivalent for the adult 100-mg dose; 6 mg/kg for 200-mg dose, and 12 mg/kg for 400-mg dose; etc.

PREGNANCY: Category C.

BREASTFEEDING: The use of fluconazole in breastfeeding mothers is not recommended.

THE ART OF ANTIMICROBIAL THERAPY

Clinical Pearls

1. Fluconazole is not active against *Candida krusei.*
2. Resistance in *Candida glabrata* is caused by efflux of the azoles. If fluconazole is used against this species, the highest dosage is recommended.
3. Fluconazole does not have activity against molds, *Blastomyces* species, or *Histoplasma* species.
4. Fluconazole is an inhibitor of cytochrome P450 and can enhance the activity of many commonly used drugs, including oral hypoglycemics and anticoagulants.
5. Fluconazole should be administered with caution to patients with potentially proarrhythmic conditions.

BASIC CHARACTERISTICS

Class: Fluorinated pyrimidine analogue

Mechanism of Action: Flucytosine is taken up by fungal organisms and is rapidly converted to fluorouracil. Fluorouracil is converted into several active metabolites that inhibit protein synthesis by being falsely incorporated into fungal RNA or interfere with the biosynthesis of fungal DNA through the inhibition of the enzyme thymidylate synthetase. Flucytosine exhibits in vitro activity against *Candida* species and *Cryptococcus neoformans.*

Mechanism of Resistance: Flucytosine resistance may arise from a mutation of an enzyme necessary for the cellular uptake or metabolism of flucytosine or from increased synthesis of pyrimidines, which compete with the active metabolites of flucytosine. Resistance to flucytosine has been shown to develop during monotherapy after prolonged exposure to the drug.

Metabolic Route: Flucytosine is excreted via the kidneys.

FDA FDA-APPROVED INDICATIONS

FDA-Approved Indications: Serious infections caused by susceptible strains of *Candida* (septicemia, endocarditis, urinary tract infection, and pneumonia) or *Cryptococcus* (meningitis, pneumonia). Flucytosine should be used in combination with amphotericin B because of the emergence of resistance to flucytosine when it is used alone.

SIDE EFFECTS/TOXICITY

> **WARNING:** Use with extreme caution in patients with impaired renal function, and monitor renal, hematologic, and hepatic status of all patients.

Flucytosine should not be used in patients with a known hypersensitivity to the drug.

Flucytosine must be given with extreme caution to patients with bone marrow depression. Bone marrow toxicity with anemia, leukopenia, or granulocytopenia can be irreversible and may lead to death in immunosuppressed patients.

Other side effects/toxicities include nausea, vomiting, diarrhea, hepatitis, renal failure, cardiac arrest, respiratory arrest, chest pain, rash, photosensitivity, ataxia, peripheral neuropathy, seizure, psychosis, hypoglycemia, and hypokalemia.

DRUG INTERACTIONS/FOOD INTERACTIONS

Cytosine arabinoside can inactivate the antifungal activity of flucytosine by competitive inhibition. Drugs that impair glomerular filtration may prolong the biological half-life of flucytosine.

FLUCYTOSINE (Ancobon)

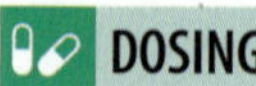

DOSING

Flucytosine is administered in 250-mg and 500-mg capsules.

Usual dosage is 50 mg/kg/day to 150 mg/kg/day administered in divided doses at 6-hour intervals.

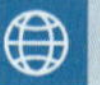

SPECIAL POPULATIONS

RENAL IMPAIRMENT: Use with extreme caution in patients with impaired renal function.

CrCl Measurement/Hemodialysis	*Dosage*
50 mL/min to 80 mL/min	500 mg every 12 hours
10 mL/min to 49 mL/min	500 mg every 18 hours
< 10 mL/min	500 mg/day
Chronic ambulatory peritoneal dialysis	0.5 g to 1.0 g every 24 hours
Hemodialysis	Give additional dose after dialysis

Note: CrCl = Creatinine Clearance

HEPATIC IMPAIRMENT: Monitor liver function tests routinely.

PEDIATRIC PATIENTS: Safety and dosing has not been systematically studied in children.

PREGNANCY: Category C.

BREASTFEEDING: Discontinue breastfeeding or discontinue the drug.

THE ART OF ANTIMICROBIAL THERAPY

Clinical Pearls

1. Flucytosine should be used in combination with amphotericin B compounds to minimize resistance.
2. Flucytosine is active only against *Candida* and *Cryptococcus.*
3. Nausea or vomiting may be reduced or avoided if the capsules are given a few at a time over a 15-minute period.
4. Frequent monitoring of hepatic, renal, and hematopoietic function is indicated during therapy.
5. Serum levels should be between 25 µg/mL and 100 µg/mL.

BASIC CHARACTERISTICS

Class: Protease inhibitor

Mechanism of Action: Amprenavir, the active drug, reversibly binds the active site of the enzyme protease. Inhibition of protease prevents cleavage of the *gag* and *gag-pol* polyprotein resulting in the production of immature, noninfectious virus.

Mechanism of Resistance: Development of mutations on the enzyme protease causes a conformational change that prevents amprenavir from binding the active site, allowing protease activity to continue. The most frequent resistance mutations include I50V, I54 L/M, and I84V.

Metabolic Route: After oral administration, fosamprenavir is hydrolyzed to amprenavir and inorganic phosphate. Amprenavir is metabolized in the liver and excreted in the feces.

FDA-APPROVED INDICATIONS

FDA-Approved Indication: Treatment of HIV-1 in combinations with other antiretroviral agents.

SIDE EFFECTS/TOXICITY

Side effects/toxicities include new-onset diabetes mellitus, exacerbation of preexisting diabetes mellitus, and hyperglycemia; increased bleeding including spontaneous skin hematomas and hemarthrosis in patients with hemophilia type A or B; redistribution or accumulation of body fat including central obesity, dorsocervical fat enlargement (buffalo hump), peripheral wasting, facial wasting, and breast enlargement; cushingoid appearance; immune reconstitution syndrome; mouth ulceration; diarrhea; nausea; vomiting; anorexia; dyspepsia; epigastric pain; hepatitis; pancreatitis; headache; QTc prolongation and torsades de pointes; (hemolytic) anemia; leukopenia; thrombocytopenia; increased amylase; increased CPK; hyperlipemia; hyperuricemia; hypoglycemia; and dehydration.

DRUG INTERACTIONS/FOOD INTERACTIONS

Fosamprenavir tablets may be taken with or without food. The oral suspension must be taken without food. Drugs that **should not be coadministered** with fosamprenavir include amiodarone, flecainide, propafenone, quinidine, rifampin, ergot derivatives, Saint-John's-wort, HMG-CoA reductase inhibitors simvastatin or lovastatin, pimozide, cisapride, benzodiazepines, oral contraceptives, lopinavir/ritonavir, tipranavir, delavirdine, and etravirine.

Fosamprenavir is an inhibitor of the CYP3A enzyme; coadministration of fosamprenavir and drugs primarily metabolized by CYP3A may result in increased plasma concentrations of the other drug that could increase or prolong its therapeutic and adverse effects.

Fosamprenavir is metabolized by CYP3A; coadministration of fosamprenavir and drugs that induce CYP3A may decrease fosamprenavir plasma concentrations and reduce its therapeutic effect. Coadministration of fosamprenavir and drugs that inhibit CYP3A may increase fosamprenavir plasma concentrations. Because of these metabolic effects, potential drug interactions that may require dosage change or clinical/laboratory monitoring are:

Medication	*Adjustment or Action*
Itraconzole	Dosage adjustments for those taking > 400 mg/day
Ketoconazole	Do not exceed 200 mg daily
Voriconazole	Monitor for toxicity
Rifabutin	Decrease rifabutin to 150 mg every other day or three times per week
Atorvastatin or rosuvastatin	Use lowest possible dosage with close monitoring
Phenobarbital, phenytoin, or carbamazepine	Monitor anticonvulsant level; consider alternative
Methadone	Monitor; may require higher methadone dose
Sildenafil	25 mg every 48 hours
Tadalafil	5 mg; no more than 10 mg in 72 hours
Vardenafil	no more than 2.5 mg in 24 hours
H2 blockers	May decrease fosamprenavir activity
Proton pump inhibitors	May be given simultaneously
Maraviroc	Maraviroc dosage of 150 mg twice a day

DOSING

Fosamprenavir is supplied as 700-mg tablets and a white-to-off-white grape-bubblegum-peppermint-flavored suspension that contains 50 mg/ml.

For antiretroviral-naïve patients, fosamprenavir can be administered:

- 1400 mg twice daily (without ritonavir),
- 1400 mg once daily plus ritonavir 200 mg once daily, or
- 1400 mg once daily plus ritonavir 100 mg once daily.

For naive or protease inhibitor–experienced patients, the dose is 700 mg twice daily plus ritonavir 100 mg twice daily.

SPECIAL POPULATIONS

RENAL IMPAIRMENT: There is no dosage adjustment needed.

HEPATIC DYSFUNCTION: For patients in Child-Pugh class A, fosamprenavir should be used with caution. Some recommend administering fosamprenavir at a reduced dosage of 700 mg twice daily without ritonavir (antiretroviral therapy-naïve) or 700 mg twice daily plus ritonavir 100 mg once daily (antiretroviral therapy-naïve or protease inhibitor-experienced).

For patients in Child-Pugh class B fosamprenavir should be used with caution at a reduced dosage of 700 mg twice daily (therapy-naïve) without ritonavir, or 450 mg twice daily plus ritonavir 100 mg once daily (therapy-naïve or protease inhibitor-experienced).

In those in Child-Pugh class C fosamprenavir should be used with caution at a reduced dosage of 350 mg twice daily without ritonavir (therapy-naïve). There are no data on the use of fosamprenavir in combination with ritonavir in patients with severe hepatic impairment.

PEDIATRIC PATIENTS: The recommended dosage of fosamprenavir in patients aged 2 years and older should be calculated based on body weight (kg) and should not exceed the recommended adult dosage. The data are insufficient to recommend once-daily dosing or any dosing of fosamprenavir in therapy-experienced patients aged 2 to 5 years.

- **Therapy-naïve children aged 2 to 5 years:** Oral suspension 30 mg/kg twice daily, not to exceed the adult dosage of 1400 mg twice daily.
- **Therapy-naïve children aged 6 years or older:** Either fosamprenavir oral suspension 30 mg/kg twice daily not to exceed the adult dosage of 1400 mg twice daily, or oral suspension 18 mg/kg plus ritonavir 3 mg/kg twice daily not to exceed the adult dosage of 700 mg plus ritonavir 100 mg twice daily.
- **Therapy-experienced children aged 6 years or older:** Oral suspension 18 mg/kg plus ritonavir 3 mg/kg administered twice daily not to exceed the adult dosage of 700 mg twice daily plus ritonavir 100 mg twice daily.

PREGNANCY: Category B.

BREASTFEEDING: It is recommended that HIV-positive mothers not breastfeed their children to decrease mother-to-child transmission of HIV.

THE ART OF ANTIMICROBIAL THERAPY

Clinical Pearls

1. Fosamprenavir should always be used in combination with other antiretrovirals.
2. Fosamprenavir has a sulfa moiety and should be used with caution in patients with sulfa allergies.

3. Even though fosamprenavir can be taken with or without food, it is likely that taking boosted fosamprenavir with food may decrease gastrointestinal side effects.
4. When one is initiating boosted fosamprenavir in protease inhibitor-experienced patients, it must be given twice daily.
5. When one is assessing for resistance to fosamprenavir, a phenotype assay may be helpful.
6. Whenever initiating fosamprenavir, one should make sure to review all medications the patient is receiving to minimize drug interactions.

BASIC CHARACTERISTICS

Class: Organic pyrophosphate

Mechanism of Action: Foscarnet sodium is an organic analogue of inorganic pyrophosphate that inhibits replication of cytomegalovirus (CMV) and herpes simplex virus (HSV) types 1 and 2. Herpes simplex virus strains that are resistant to acyclovir or CMV strains that are resistant to ganciclovir may be sensitive to foscarnet sodium.

Mechanism of Resistance: Mutation in the viral DNA polymerase gene.

Metabolic Route: Most of an administered dose of foscarnet sodium is excreted unchanged in the urine.

FDA-APPROVED INDICATIONS

FDA-Approved Indications: Treatment of CMV retinitis in patients with AIDS. Foscarnet is also indicated for the treatment of acyclovir-resistant mucocutaneous HSV infections in immunocompromised patients.

Also used for: Treatment of varicella zoster virus infections and CMV infections in transplant recipients.

SIDE EFFECTS/TOXICITY

WARNING: Renal impairment is the major toxicity of foscarnet sodium injection. Frequent monitoring of serum creatinine, with dosage adjustment for changes in renal function, and adequate hydration are imperative. Also seen are seizures related to plasma minerals and electrolyte alterations.

Other side effects/toxicities include rash; genital irritation from urinary drug levels (possibly ameliorated by adequate hydration); bone marrow toxicity; rigors; paresthesia; nausea; vomiting; diarrhea; abdominal pain; depression; dementia; cough; vision abnormalities electrocardiogram abnormalities; and electrolyte disturbances (hypocalcemia, hypophosphatemia, hyperphosphatemia, hypomagnesemia, and hypokalemia) related to chelation of divalent metal ions by foscarnet; the rate of foscarnet sodium infusion may affect the decrease in ionized calcium.

DRUG INTERACTIONS/FOOD INTERACTIONS

Because foscarnet decreases serum concentrations of ionized calcium, concurrent treatment with other drugs known to influence serum calcium concentrations, including pentamidine, should be used with particular caution.

Because of foscarnet's tendency to cause renal impairment, the use of foscarnet sodium should be avoided in combination with potentially nephrotoxic drugs such as aminoglycosides, amphotericin B, and intravenous pentamidine unless the potential benefits outweigh the risks to the patient.

Abnormal renal function has been observed in clinical practice during the use of foscarnet sodium and ritonavir, or foscarnet sodium, ritonavir, and saquinavir.

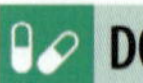

DOSING

(By controlled infusion)

For **CMV retinitis** patients: either 90 mg/kg every 12 hours or 60 mg/kg every 8 hours over 2 to 3 weeks. Following induction treatment the recommended maintenance dosage is 90 mg/kg/day to 120 mg/kg/day.

For **acyclovir-resistant HSV** patients: 40 mg/kg either every 8 or 12 hours for 2 to 3 weeks or until healed.

SPECIAL POPULATIONS

RENAL IMPAIRMENT:

CrCl, mL/min/kg	*Dosage for HSV*	*Induction Dosage for CMV*	*Maintenance Dosage for CMV*
>1.4	40 mg/kg every 12 hours	90 mg/kg every 12 hours	90 mg/kg/day
>1.0 to 1.4	30 mg/kg every 12 hours	70 mg/kg every 12 hours	70 mg/kg/day
>0.8 to 1.0	20 mg/kg every 12 hours	50 mg/kg every 12 hours	50 mg/kg/day
>0.6 to 0.8	35 mg/kg/day	80 mg/kg/day	80 mg/kg every 48 hours
>0.5 to 0.6	25 mg/kg/day	60 mg/kg/day	60 mg/kg every 48 hours
0.4 to 0.5	20 mg/kg/day	50 mg/kg/day	50 mg/kg every 48 hours
< 0.4	Not recommended	Not recommended	Not recommended
Continuous renal replacement therapy	Not recommended	Not recommended	Not recommended

Note: CrCl = Creatinine Clearance.

HEPATIC DYSFUNCTION: Caution should be used when foscarnet is administered to those with hepatic impairment.

PEDIATRIC PATIENTS: Foscarnet is not recommended for use in pediatric patients.

PREGNANCY: Category C.

BREASTFEEDING: It is not known if foscarnet is secreted in breastmilk; caution must be used.

THE ART OF ANTIMICROBIAL THERAPY

Clinical Pearls

1. The combination of foscarnet and ganciclovir has been shown to have enhanced activity for the treatment of CMV encephalitis.
2. Foscarnet is used to treat non-retinitis CMV infections in HIV patients and those who have received transplants even though it is not approved for these indications.
3. Renal impairment is most likely to become clinically evident during the second week of induction therapy.
4. Hydration is recommended with each dose of foscarnet to decrease renal toxicity.
5. The chelation of calcium is related to rate of infusion; slowing down the infusion can decrease this complication.
6. Infusion should be carefully controlled per the manufacturer's instructions.

FURAZOLIDONE (Furoxone)

BASIC CHARACTERISTICS

Class: Nitrofuran

Mechanism of Action: Unknown.

Mechanism of Resistance: Unknown.

Metabolic Route: Furazolidone is metabolized by the liver into multiple products.

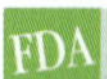

FDA-APPROVED INDICATIONS

Not FDA-approved, but used for treatment of giardiasis. Furazolidone is also active against *Klebsiella* species, *Clostridium* species, *Escherichia coli*, *Campylobacter* species, and *Staphylococcus aureus.*

SIDE EFFECTS/TOXICITY

Side effects/toxicities include nausea, vomiting, diarrhea, brown discoloration of the urine, and hemolysis in G6PDH-deficient patients. Furazolidone inhibits MAO. Furazolidone is contraindicated in infants aged younger than 1 month because of the risk of hemolytic anemia.

DRUG INTERACTIONS/FOOD INTERACTIONS

Proton pump inhibitors reduce the oral bioavailability of furazolidone.

MAO inhibitors should not be given along with furazolidone.

Alcohol should be avoided because of a possible disulfiramlike reaction.

DOSING

Furazolidone is available in both a 100-mg tablet and a suspension 50 mg/tablespoon. It is given as four doses per day in adults (100 mg per dose).

SPECIAL POPULATIONS

RENAL IMPAIRMENT: Unknown.

HEPATIC DYSFUNCTION: Unknown.

PEDIATRIC PATIENTS: Furazolidone is contraindicated in infants aged younger than 1 month. Children aged older than 1 month should receive 1.5 mg/kg four times a day for 7 to 10 days. In the pediatric suspension, two tablespoonfuls substitute for a 100-mg tablet.

PREGNANCY: Use in pregnancy is not recommended.

BREASTFEEDING: Unknown.

THE ART OF ANTIMICROBIAL THERAPY

Clinical Pearls

1. Furazolidone is not available commercially in the United States. It may be obtained from a compounding pharmacy through the National Association of Compounding Pharmacies (800–687–7850) or http://www.pccarx.com.
2. Although furazolidone has activity against bacteria, it is not used for treatment of bacterial infection.
3. Furazolidone should not be given with MAO inhibitors or alcohol.

GANCICLOVIR (Cytovene)

BASIC CHARACTERISTICS

Class: Nucleoside analogue

Mechanism of Action: Ganciclovir is a synthetic guanine nucleoside analogue of 2′-deoxyguanosine that inhibits replication of herpesviruses. Ganciclovir is active against cytomegalovirus (CMV) and herpes simplex virus (HSV). Ganciclovir is phosphorylated and it inhibits viral DNA synthesis by (1) competitive inhibition of viral DNA polymerases, and (2) incorporation into viral DNA, resulting in eventual termination of viral DNA elongation.

Mechanism of Resistance: Resistance to ganciclovir in CMV is caused by decreased ability to form the active triphosphate moiety; resistant viruses have been described that contain mutations in the UL97 gene of CMV that controls phosphorylation of ganciclovir. Mutations in the viral DNA polymerase have also been reported to confer viral resistance to ganciclovir.

Metabolic Route: Ganciclovir is excreted in the urine.

FDA-APPROVED INDICATIONS

FDA-Approved Indications: Ganciclovir IV is indicated for the treatment of CMV retinitis in immunocompromised patients and the prevention of CMV disease in transplant recipients.

Also used for: Ganciclovir IV has routinely been used for the treatment of CMV pneumonia, gastroenteritis, and disseminated disease in transplant recipients.

Ganciclovir capsules are indicated for prevention of CMV disease in transplant recipients and HIV-infected patients. It is also considered an alternative agent for treatment of stable CMV retinitis.

SIDE EFFECTS/TOXICITY

WARNING: Granulocytopenia, anemia, and thrombocytopenia have been observed in patients treated with ganciclovir. Therefore, it should be used with caution in patients with preexisting cytopenias and should not be administered if the absolute neutrophil count is less than 500 cells/μL or the platelet count is less than 25,000 cells/μL. Granulocytopenia usually occurs during the first or second week of treatment but may occur at any time during treatment. Cell counts usually begin to recover within 3 to 7 days of discontinuing drug. Colony-stimulating factors have been shown to increase neutrophil and white blood cell counts in patients receiving ganciclovir. Also, in animal studies, ganciclovir was carcinogenic, teratogenic, and caused aspermatogenesis.

Other side effects/toxicities include fever, hepatic and renal dysfunction, stomatitis, diarrhea, vomiting, intestinal perforation, pancreatitis, pulmonary fibrosis, seizures, neuropathy, tinnitus, torsades de pointes, sweating, and pruritus.

 DRUG INTERACTIONS/FOOD INTERACTIONS

Ganciclovir capsules are poorly absorbed and should be administered with food.

Both zidovudine and ganciclovir have the potential to cause neutropenia and anemia; some patients may not tolerate concomitant therapy with these drugs at full dosage. Generalized seizures have been reported in patients who received ganciclovir and imipenem plus cilastatin. These drugs should not be used concomitantly unless the potential benefits outweigh the risks.

Because of the possibility of additive toxicity, drugs such as dapsone, pentamidine, flucytosine, vincristine, vinblastine, adriamycin, amphotericin B, trimethoprim plus sulfamethoxazole combinations, or other nucleoside analogues, should be considered for concomitant use with ganciclovir only if the potential benefits are judged to outweigh the risks.

Increases in serum creatinine were observed in patients treated with ganciclovir plus either cyclosporine or amphotericin B, drugs with known potential for nephrotoxicity.

 DOSING

Ganciclovir IV

For Treatment of CMV Retinitis in Patients with Normal Renal Function

Induction treatment: The drug is given as a constant rate infusion over 1 hour. The recommended initial dosage for patients with normal renal function is 5 mg/kg intravenously every 12 hours for 14 to 21 days.

Maintenance treatment: Following induction treatment, the recommended maintenance dosage of ganciclovir is 5 mg/kg intravenously given once daily, 7 days per week, or 6 mg/kg once daily, 5 days per week.

For the Prevention of CMV Disease in Transplant Recipients with Normal Renal Function: The recommended initial dosage of ganciclovir for patients with normal renal function is 5 mg/kg intravenously every 12 hours for 7 to 14 days, followed by 5 mg/kg once daily, 7 days per week or 6 mg/kg once daily, 5 days per week. The duration of treatment in transplant recipients is dependent upon the duration and degree of immunosuppression.

Ganciclovir Capsules

Ganciclovir is supplied as 250-mg and 500-mg capsules. The usual dosage is 1000 mg three times a day.

 SPECIAL POPULATIONS

RENAL IMPAIRMENT:

Ganciclovir IV:

CrCl Measurement/ Hemodialysis	*Induction Dosage*	*Maintenance Dosage*
≥70 mL/min	5 mg/kg every 12 hours	5 mg/kg/day
50 mL/min to 69 mL/min	2.5 mg/kg every 12 hours	2.5 mg/kg/day
25 mL/min to 49 mL/min	2.5 mg/kg/day	1.25 mg/kg/day
10 mL/min to 24 mL/min	1.25 mg/kg/day	0.625 mg/kg/day
Hemodialysis	1.25 mg/kg/after hemodialysis	0.625 mg/kg after hemodialysis
Continuous renal replacement therapy	2.5 mg/kg every 12 hours	2.5 mg/kg/day

Note: CrCl = Creatinine Clearance.

Ganciclovir Capsules:

CrCl Measurement/Hemodialysis	*Dosage*
≥ 80 mL/min	1000 mg three times a day
50 mL/min to 79 mL/min	500 mg three times a day
25 mL/min to 49 mL/min	500 mg twice a day
10 mL/min to 24 mL/min	500 mg daily
Hemodialysis	500 mg three times a week administered after dialysis

Note: CrCl = Creatinine Clearance.

HEPATIC DYSFUNCTION: No dosage adjustment is needed.

PEDIATRIC PATIENTS: Ganciclovir has not been studied in pediatric patients.

PREGNANCY: Category C.

BREASTFEEDING: Mothers should be told to stop breastfeeding while receiving ganciclovir.

 THE ART OF ANTIMICROBIAL THERAPY

Clinical Pearls

1. Ganciclovir should not be administered if the absolute neutrophil count is less than 500 cells/μL or the platelet count is less than 25,000 cells/μL.

2. Ganciclovir is effective against HSV, varicella zoster virus, and CMV. It may also have activity against Epstein-Barr virus and human herpesvirus 8, although its FDA-approved indications are for specific CMV infections.
3. Oral ganciclovir is not well absorbed; if one is using an oral therapy, valganciclovir is more reliable.

GEMIFLOXACIN (Factive)

BASIC CHARACTERISTICS

Class: Fluoroquinolone

Mechanism of Action: Inhibits bacterial topoisomerase IV and DNA gyrase.

Mechanisms of Resistance: Mutations in DNA gyrase and/or topoisomerase IV.

Metabolic Route: Approximately two thirds of the gemifloxacin is excreted in the feces with the remainder excreted in the urine.

FDA-APPROVED INDICATIONS

FDA-Approved Indications: Treatment of the following serious infections caused by susceptible strains of microorganisms: acute bacterial exacerbation of chronic bronchitis and community-acquired pneumonia of mild-to-moderate severity.

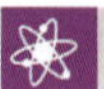

SIDE EFFECTS/TOXICITY

> **WARNING:** Fluoroquinolones, including gemifloxacin, are associated with an increased risk of **tendinitis and tendon rupture** in all ages. This risk is further increased in older patients usually aged older than 60 years, in patients taking corticosteroid drugs, and in patients with kidney, heart, and lung transplants.

Gemifloxacin is **contraindicated** in persons with a history of hypersensitivity associated with the use of gemifloxacin or any quinolone.

Other side effects/toxicities include anaphylactic reactions with cardiovascular collapse; angioedema; allergic skin reactions including toxic epidermal necrolysis and Stevens-Johnson syndrome; photosensitivity; renal toxicity; hepatotoxicity (sometimes fatal); central nervous system effects including headache, dizziness, seizures, anxiety, confusion, depression, and insomnia (use with caution in patients at risk of seizures); peripheral neuropathy; nausea; diarrhea; constipation; *Clostridium difficile*–associated colitis; prolongation of the QT interval and torsade de pointes (avoid use in patients with known prolongation of QT, hypokalemia, and with other drugs that prolong the QT interval); and pancytopenia.

DRUG INTERACTIONS/FOOD INTERACTIONS

Gemifloxacin can be taken with or without food.

Antacids containing calcium, magnesium, or aluminum; sucralfate; divalent or trivalent cations such as iron; or multivitamins containing zinc should not be taken within the 3-hour period before or within the 2-hour period after taking gemifloxacin.

The concomitant administration of a nonsteroidal antiinflammatory drug with a quinolone may increase the risk of seizures.

The concomitant use of probenecid with quinolones decreases renal tubular secretion.

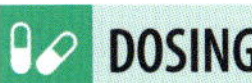

DOSING

Gemifloxacin is administered as a 320-mg tablet once daily.

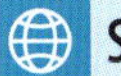

SPECIAL POPULATIONS

RENAL IMPAIRMENT: If creatinine clearance is less than 40 mL/min, the dosage should be 160 mg daily.

HEPATIC DYSFUNCTION: No dosage adjustment is necessary.

PEDIATRIC PATIENTS: Safety and efficacy in pediatric patients aged younger than 18 years have not yet been established.

PREGNANCY: Category C.

BREASTFEEDING: Gemifloxacin should not be administered to breastfeeding mothers.

THE ART OF ANTIMICROBIAL THERAPY

Clinical Pearls

1. Gemifloxacin should be given should be given at least 3 hours after or 2 hours before cations.
2. All fluoroquinolones can lead to tendon rupture, especially in patients aged older than 60 years.
3. All fluoroquinolones can prolong QT intervals, and caution should be used when given with medications that affect QT intervals.
4. All fluoroquinolones can cause phototoxicity.
5. All fluoroquinolones can lower seizure threshold.
6. Fluoroquinolones should be avoided if possible in children, pregnant women, and breastfeeding mothers, because of possible disturbance in cartilage development.
7. Fluoroquinolones have activity against mycobacteria; therefore, gemifloxacin monotherapy (e.g., for pneumonia) should be avoided if mycobacterial infection is possible.
8. Gemifloxacin is not recommended for treatment of urinary tract infections.

GENTAMICIN (Garamycin)

BASIC CHARACTERISTICS

Class: Aminoglycoside

Mechanisms of Action:

1. Rearranges lipopolysaccharide in the outer membrane of the bacterial cell wall, resulting in disruption of the cell wall, and
2. binds the 30S subunit of the bacterial ribosome, which terminates protein synthesis.

Mechanisms of Resistance:

1. Gram-negative bacteria inactivate aminoglycosides by acetylation,
2. some bacteria alter the 30S ribosomal subunit, which prevents gentamicin's interference with protein synthesis, and
3. low-level resistance may result from inhibition of gentamicin uptake by the bacteria.

Metabolic Route: Gentamicin is excreted unchanged in the urine.

FDA FDA-APPROVED INDICATIONS

FDA-Approved Indications: Treatment of susceptible gram-negative bacteria causing bacteremia, pneumonia, osteomyelitis, arthritis, meningitis, skin and soft tissue infection, intraabdominal infections, in burns, postoperative infections, and urinary tract infections.

Also used for: Combination therapy with β-lactams for the treatment of gram-positive endovascular infections.

SIDE EFFECTS/TOXICITY

WARNINGS: Ototoxicity: vestibular toxicity and auditory ototoxicity, especially in patients with renal damage, those treated with higher doses, and those with prolonged treatment. Avoid use with potent diuretics such as ethacrynic acid because of additive ototoxicity.

Nephrotoxicity: especially in patients with impaired renal function and those treated with higher doses or prolonged treatment. Avoid concurrent use with other nephrotoxic agents and potent diuretics, which can cause dehydration.

Neuromuscular blockade: especially in those receiving anesthetics, neuromuscular blocking agents or massive transfusions.

Other side effects/toxicities include fever, rash, anaphylactoid reactions, encephalopathy, pseudotumor cerebri, peripheral neuropathy, nausea, vomiting, abnormal liver function tests, myasthenia gravis–like syndrome, leukopenia, thrombocytopenia, and decreased serum calcium, magnesium, sodium, and potassium.

DRUG INTERACTIONS

Gentamicin should not be administered with other medications that are nephrotoxic or ototoxic.

DOSING

After a loading dose of 2 mg/kg, give 3 mg/kg/day to 5 mg/kg/day IM or IV in divided doses every 8 hours; desired serum levels are peak 6 µg/mL to 12 µg/mL and trough less than 2 µg/mL. Can also be given once daily as 5 mg/kg/day to 7 mg/kg/day; desired serum levels are peak 16 µg/mL to 24 µg/mL, trough less than 1 µg/mL. Infuse over 60 minutes to avoid neuromuscular blockade.

Intrathecal dosage: 4 mg/day to 8 mg/day.

Synergistic dosage: 1 mg/kg every 8 hours.

SPECIAL POPULATIONS

RENAL IMPAIRMENT: Adjust dosage either by increased interval (serum creatinine multiplied by 8, or usual dose every 12-24 hours for CrCl 10-50 and every 48 hours for CrCl less than or equal to 10.), or by lowering the dose by dividing the dose by the serum creatinine. With either approach, give an initial dose as for normal renal function, and then subsequent adjustments should be made by following serum assays. (See Dosing, above, for desired levels.)

- **Hemodialysis**: One-half of normal renal function dose after hemodialysis, and then follow assays.
- **Peritoneal dialysis**: 3-4 mg/L are removed in dialysate daily and should be replaced.
- **Continuous renal replacement therapy**: 3 mg/kg loading dose followed by 2 mg/kg every 24 to 48 hours or 1 mg/kg every 24 to 36 hours for gram-positive synergy.

HEPATIC DYSFUNCTION: No dosage adjustment necessary.

PEDIATRIC PATIENTS: 3 mg/kg/day to 7.5 mg/kg/day; divide IV every 8 hours (newborn aged 0 to 7 days: 2.5 mg/kg every 12 hours; aged 1 to 4 weeks: 7.5 mg/kg/day divided every 8 hours)

PREGNANCY: Category D.

BREASTFEEDING: It is not known if gentamicin is secreted in human milk.

THE ART OF ANTIMICROBIAL THERAPY

Clinical Pearls

1. Gentamicin is more likely to be active against gram-positive cocci compared with the other aminoglycosides when used synergistically with cell-wall active antibiotics.
2. Aminoglycosides require oxygen to be active and thus are less effective in anaerobic environments such as an abscess or infected bone.
3. Aminoglycosides have decreased activity in low-pH environments such as respiratory secretions or abscesses.
4. When dosing aminoglycosides, one should use the ideal body weight, not true body weight.
5. Gentamicin has a postantibiotic effect that allows it to be used once daily.

GRISEOFULVIN (Grifulvin V [microcrystalline]; Gris-Peg [ultramicrocrystalline])

 BASIC CHARACTERISTICS

Class: Antifungal

Mechanism of Action: Griseofulvin is deposited in the keratin precursor cells and has a greater affinity for diseased tissue. The drug is tightly bound to the new keratin, which becomes highly resistant to fungal invasion.

Mechanism of Resistance: Data incomplete.

Metabolic Route: Griseofulvin is metabolized in the liver and excreted in the feces and urine.

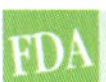 FDA-APPROVED INDICATIONS

FDA-Approved Indications: Tinea capitis, tinea corporis, tinea pedis, tinea unguium, tinea cruris, and tinea barbae, when caused by one or more of the following genera of fungi: *Trichophyton rubrum, Trichophyton tonsurans, Trichophyton mentagrophytes, Trichophyton interdigitalis, Trichophyton verrucosum, Trichophyton megnini, Trichophyton gallinae, Trichophyton crateriform, Trichophyton sulphureum, Trichophyton schoenleinii, Microsporum audouini, Microsporum canis, Microsporum gypseum,* and *Epidermophyton floccosum.*

 SIDE EFFECTS/TOXICITY

Contraindicated in pregnancy, porphyria, hepatocellular failure, and in patients with a history of hypersensitivity to griseofulvin. Cross-sensitivity with penicillin exists.

Side effects/toxicities include photosensitivity, paresthesias, oral thrush, nausea, vomiting, epigastric distress, diarrhea, headache, fatigue, dizziness, insomnia, confusion and impairment of performance of routine activities, lupuslike syndrome, proteinuria, and leukopenia. Administration of the drug should be discontinued if granulocytopenia occurs. Periodic monitoring of renal, hepatic, and hematopoietic function is recommended.

 DRUG INTERACTIONS/FOOD INTERACTIONS

Patients on warfarin therapy may require dosage adjustment of the anticoagulant during and after griseofulvin therapy.

Concomitant use of barbiturates usually depresses griseofulvin activity and may necessitate raising the dosage.

Griseofulvin has been reported to reduce the efficacy of oral contraceptives and to increase the incidence of breakthrough bleeding.

The effects of ethanol ingestion may be potentiated.

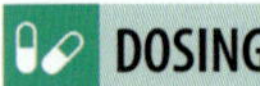

DOSING

Disease	*Oral Dosage Ultramicrosize Crystals*	*Oral Dosage Microsize Crystals*	*Duration*
Tinea capitis	375 mg	500 mg	4 to 6 weeks
Tinea corporis	375 mg	500 mg	2 to 4 weeks
Tinea pedis	750 mg divided	1 g	4 to 8 weeks
Tinea unguium of fingernails	750 mg divided	1 g	> 4 months
Tinea unguium of toenails	750 mg divided	1 g	> 6 months

SPECIAL POPULATIONS

RENAL IMPAIRMENT: Monitoring of renal function is recommended.

HEPATIC IMPAIRMENT: Griseofulvin should not be administered to those with severe hepatic impairment; hepatic function should be monitored.

PEDIATRIC PATIENTS:

Ultramicrosize Crystals:

- Children weighing 30 to 60 pounds: 125 mg to 187.5 mg daily
- Children weighing more than 60 pounds: 187.5 mg to 375 mg daily

Microsize Crystals:

- Children weighing 30 to 50 pounds: 125 mg to 250 mg daily
- Children weighing more than 50 pounds: 250 mg to 500 mg daily

PREGNANCY: Griseofulvin should not be prescribed to pregnant women.

BREASTFEEDING: Breastfeeding mothers should not be prescribed griseofulvin.

THE ART OF ANTIMICROBIAL THERAPY

Clinical Pearls

1. Griseofulvin should be used only for tinea infections.
2. Griseofulvin is better absorbed with a high-fat diet.
3. Periodic monitoring of renal, hepatic, and hematopoietic function is recommended.

BASIC CHARACTERISTICS

Class: Arylaminoalcohol

Mechanism of Action: Unknown.

Metabolic Route: Metabolized by the liver cytochrome P450.

FDA-APPROVED INDICATIONS

Not FDA-approved, but used for treatment of *Plasmodium falciparum* malaria. However, it has no activity against the hypnozoites and may not cure those with *Plasmodium vivax* malaria.

SIDE EFFECTS/TOXICITY

Side effects/toxicities include QTc prolongation leading to torsade de pointes or sudden death.

DRUG INTERACTIONS/FOOD INTERACTIONS

Halofantrine should be administered with food.

Halofantrine should not be used with mefloquine.

DOSING

Halofantrine is available in 250-mg tablets and a suspension, 20 mg/mL.

The recommended dosage is 8 mg/kg every 6 hours for three doses. For those who weigh less than 40 kg, the dosage is 500 mg every 6 hours for three doses. For nonimmune patients a second dose is recommended after 7 days.

SPECIAL POPULATIONS

RENAL IMPAIRMENT: No dosage adjustment necessary.

HEPATIC DYSFUNCTION: Unknown.

PEDIATRIC PATIENTS: 8 mg/kg in flavored suspension (20 mg/mL) every 6 hours for three doses.

PREGNANCY: Halofantrine should not be given in pregnancy.

BREASTFEEDING: Unknown.

THE ART OF ANTIMICROBIAL THERAPY

Clinical Pearls

1. Halofantrine is not recommended for first-line therapy of malaria because of QTc prolongation.
2. Halofantrine is not available in the United States or the United Kingdom.

IMIPENEM PLUS CILASTATIN SODIUM (Primaxin)

BASIC CHARACTERISTICS

Class: Carbapenem.

Mechanism of Action: Binds penicillin-binding protein (PBP), disrupting cell wall synthesis.

Mechanisms of Resistance:

1. The PBP can be altered, with reduced affinity,
2. production of a β-lactamase resulting in hydrolysis of the β-lactam ring,
3. decreased ability of the antibiotic to reach the PBP when bacteria decrease porin production, resulting in a decrease of the drug concentration within the cell, and
4. increased expression of efflux pump components.

Metabolic Route: Imipenem is metabolized in the kidneys by dehydropeptidase I resulting in relatively low levels. Cilastatin sodium, an inhibitor of this enzyme, prevents renal metabolism; approximately 70% of both imipenem and cilastatin are recovered in the urine.

FDA-APPROVED INDICATIONS

FDA-Approved Indications: Treatment of serious infections caused by susceptible strains of microorganisms in: lower respiratory tract infections, urinary tract infections (complicated and uncomplicated), intraabdominal infections, gynecological infections, bacterial septicemia, bone and joint infections, skin and skin structure infections, endocarditis, and polymicrobic infections.

SIDE EFFECTS/TOXICITY

Imipenem is **contraindicated** in patients with known hypersensitivity to any component of this product or to other drugs in the same class or in patients who have demonstrated anaphylactic reactions to β-lactams. Before initiation of therapy with imipenem, careful inquiry should be made concerning previous hypersensitivity reactions to penicillins, cephalosporins, other β-lactams, and other allergens, because of the slightly increased possibility of hypersensitivity.

Side effects/toxicities include seizures; phlebitis; fever; anaphylaxis; rash including Stevens-Johnson syndrome, erythema multiforme, and toxic epidermal necrolysis; angioedema; hypotension; encephalopathy; hearing loss; diarrhea; *Clostridium difficile*–associated diarrhea and pseudomembranous colitis; oral candidiasis; glossitis; anorexia; nausea; vomiting; stomach cramps; hepatitis; renal impairment; genital pruritis; dyspnea; polyarthralgia; pyuria; hematuria; prolonged prothrombin time; pancytopenia; positive Coombs' test; decreased serum sodium; and increased potassium and chloride.

DRUG INTERACTIONS/FOOD INTERACTIONS

Ganciclovir should not be used with imipenem unless the potential benefits outweigh the risks.

Imipenem may reduce serum valproic acid concentrations; levels should be monitored.

It is not recommended that probenecid be given with imipenem.

DOSING

INTRAVENOUS DOSAGE SCHEDULE:

For Adults with Normal Renal Function and Body Weight ≥ 70 kg

Type of Infection	*Susceptible*	*Moderately Susceptible*
Mild	250 mg every 6 hours	500 mg every 6 hours
Moderate	500 mg every 6 or 8 hours	500 mg every 6 hours or 1 g every 8 hours
Severe	500 mg every 6 hours	1 g every 6 or 8 hours
Uncomplicated urinary tract infection	250 mg every 6 hours	250 mg every 6 hours
Complicated urinary tract infection	500 mg every 6 hours	500 mg every 6 hours

SPECIAL POPULATIONS

RENAL IMPAIRMENT:

CrCl Measurement or Hemodialysis	*Dosage*
50 mL/min to 80 mL/min	500 mg every 6 hours
10 mL/min to 49 mL/min	500 mg every 8 hours
5 mL/min to < 10 mL/min	250 mg every 12 hours
< 5 mL/min	Avoid
After hemodialysis or peritoneal dialysis	250 mg
Continuous renal replacement therapy	500 mg every 8 hours

HEPATIC DYSFUNCTION: No dosage adjustment is necessary.

PEDIATRIC PATIENTS:

Age	*Dosage*
< 1 week	25 mg/kg every 12 hours
1 to <4 weeks	25 mg/kg every 8 hours

Age	*Dosage*
4 weeks to <3 months	25 mg/kg every 6 hours
3 months to < 3 years	25 mg/kg every 6 hours
3 to 12 years	15 mg/kg every 6 hours

Imipenem is not recommended in pediatric patients who weigh less than 30 kg with impaired renal function.

PREGNANCY: Category C.

BREASTFEEDING: Imipenem should be used with caution in breastfeeding mothers.

THE ART OF ANTIMICROBIAL THERAPY

Clinical Pearls

1. Dosage of imipenem must be adjusted for patients with renal dysfunction.
2. Cross-allergy with penicillins is less than 10%.
3. Imipenem is not indicated in patients with meningitis because safety and efficacy have not been established, and seizure potential is increased in the presence of central nervous system inflammation.
4. Imipenem is active against many organisms that carry extended-spectrum β-lactamases.

 BASIC CHARACTERISTICS

Class: Protease inhibitor

Mechanism of Action: Reversibly binds the active site of the enzyme protease. Inhibition of protease prevents cleavage of the *gag* and *gag-pol* polyprotein resulting in the production of immature, noninfectious virus.

Mechanism of Resistance: Development of mutations on the enzyme protease causes a conformational change that prevents indinavir from binding the active site, allowing protease activity to continue. The most frequent resistance mutations include 46I, 82A, 84V, and L90M. However, other mutations may confer resistance to indinavir.

Metabolic Route: Indinavir is metabolized in the liver; however, 20% may be excreted in the urine unchanged.

 FDA-APPROVED INDICATIONS

FDA-Approved Indication: Treatment of HIV-1 in combinations with other antiretroviral agents.

 SIDE EFFECTS/TOXICITY

Side effects/toxicities include diarrhea; indirect hyperbilirubinemia; nephrolithiasis/urolithiasis; renal insufficiency; pyelonephritis; tubulointerstitial nephritis with medullary calcification and cortical atrophy; new-onset diabetes mellitus; exacerbation of preexisting diabetes mellitus; hyperglycemia; increased bleeding including spontaneous skin hematomas and hemarthrosis in patients with hemophilia type A or B; redistribution/accumulation of body fat including central obesity, dorsocervical fat enlargement (buffalo hump), peripheral wasting, facial wasting, and breast enlargement; cushingoid appearance; immune reconstitution syndrome; headache; QTc prolongation; torsade de pointes; mouth ulceration; anorexia; dyspepsia; epigastric pain; hepatitis; pancreatitis; vomiting; anemia; leukopenia; thrombocytopenia; increases in alkaline phosphatase, amylase, creatine phosphokinase, and lactic dehydrogenase; hyperlipemia; hyperuricemia; hypoglycemia; and dehydration.

 DRUG INTERACTIONS/FOOD INTERACTIONS

When indinavir is administered without ritonavir, it should be taken on an empty stomach. However, when administered with ritonavir, indinavir should be taken with food to decrease toxicity.

Drugs that **should not be coadministered** with indinavir include amiodarone, quinidine, ergot derivatives, Saint-John's-wort, HMG-CoA reductase inhibitors, (simvastatin, lovastatin, rosuvastatin), pimozide, cisapride, benzodiazepines, rifampin, atazanavir, etravirine, or tipranavir.

INDINAVIR (Crixivan)

Indinavir is an inhibitor of the CYP3A enzyme; coadministration of indinavir and drugs primarily metabolized by CYP3A may result in increased plasma concentrations of the other drug that could increase or prolong its therapeutic and adverse effects.

Indinavir is metabolized by CYP3A and CYP2C19; coadministration of indinavir and drugs that induce CYP3A or CYP2C19 may decrease indinavir plasma concentrations and reduce its therapeutic effect. Coadministration of indinavir and drugs that inhibit CYP3A or CYP2C19 may increase indinavir plasma concentrations. Because of these metabolic affects, potential drug interactions that may require dosage change or clinical/laboratory monitoring are listed below:

Medication	*Adjustment or Action*
Itraconzole	Indinavir 600 mg every 8 hours; itraconazole 200 mg twice a day
Ketoconazole	Indinavir 600 mg every 8 hours
Rifabutin	Rifabutin 150 mg/day or 300 mg three times a week and indinavir 1000 mg every 8 hours; if using ritonavir, 150 mg every other day or three times a week
Atorvastatin	Use lowest possible dose with close monitoring
Phenobarbital, phenytoin, or carbamazepine	Monitor anticonvulsant level; consider alternative; dose indinavir with ritonavir
Sildenafil	25 mg every 48 hours
Tadalafil	5 mg; no more than 10 mg in 72 hours
Vardenafil	Consider sildenafil if indinavir is not boosted with ritonavir; if boosted, no more than 2.5 mg in 24 hours
Grapefruit juice, vitamin C, amlodipine	Use indinavir with ritonavir
Delavirdine	Indinavir 600 mg every 8 hours
Efavirenz or nevirapine	Indinavir 1000 mg every 8 hours or dose with ritonavir
Maraviroc	Maraviroc dosage 150 mg twice a day

DOSING

Indinavir comes in 100-mg, 200-mg, and 400-mg tablets. The recommended dosage of indinavir is 800 mg (usually **two** 400-mg capsules) orally every 8 hours. Indinavir must be taken at intervals of 8 hours. To ensure adequate hydration, it is recommended that adults drink at least 1.5 liters (approximately 48 ounces) of liquids during the course of 24 hours.

In addition, indinavir can be administered with ritonavir. The recommended dosage is 800 mg every 12 hours with ritonavir 100 mg twice daily. The ritonavir must be taken at the same time as the indinavir.

SPECIAL POPULATIONS

RENAL IMPAIRMENT: There is no dosage adjustment needed.

HEPATIC DYSFUNCTION: The dosage of indinavir should be reduced to 600 mg every 8 hours in patients with mild-to-moderate hepatic insufficiency caused by cirrhosis.

PEDIATRIC PATIENTS: The optimal dosing regimen for use of indinavir in pediatric patients has not been established.

PREGNANCY: Category C.

BREASTFEEDING: It is recommended that HIV-positive mothers not breastfeed their children to decrease mother-to-child transmission of HIV.

THE ART OF ANTIMICROBIAL THERAPY

Clinical Pearls

1. Indinavir should always be used in combination with other antiretrovirals.
2. Indinavir should be taken on an empty stomach to increase absorption.
3. Indinavir can be coadministered with ritonavir to increase the dosing interval and allow administration with food.
4. If boosting indinavir with ritonavir, both medications should be taken at the same time.
5. When one is evaluating resistance to ritonavir-boosted protease inhibitors, phenotypic resistance testing is extremely helpful.
6. Because indinavir can cause nephrolithiasis, adequate hydration is necessary.
7. Indinavir can cause hyperbilirubinemia.
8. Whenever initiating indinavir, one should make sure to review all medications the patient is receiving to minimize drug interactions.

INTERFERON ALFA (Infergen [interferon alfacon-1] injection and Roferon-A [interferon alfa-2a] injection)

BASIC CHARACTERISTICS

Class: Alpha interferon

Mechanism of Action: After interferon binds to the cell-surface receptor, production of several interferon-stimulated gene products leads to antiviral, antiproliferative, and immunomodulatory effects; regulation of cell surface major histocompatibility antigen (HLA class I and class II) expression; and regulation of cytokine expression.

Mechanism of Resistance: Unknown.

Metabolic Route: Interferon is metabolized into amino acids.

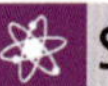

FDA-APPROVED INDICATIONS

FDA-Approved Indications: Both Infergen and Roferon-A are indicated for treatment of chronic hepatitis C in patients aged 18 years and older. Roferon-A is also indicated for hairy cell leukemia and chronic myelogenous leukemia.

Also Used for: Hepatitis B.

SIDE EFFECTS/TOXICITY

Interferon is **contraindicated** in patients with known hypersensitivity to alfa interferons or to any component of the product, decompensated hepatic disease, or autoimmune hepatitis.

Other side effects/toxicities include fever, hypersensitivity, depression, suicide, psychosis, aggressive behavior, nervousness, anxiety, emotional lability, abnormal thinking, agitation, apathy, relapse of drug addiction, bone marrow suppression, hypertension, tachycardia, palpitation, tachyarrhythmias, supraventricular arrhythmias, chest pain, myocardial infarction, hyperthyroidism, hypothyroidism, hyperglycemia, diabetes mellitus, elevated serum triglycerides, autoimmune thrombocytopenia, idiopathic thrombocytopenic purpura, psoriasis, systemic lupus erythematosus, thyroiditis, rheumatoid arthritis, pneumonia, interstitial pneumonitis, hemorrhagic/ischemic gastrointestinal disorders, ulcerative colitis, pancreatitis, hepatic decompensation, decrease or loss of vision, macular edema, retinal artery or vein thrombosis, retinal hemorrhages, cotton wool spots, optic neuritis, papilledema, and ischemic and hemorrhagic cerebrovascular events.

DRUG INTERACTIONS/FOOD INTERACTIONS

None.

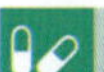

DOSING

Infergen (interferon alfacon-1): 9 μg three times weekly administered subcutaneously as a single injection for 24 weeks. At least 48 hours should elapse between doses.

Patients who do not respond or who relapse following its discontinuation may be subsequently treated with 15 μg three times a week administered subcutaneously as a single injection for up to 48 weeks.

Dose reduction to 7.5 μg may be necessary following an intolerable adverse event.

Roferon-A: Three million units (3 MIU) three times a week administered subcutaneously for 12 months (48 to 52 weeks). Temporary dose reduction by 50% is recommended in patients who do not tolerate the prescribed dose.

SPECIAL POPULATIONS

RENAL IMPAIRMENT: Interferon should be used with caution in patients with renal insufficiency.

HEPATIC DYSFUNCTION: Interferon should not be administered to those with decompensated liver disease. Liver function tests should be monitored closely.

PEDIATRIC PATIENTS: Interferon is not recommended for those aged younger than 18 years.

PREGNANCY: Category C.

BREASTFEEDING: Caution should be exercised when interferon is administered to a breastfeeding woman.

THE ART OF ANTIMICROBIAL THERAPY

Clinical Pearls

1. Interferon alfa is not indicated for multiple sclerosis (MS); interferon **beta** is used for MS.
2. Before initiation of interferon alfa, evaluate for psychiatric issues including depression.
3. Hepatitis C genotypes 2 and 3 respond better to therapy compared with types 1 and 4.
4. It is current standard of care to administer pegylated interferon in combination with ribavirin for hepatitis C.
5. If a 2-log drop of hepatitis C RNA is not noticed by 12 weeks, treatment can be stopped because the patient is most likely going to be a nonresponder.
6. Complete blood counts should be monitored during therapy. Alfa interferon therapy should be discontinued in patients who develop severe decreases in neutrophil counts ($< 0.5 \times 10^9$/L) or platelet counts ($< 50 \times 10^9$/L).
7. Hepatic function should be closely monitored, and interferon treatment should be immediately discontinued for signs of hepatic decompensation, such as jaundice, ascites, coagulopathy, or decreased serum albumin.

IODOQUINOL (Yodoxin)

BASIC CHARACTERISTICS

Class: Halogenated hydroxyquinoline

Mechanism of Action: Unknown.

Metabolic Route: Iodoquinol is poorly absorbed from the gastrointestinal tract and most of it is excreted in the feces.

FDA-APPROVED INDICATIONS

Not FDA-approved, but used for treatment of intestinal amebiasis (for those with asymptomatic disease, it is given as monotherapy; if the patient has invasive disease, it should be used with metronidazole or nitroimidazole), balantidiasis, *Blastocystis hominis,* and *Dientamoeba fragilis.*

SIDE EFFECTS/TOXICITY

Iodoquinol is contraindicated in patients with known hypersensitivity to iodine and halogenated hydroxyquinolines.

Side effects/toxicities include rash, hypersensitivity, nausea, vomiting, diarrhea, rare optic atrophy, neuritis, and blindness.

DRUG INTERACTIONS/FOOD INTERACTIONS

None reported.

Iodoquinol may interfere with thyroid function tests because of its high iodine content.

DOSING

650 mg three times a day for 20 days for intraluminal amebic infection.

SPECIAL POPULATIONS

RENAL IMPAIRMENT: Contraindicated.

HEPATIC DYSFUNCTION (not attributable to amebiasis): Contraindicated.

PEDIATRIC PATIENTS: 10 mg/kg every 8 hours for 20 days with a maximum of 2 g per day. However, the World Health Organization does not recommend the use of iodoquinol because of the neurological complications it may cause.

PREGNANCY: Iodoquinol can be used in pregnancy.

BREASTFEEDING: Unknown.

THE ART OF ANTIMICROBIAL THERAPY

Clinical Pearls

1. Iodoquinol should be avoided in children if possible.
2. For extraluminal or severe cases of amebiasis, iodoquinol should be used with another agent such as metronidazole.
3. Iodoquinone is not available commercially in the United States. It may be obtained from a compounding pharmacy through the National Association of Compounding Pharmacies (800-687-7850 or http://www.pccarx.com).

Note: Isoniazid is also available in combination with rifampin as Rifamate and in combination with rifampin plus pyrazinamide as Rifater.

BASIC CHARACTERISTICS

Class: Isonicotinic acid hydrazide

Mechanisms of Action: Inhibits the synthesis of mycolic acid, a constituent of the cell wall of the mycobacterium, and inhibits catalase-peroxidase.

Mechanisms of Resistance: Point mutations in the catalase-peroxidase gene, and mutations of the regulatory genes involved in mycolic acid synthesis.

Metabolic Route: Isoniazid is metabolized by acetylation and dehydrazination. The rate of acetylation is genetically determined.

FDA-APPROVED INDICATIONS

FDA-Approved Indications: Treatment of active tuberculosis in combination with other antimycobacterials, and latent tuberculosis.

SIDE EFFECTS/TOXICITY

WARNING: Severe and sometimes fatal **hepatitis** has been associated with isoniazid. The risk of hepatitis is greatest in older and peripartum patients and Asian males, and risk is increased with acetaminophen, alcohol, elevated baseline transaminases, chronic hepatitis B and hepatitis C virus infection, and possibly HIV.

Other side effects/toxicities include peripheral neuropathy, hypersensitivity, fever, skin eruptions, vasculitis, a systemic lupus erythematosus–like syndrome, nausea, vomiting, epigastric distress, seizures, encephalopathy, psychosis, metabolic acidosis, gynecomastia, optic neuritis, arthralgias, agranulocytosis, hemolytic or sideroblastic anemia, and thrombocytopenia.

DRUG INTERACTIONS/FOOD INTERACTIONS

When isoniazid is taken with food, the absorption of isoniazid is reduced but still adequate for most patients and is much better tolerated. Foods rich in histamine (e.g., cheese, wine, tuna) or tyramine (e.g., cured meats, soybeans, aged cheese) may produce flushing and headache. Antacids may impair absorption and should be separated from isoniazid (INH) ingestion by 2 hours.

Isoniazid inhibits the metabolism of many drugs, potentially increasing their serum levels; patients on anticoagulants, anticonvulsants, benzodiazepines, haloperidol, theophylline, and cycloserine should be monitored for toxic effects; levels of carbamazepine, phenytoin, and valproate should be measured.

Acetaminophen and alcohol should be avoided, as they may increase hepatotoxicity, as should disulfiram, enflurane, stavudine, and vincristine.

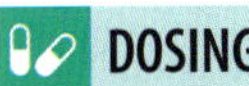

DOSING

Note: Dose should never be divided, but should be given a single dose.

Isoniazid is available as an elixir and for oral, intravenous, and intramuscular administration; the dosage is 5 mg/kg/day up to 300 mg daily. It may also be given twice- or thrice-weekly, 15 mg/kg up to 900 mg per dose.

SPECIAL POPULATIONS

RENAL IMPAIRMENT: No dosage adjustment is necessary.

HEPATIC DYSFUNCTION: No dosage adjustment, but use with caution.

PEDIATRIC PATIENTS: 10 mg/kg/day to 15 mg/kg/day with a maximum of 300 mg daily. Twice- or thrice-weekly dosage is 20 mg/kg/dose to 30 mg/kg/dose, with a maximum of 900 mg per dose.

PREGNANCY: Category C. However, INH is used routinely to treat tuberculosis in pregnancy, as the benefit is felt to justify potential risk.

BREASTFEEDING: May be given; both mother and baby should receive supplemental pyridoxine.

THE ART OF ANTIMICROBIAL THERAPY

Clinical Pearls

1. Isoniazid should not be used alone in the treatment of active tuberculosis.
2. Liver function tests, symptoms of gastrointolerance, and complete blood count should be monitored at least monthly in all patients receiving isoniazid.
3. Pyroxidine (25 mg/day) should be given to prevent B6 deficiency in those at risk for peripheral neuropathy, (i.e., those with nutritional deficiency, diabetes, HIV infection, renal failure, alcoholism, pregnancy, and in breastfeeding mothers).
4. When used to treat latent tuberculosis in pregnant patients, INH therapy should be deferred 2 to 3 months after delivery because of increased hepatotoxicity. Exceptions, whose treatment should not be deferred, are women with recently acquired infection and those who are HIV-positive.
5. INH dosage should never be split but should be given as a single dose.

ITRACONAZOLE (Sporanox capsules, oral solution, and IV infusion)

BASIC CHARACTERISTICS

Class: Triazole

Mechanism of Action: Inhibits lanosterol 14-α-demethylase, which is involved in the synthesis of ergosterol, an essential component of fungal cell membranes.

Mechanisms of Resistance:

1. Point mutations in the gene (*ERG11*) encoding for the target enzyme lead to an altered target with decreased affinity for azoles,
2. overexpression of *ERG11* results in the production of high concentrations of the target enzyme, creating the need for higher intracellular drug concentrations to inhibit all of the enzyme molecules in the cell, and
3. active efflux of itraconazole out of the cell through the activation of two types of multidrug efflux transporters.

Metabolic Route: Itraconazole is metabolized predominantly by the cytochrome P450 3A4 isoenzyme system resulting in the formation of several metabolites, including hydroxyitraconazole, the major metabolite.

FDA FDA-APPROVED INDICATIONS

FDA-Approved Indications: Itraconazole injection/oral solution is indicated for empirical therapy of febrile neutropenic patients with suspected fungal infections.

For **immunocompromised or nonimmunocompromised** hosts, itraconazole capsules and intravenous infusion are indicated for primary therapy of blastomycosis, nonmeningeal histoplasmosis, and aspergillosis in patients who are intolerant of or refractory to amphotericin B therapy.

In **nonimmunocompromised** patients, itraconazole capsules are indicated for onychomycosis caused by dermatophytes (tinea unguium).

SIDE EFFECTS/TOXICITY

WARNING: Itraconazole should not be administered for the treatment of onychomycosis in patients with evidence of ventricular dysfunction such as congestive heart failure (CHF) or a history of CHF.

Drug interactions: Coadministration of cisapride, pimozide, quinidine, dofetilide, or levacetylmethadol (levomethadyl) with itraconazole capsules, injection, or oral solution is contraindicated. Itraconazole, a potent cytochrome P450 3A4 isoenzyme system (CYP3A4) inhibitor, may increase plasma concentrations of

WARNINGS: (cont.)

WARNINGS: (cont.)

drugs metabolized by this pathway. Serious cardiovascular events, including QT prolongation, torsade de pointes, ventricular tachycardia, cardiac arrest, and/or sudden death have occurred in patients using cisapride, pimozide, levacetylmethadol (levomethadyl), or quinidine concomitantly with itraconazole and/or other CYP3A4 inhibitors.

Other side effects/toxicities include fever, rash, rhinitis, pharyngitis, sinusitis, increased appetite, nausea, diarrhea, constipation, dyspepsia, flatulence, abdominal pain, dizziness, cystitis, urinary tract infection, gastritis, gastroenteritis, headache, tremor, myalgia, abnormal dreams, and hearing loss that usually resolves when treatment is stopped.

DRUG INTERACTIONS/FOOD INTERACTION

Itraconazole capsules should be administered after a full meal. The absorption of itraconazole may be decreased with the concomitant administration of antacids or gastric acid secretion suppressors.

Itraconazole, a potent cytochrome P450 3A4 isoenzyme system (CYP3A4) inhibitor, may increase plasma concentrations of drugs metabolized by this pathway. In addition, drugs that enhance or inhibit CYP3A4 activity may decrease or elevate levels of itraconazole, respectively. The following list includes significant drug interactions with itraconazole:

Benzodiazepines – alprazolam and diazepam levels increased; midazolam and triazolam **contraindicated**.

Calcium channel blockers – dihydropyridines (including nisoldipine) are **contraindicated**; others may have elevated levels of calcium channel blockers.

Carbamazepine – carbamazepine levels increased; also decrease in itraconazole.

Cisapride – contraindicated.

Cyclosporine, tacrolimus, sirolimus – levels of these elevated.

Dexamethasone – dexamethasone levels elevated.

Digoxin – digoxin levels increased.

Disopyramide – disopyramide levels increased.

Docetaxel – docetaxel levels increased.

Dofetilide – contraindicated.

Ergot alkaloids – contraindicated.

Fentanyl – fentanyl levels elevated.

H2-receptor antagonists – decrease itraconazole levels.

HMG CoA-reductase inhibitors (statins) – lovastatin and simvastatin **contraindicated**; atorvastatin and cerivastatin may have elevated levels.

Isoniazid – decrease itraconazole levels.

Macrolides – clarithromycin, erythromycin – increase itraconazole levels.

NNRTIs – decrease itraconazole levels.

Oral hypoglycemics – oral hypoglycemics levels elevated.

Phenobarbitol – decrease itraconazole levels.

Phenytoin – decrease itraconazole levels.

Pimozide – **contraindicated.**

Protease inhibitors – indinivir, ritonavir, and saquinavir levels elevated; also, itraconazole levels elevated.

Proton pump inhibitors – decrease itraconazole levels.

Quinidine – **contraindicated.**

Rifabutin – rifabutin levels increased; also decrease itraconazole levels.

Rifampin – decrease itraconazole levels.

Trimetraxate – trimetraxate levels elevated.

Vinca alkaloids – vinca alkaloics levels increased.

Warfarin – warfarin levels elevated.

DOSING

Itraconazole is available as a 100-mg capsule and in an oral solution containing 10 mg of itraconazole per mL. Intravenous solution is supplied as 10 mg/mL.

Blastomycosis and histoplasmosis: The recommended oral dosage is 200 mg once daily. The dosage can be increased in 100-mg increments to a maximum of 400 mg daily if no response is noted. Dosages above 200 mg/day should be given in two divided doses.

The recommended intravenous dosage is 200 mg twice a day for four doses, followed by 200 mg/day.

Treatment of aspergillosis: The recommended oral dosage is 200 mg to 400 mg daily. In life-threatening situations it is recommended that a loading dose of 200 mg three times daily be given for the first 3 days of treatment.

The recommended intravenous dosage is 200 mg twice a day for four doses, followed by 200 mg/day. Each intravenous dose should be infused over 1 hour.

Treatment of onychomycosis: Toenails: 200 mg once daily for 12 consecutive weeks.

Fingernails only: two treatment regimen pulses, each consisting of 200 mg twice a day for 1 week. The pulses are separated by a 3-week period.

SPECIAL POPULATIONS

RENAL IMPAIRMENT: Use caution when itraconazole is administered in patients with renal impairment. Intravenous form should not be used in patients with creatinine clearance less than 30 mL/min.

The oral formulation should be used during chronic renal replacement therapy at the usual dosage.

HEPATIC IMPAIRMENT: Caution should be used when itraconazole is used in patients with hepatic impairment. Liver function tests should be monitored.

PEDIATRIC PATIENTS: The efficacy and safety of itraconazole have not been established in pediatric patients. If used, 100 mg/day of itraconazole capsules for systemic fungal infections can be given.

PREGNANCY: Category C. Itraconazole should not be administered for the treatment of onychomycosis to pregnant patients or to women contemplating pregnancy.

BREASTFEEDING: The expected benefits of itraconazole therapy for the mother should be weighed against the potential risk from exposure of itraconazole to the infant.

THE ART OF ANTIMICROBIAL THERAPY

Clinical Pearls

1. Itraconazole requires a low pH for absorption. In achlorhydric patients, administration of a cola beverage increases absorption.
2. Drug exposure is greater with the oral solution than with the capsules when the same dose of drug is given.
3. Only the oral solution has been demonstrated to be effective for oral and/or esophageal candidiasis.
4. Itraconazole is an inhibitor of cytochrome P450 and can enhance the activity of many commonly used drugs, including oral hypoglycemics and anticoagulants.

IVERMECTIN (Stromectol)

BASIC CHARACTERISTICS

Class: Avermectin antiparasitic

Mechanism of Action: Ivermectin selectively binds to glutamate-gated chloride ion channels, which occur in invertebrate nerve and muscle cells. This leads to an increase in the permeability of the cell membrane to chloride ions with hyperpolarization of the nerve or muscle cell, resulting in paralysis and death of the parasite.

Metabolic Route: Ivermectin is metabolized by the liver and excreted in the feces.

FDA-APPROVED INDICATIONS

FDA-Approved Indications: The treatment of strongyloidiasis of the intestinal tract and onchocerciasis (river blindness),

Also Used for: Cutaneous larva migrans, scabies, body lice, trichostrongyliasis, ascariasis, and trichuriasis.

SIDE EFFECTS/TOXICITY

Side effects/toxicities include hypotension, dizziness, pruritus, worsening of bronchial asthma, toxic epidermal necrolysis, Stevens-Johnson syndrome, seizures, and hepatotoxicity. If patients with onchocerciasis are co-infected with *Loa loa* and receive ivermectin, encephalopathy and other neurologic and ophthalmologic side effects are rarely seen.

Mazzotti reaction (fever, rash, adenopathy, arthralgia, etc.) may be seen in patients treated for onchocerciasis; though the Mazzotti reaction is not a direct toxic effect of ivermectin and probably results from antigenic products of the treated parasite, it may resemble drug toxicity and should be anticipated.

DRUG INTERACTIONS/FOOD INTERACTIONS

Ivermectin should be taken on an empty stomach with a glass of water.

Increased INR may occur when ivermectin is administered with warfarin.

DOSING

Strongyloidiasis and scabies: A single oral dose of 200 μg of ivermectin per kg of body weight.

Onchocerciasis: A single oral dose of 150 μg of ivermectin per kg of body weight.

SPECIAL POPULATIONS

RENAL IMPAIRMENT: There is no dosage adjustment for patients with renal insufficiency.

HEPATIC DYSFUNCTION: There is no dosage adjustment for patients with hepatic dysfunction.

PEDIATRIC PATIENTS: Not studied in children who weigh less than 15 kg. Otherwise, use adult dose per body weight.

PREGNANCY: Category C.

BREASTFEEDING: Mothers should not breastfeed while taking ivermectin.

THE ART OF ANTIMICROBIAL THERAPY

Clinical Pearls

1. Although ivermectin is indicated only for the treatment of strongyloidiasis and onchocerciasis, it is also used for multiple additional parasitic infections.
2. Although not approved for use in scabies, ivermectin has been found particularly helpful in Norwegian or crusted scabies, in view of the difficulty of penetrating the crusts with topical therapy alone.
3. When one is treating strongyloidiasis in HIV-infected patients, more than one course of therapy may be needed.
4. Follow-up stool examinations should be performed to verify eradication of infection.
5. Mazzotti reaction is a possible complication of therapy for onchocerciasis.

KANAMYCIN (Kantrex)

BASIC CHARACTERISTICS

Class: Aminoglycoside

Mechanism of Action: Binds the 30S subunit of the bacterial ribosome, which terminates protein synthesis.

Mechanisms of Resistance:

1. Gram-negative bacteria inactivate aminoglycosides by acetylation,
2. some bacteria alter the 30S ribosomal subunit, which prevents kanamycin's interference with protein synthesis, and
3. low-level resistance may result from inhibition of kanamycin uptake by the bacteria.

Metabolic Route: Kanamycin is excreted unchanged in the urine.

FDA-APPROVED INDICATIONS

FDA-Approved Indications: Treatment of serious infections caused by susceptible strains of gram-negative bacteria.

Also Used for: Treatment of *Mycobacterium tuberculosis.*

SIDE EFFECTS/TOXICITY

WARNINGS: Ototoxicity: vestibular toxicity and auditory ototoxicity, especially in patients with renal damage, those treated with higher doses, and those with prolonged treatment. Avoid use with potent diuretics such as ethacrynic acid because of additive ototoxicity.

Nephrotoxicity: especially in patients with impaired renal function and those treated with higher doses or prolonged treatment. Avoid concurrent use with other nephrotoxic agents and potent diuretics, which can cause dehydration.

Neuromuscular blockade: especially in those receiving anesthetics, neuromuscular blocking agents, or massive transfusions.

Other side effects/toxicities: Other neurotoxic reactions include numbness, skin tingling, muscle twitching, and seizures. Also reported are rash, fever, headache, nausea, vomiting, and diarrhea. The "malabsorption syndrome" characterized by an increase in fecal fat, decrease in serum carotene, and fall in xylose absorption, reportedly has occurred with prolonged therapy.

DRUG INTERACTIONS/FOOD INTERACTIONS

Kanamycin should not be administered with other medications that are nephrotoxic or ototoxic.

DOSING

Kanamycin may be given intramuscularly, intravenously, or by aerosol.

Intramuscular or intravenous route: 7.5 mg/kg every 12 hours.

For tuberculosis: (All doses once daily) 15 mg/kg/day (maximum 1 g), reduced to 15 mg/kg/dose two or three times per week after initial period of daily administration. For patients aged older than 59 years, dosage is 10 mg/kg/day (maximum 750 mg).

Aerosol treatment: 250 mg two to four times a day.

SPECIAL POPULATIONS

RENAL IMPAIRMENT: Creatinine clearance less than 30 mL/min or in dialysis patients: 12 mg/kg to 15 mg/kg two or three times a week.

HEPATIC DYSFUNCTION: No adjustment necessary.

PEDIATRIC PATIENTS: 7.5 mg/kg every 12 hours.

PREGNANCY: Category D.

BREASTFEEDING: In general, kanamycin should be avoided in breastfeeding mothers but is used in treating tuberculosis in mothers in whom the benefit is judged to outweigh the risks.

THE ART OF ANTIMICROBIAL THERAPY

Clinical Pearls

1. When dosing aminoglycosides, one should use the ideal body weight, not true body weight.
2. Peak concentrations should be between 35 μg/mL and 45 μg/mL.
3. Kanamycin should be used in combination with other medications when it is being used to treat tuberculosis.
4. Monitor renal function and hearing and auditory function of a patient who is receiving kanamycin.
5. *M. tuberculosis* cross-resistance is seen with amikacin and possibly with capreomycin.

 BASIC CHARACTERISTICS

Class: Imidazole

Mechanism of Action: Inhibition of lanosterol 14-α-demethylase, which is involved in the synthesis of ergosterol, an essential component of fungal cell membranes.

Mechanisms of Resistance:

1. Point mutations in the gene (*ERG11*) encoding for the target enzyme lead to an altered target with decreased affinity for azoles,
2. overexpression of *ERG11* results in the production of high concentrations of the target enzyme, creating the need for higher intracellular drug concentrations to inhibit all of the enzyme molecules in the cell, and
3. active efflux of itraconazole out of the cell through the activation of two types of multidrug efflux transporters.

Metabolic Route: Ketoconazole is metabolized in the liver and excreted in the bile.

FDA FDA-APPROVED INDICATIONS

FDA-Approved Indications: Treatment of candidiasis, chronic mucocutaneous candidiasis, oral thrush, candiduria, blastomycosis, coccidioidomycosis, histoplasmosis, chromomycosis, and paracoccidioidomycosis. Treatment of patients with severe recalcitrant cutaneous dermatophyte infections who have not responded to topical therapy or oral griseofulvin, or who are unable to take griseofulvin.

 SIDE EFFECTS/TOXICITY

WARNING: Ketoconazole has been associated with hepatic toxicity, including some fatalities. Coadministration of terfenadine, astemizole, and cisapride is **contraindicated** because of serious cardiovascular adverse events, including death, ventricular tachycardia, QTc prolongation, and torsade de pointes.

Other side effects/toxicities include hypersensitivity, fever and chills, pruritus, hepatotoxicity, suppression of adrenal corticosteroid and testosterone secretion, nausea, vomiting, diarrhea, abdominal pain, headache, photophobia, gynecomastia, impotence, dizziness, somnolence, suicidal tendencies, severe depression, bulging fontanelles, thrombocytopenia, leukopenia, and hemolytic anemia.

DRUG INTERACTIONS/FOOD INTERACTIONS

Ketoconazole can be taken with or without food; however, in studies, ketoconazole was administered with meals. Ketoconazole requires a low pH for absorption; if concomitant antacids, anticholinergics, and H2-blockers are needed, they should be given at least 2 hours after administration of ketoconazole.

Ketoconazole is an inhibitor of the cytochrome P450 3A4 enzyme system. Coadministration of ketoconazole tablets and drugs primarily metabolized by the cytochrome P450 3A4 enzyme system may result in increased plasma concentrations of the latter drugs, possibly requiring dosage adjustments. The following list includes significant drug interactions with ketoconazole:

Astemizole – contraindicated

Cisapride – contraindicated

Cyclosporine, tacrolimus – levels of cyclosporine and tacrolimus may be elevated

Digoxin – levels of digoxin may be elevated

Ethanol – may see disulfiramlike reaction

Isoniazid – may lower ketoconazole concentrations

Methylprednisolone – levels of methylprednisolone may be elevated

Midazolam or triazolam – contraindicated

Oral hypoglycemics – may increase levels of oral hypoglycemics

Phenytoin – monitor for altered levels of both phenytoin and ketoconazole

Rifampin – may lower ketoconazole levels

Terfenadine – contraindicated

Warfarin – elevated levels of warfarin

DOSING

Adults: Ketoconazole is available in 200-mg tablets. Ketoconazole should be started at 200 mg daily; in very serious infections or if clinical responsiveness is insufficient within the expected time, the dosage may be increased to 400 mg once daily.

SPECIAL POPULATIONS

RENAL IMPAIRMENT: No dosage adjustment.

HEPATIC DYSFUNCTION: Caution should be used when used in patients with hepatic dysfunction. Liver function tests should be monitored.

PEDIATRIC PATIENTS: Ketoconazole should not be used in pediatric patients unless the potential benefit outweighs the risks. In pediatric patients aged 2 years and older, a single daily dose of 3.3 mg/kg to 6.6 mg/kg has been used. Ketoconazole tablets have not been studied in patients aged younger than 2 years.

PREGNANCY: Category C.

BREASTFEEDING: Not recommended.

THE ART OF ANTIMICROBIAL THERAPY

Clinical Pearls

1. Ketoconazole requires a low pH for absorption. If concomitant antacids, anticholinergics, or H2-blockers are needed, they should be given at least 2 hours after administration of ketoconazole tablets. In achlorhydric patients, dissolve each tablet in 4 mL aqueous solution of 0.2 N HCl. For ingesting the resulting mixture, they should use a drinking straw to avoid contact with the teeth. This administration should be followed with a cup of tap water.
2. Ketoconazole should not be used for fungal meningitis because it penetrates poorly into the cerebrospinal fluid.
3. Ketoconazole is an inhibitor of cytochrome P450 and can enhance the activity of many commonly used drugs (e.g., oral hypoglycemics and anticoagulants).

Note: Also available combined with abacavir as Epzicom, combined with zidovudine as Combivir and combined with both zidovudine and abacavir as Trizivir.

BASIC CHARACTERISTICS

Class: Nucleoside reverse transcriptase inhibitor (NRTI).

Mechanism of Action: Converted by cellular enzymes to its active drug, lamivudine triphosphate, an analogue of cytosine triphosphate. Lamivudine triphosphate competes with the naturally occurring nucleotide for incorporation in newly forming HIV DNA. Because lamivudine triphosphate does not have a terminal hydroxyl group, it halts transcription and replication of the virus.

Mechanism of Resistance: Changes in the structure of HIV reverse transcriptase leads to preferred incorporation of cytosine triphosphate and decreased incorporation of lamivudine triphosphate, which allows transcription of DNA to continue. Resistance mutations include M184V.

Metabolic Route: The majority of lamivudine is eliminated unchanged in urine by active organic cationic secretion.

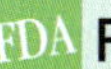

FDA-APROVED INDICATIONS

FDA-Approved Indications: Treatment of HIV infection, in combination with other antiretrovirals, and treatment of HBV.

SIDE EFFECTS/TOXICITY

WARNING: Lactic acidosis and hepatomegaly with steatosis have been reported with nucleoside analogues, including lamivudine. If this syndrome occurs, the drug should be discontinued.

Severe acute exacerbations of HBV have been reported in patients who are co-infected with HBV and HIV and have discontinued lamivudine. Hepatic function should be monitored closely with both clinical and laboratory follow-up for at least several months in patients who discontinue lamivudine and are co-infected with HIV and HBV. If appropriate, initiation of anti-HBV therapy may be warranted.

Other side effects/toxicities: Immune reconstitution inflammatory syndrome; fat redistribution including central obesity and dorsocervical fat enlargement, peripheral wasting, facial wasting, and breast enlargement; headache; nausea; malaise and fatigue; nasal signs and symptoms; diarrhea; and cough.

DRUG INTERACTIONS/FOOD INTERACTIONS

Lamivudine can be taken with or without food and is unaffected by pH.

Lamivudine should not be co-administered with emtricitabine, because they are both cytosine analogues and may be antagonistic.

DOSING

Lamivudine is administered in 100-mg, 150-mg, and 300-mg tablets, and a yellow strawberry-banana–flavored liquid, which contains 10 mg/mL. The recommended adult dosage is 300 mg once daily or 150 mg twice daily for HIV and 100 mg once daily for HBV.

SPECIAL POPULATIONS

RENAL IMPAIRMENT: Lamivudine dosage must be reduced in patients with renal insufficiency. When creatinine clearance (CrCl) drops below 50 mL/min, the recommended doses are as follows:

- CrCl 30 mL/min to 49 mL/min: 150 mg once daily
- CrCl 15 mL/min to 29 mL/min: 150 mg first dose, then 100 mg once daily
- CrCl 5 mL/min to 14 mL/min: 150 mg first dose, then 50 mg once daily
- CrCl < 5mL/min: 50 mg first dose, then 25 mg once daily

HEPATIC DYSFUNCTION: No dosage adjustment is necessary.

PEDIATRIC PATIENTS: The recommended dosage is 4 mg/kg twice daily (up to a maximum of 150 mg twice a day), administered in combination with other antiretroviral agents.

PREGNANCY: Category C.

BREASTFEEDING: It is recommended that HIV-positive mothers not breastfeed their children, to decrease mother-to-child transmission of HIV.

THE ART OF ANTIMICROBIAL THERAPY

Clinical Pearls

1. Lamivudine should be used in combination with other antiretroviral agents.
2. Lamivudine is present in four different medications: Epivir, Trizivir, Combivir, and Epzicom.

3. If lamivudine is used in HBV-infected patients, it is important to check for HIV, because using lamivudine alone in HIV-infected individuals leads to rapid resistance to lamivudine.
4. If lamivudine is used in HIV-infected patients, it is important to check for hepatitis B, since lamivudine monotherapy in Hepatitis B leads to the YMDD mutation and resistance.

■ LAMIVUDINE PLUS ABACAVIR (Epzicom)

Note: Lamivudine plus zidovudine plus abacavir is available as Trizivir.

BASIC CHARACTERISTICS

Class: Nucleoside reverse transcriptase inhibitors (NRTI) with activity against HIV.

Mechanism of Action: Converted by cellular enzymes to its active drugs lamivudine triphosphate (a cytosine analogue), and carbavir triphosphate (a guanosine triphosphate). These triphosphate analogues compete with the naturally occurring nucleotides for incorporation in newly forming HIV DNA. Because the triphosphate analogues do not have terminal hydroxyl groups, they halt transcription and replication of the virus.

Mechanism of Resistance: Lamivudine and abacavir lead to changes in the structure of HIV reverse transcriptase, leading to preferred incorporation of cytosine and guanosine triphosphate; this results in decreased incorporation of lamivudine and carbavir triphosphate, which allows transcription of DNA to continue. Resistance mutations that emerge in those on lamivudine plus abacavir include M184V, K65R, and L74V.

Metabolic Route: The majority of lamivudine is eliminated unchanged in urine by active organic cationic secretion. Abacavir is metabolized by alcohol dehydrogenase and glucuronyl transferase into inactive metabolites that are eliminated primarily in the feces.

FDA-APPROVED INDICATIONS

FDA-Approved Indication: Treatment of HIV infection, in combination with other antiretrovirals.

SIDE EFFECTS/TOXICITY

WARNINGS: Hypersensitivity to Epzicom or any agents containing abacavir can be fatal. The hypersensitivity syndrome is a multiorgan clinical syndrome with two or more of the following: fever, rash, gastrointestinal symptoms, constitutional symptoms, and respiratory symptoms. If hypersensitivity occurs, epzicom or any agents containing abacavir should be discontinued immediately and never restarted. Reintroduction can lead to serious or fatal reactions. Hypersensitivity occurs in up to 8% of patients, usually within the first month of therapy. Determining the patient's HLA-B5701 status may screen for the risk of reaction: if HLA-B5701 test is negative, the risk of hypersensitivity is near zero; if positive, the risk is 50%.

WARNINGS: (cont.)

WARNINGS: (cont.)

Lactic acidosis and severe hepatomegaly with steatosis, including fatal cases, have been reported with the use of nucleoside analogues alone or in combination, including abacavir and lamivudine.

Severe acute exacerbations of hepatitis B (HBV) have been reported in patients who are co-infected with HBV and HIV and have discontinued Epzicom or any medication containing lamivudine. Hepatic function should be monitored closely with both clinical and laboratory follow-up for at least several months in patients who discontinue Epzicom or any medication containing lamivudine and are co-infected with HIV and HBV. If appropriate, initiation of anti–hepatitis B therapy may be warranted.

Other side effects/toxicities: Immune reconstitution inflammatory syndrome; fat redistribution including central obesity and dorsocervical fat enlargement, peripheral wasting, facial wasting, and breast enlargement; GGT elevation; and pancreatitis.

DRUG INTERACTIONS/FOOD INTERACTIONS

Epzicom can be taken with or without food and is unaffected by pH.

Epzicom should not be used with emtricitabine because both lamivudine and emtricitabine are cytosine analogues and may be antagonistic.

Epzicom should not be given with other antiretrovirals containing lamivudine or abacavir. These include Epivir, Combivir, Ziagen, and Trizivir.

DOSING

Epzicom is administered in a fixed-dose combination of lamivudine 300 mg and abacavir 600 mg. The recommended adult dosage is one tablet daily.

SPECIAL POPULATIONS

RENAL IMPAIRMENT: In patients with renal insufficiency, this formulation should not be used.

HEPATIC DYSFUNCTION: In patients with hepatic insufficiency, this formulation should not be used.

PEDIATRIC PATIENTS: Not recommended for those aged younger than 12 years.

PREGNANCY: Category C.

BREASTFEEDING: It is recommended that HIV-positive mothers not breastfeed their children to decrease mother-to-child transmission of HIV.

THE ART OF ANTIMICROBIAL THERAPY

Clinical Pearls

1. Epzicom should be used in combination with other antiretroviral agents.
2. Epzicom contains lamivudine and abacavir and should not be used with medications containing these components, including Trizivir, Combivir, Ziagen, and Epivir.
3. An HLA-B5701 test should be done before starting any medication containing abacavir; if positive, abacavir should be avoided.
4. If a person has suspected hypersensitivity, abacavir and any medication containing abacavir should not be used.
5. Lamivudine has activity against HBV; therefore, it is important to check for HBV because using lamivudine or any medication containing lamivudine alone in HBV–infected individuals leads to rapid resistance to lamivudine.

LAMIVUDINE PLUS ZIDOVUDINE (Combivir)

Note: Lamivudine plus zidovudine are also combined with abacavir as Trizivir.

BASIC CHARACTERISTICS

Class: Nucleoside reverse transcriptase inhibitors (NRTI).

Mechanism of Action: Converted by cellular enzymes to its active drugs lamivudine triphosphate (a cytosine analogue) and zidovudine triphosphate (a thymidine analogue). These triphosphate analogues compete with the naturally occurring nucleotides for incorporation in newly forming HIV DNA. Because the triphosphate analogues do not have terminal hydroxyl groups, they halt transcription and replication of the virus.

Mechanisms of Resistance: Zidovudine resistance mutations change the structure of HIV reverse transcriptase, leading to pyrophosphorolysis of the nucleoside analogues, which allows transcription of DNA to continue. Resistance mutations include the "TAMS": 41L, 67N, 70R, 210W, 215F, and 219E.

Lamivudine resistance mutations change the structure of HIV reverse transcriptase, leading to preferred incorporation of cytosine triphosphate and decreased incorporation of lamivudine triphosphate, which allows transcription of DNA to continue. Resistance mutations include M184V.

Metabolic Route: Zidovudine is primarily eliminated by hepatic metabolism. The major metabolite of zidovudine is 3′-azido-3′-deoxy-5′-*O*-β-*D*-glucopyranuronosylthymidine.

The majority of lamivudine is eliminated unchanged in urine by active organic cationic secretion.

FDA-APPROVED INDICATIONS

FDA-Approved Indications: Treatment of HIV infection, in combinations with other antiretrovirals.

SIDE EFFECTS/TOXICITY

> **WARNING:** Combivir or any medication containing zidovudine is associated with **hematologic toxicity** including neutropenia and severe anemia particularly in patients with advanced HIV.
>
> Prolonged use of Combivir or any medication containing zidovudine has been associated with symptomatic **myopathy**.
>
> **Lactic acidosis and severe hepatomegaly** with steatosis, including fatal cases, have been reported with the use of nucleoside analogues alone or in combination, including zidovudine and lamivudine.

WARNINGS: (cont.)

WARNINGS: (cont.):

> Severe acute **exacerbations of hepatitis B** have been reported in patients who are coinfected with hepatitis B virus (HBV) and HIV and have discontinued Combivir or any medication containing lamivudine. Hepatic function should be monitored closely with both clinical and laboratory follow-up for at least several months in patients who discontinue Combivir or any medication containing lamivudine and are coinfected with HIV and HBV. If appropriate, initiation of anti-HBV therapy may be warranted.

Other side effects/toxicities: Immune reconstitution inflammatory syndrome; fat redistribution including central obesity and dorsocervical fat enlargement, peripheral wasting, facial wasting, and breast enlargement; headache; nausea; malaise and fatigue; nasal symptoms; diarrhea; and cough.

DRUG INTERACTIONS/FOOD INTERACTIONS

Combivir can be taken with or without food and is unaffected by pH.

Combivir should not be used with stavudine, because zidovudine and stavudine are both thymidine analogues and may be antagonistic.

Combivir should not be administered with ribavirin because of additive effects on anemia.

Combivir should not be used with emtricitabine because both lamivudine and emtricitabine are cytosine analogues and may be antagonistic.

Combivir should not be given with other antiretrovirals containing lamivudine or zidovudine. These include Epivir, Trizivir, Epzicom, and Retrovir.

DOSING

Combivir is administered in a fixed-dose combination of zidovudine 300 mg and lamivudine 150 mg. The recommended adult dosage is one tablet twice daily.

SPECIAL POPULATIONS

RENAL IMPAIRMENT: This formulation should not be used.

HEPATIC DYSFUNCTION: No dosage adjustment is necessary.

PEDIATRIC PATIENTS: Not recommended for those aged younger than 12 years.

PREGNANCY: Category C.

BREASTFEEDING: It is recommended that HIV-positive mothers not breastfeed their children, to decrease mother-to-child transmission of HIV.

THE ART OF ANTIMICROBIAL THERAPY

Clinical Pearls:

1. Combivir should be used in combination with other antiretroviral agents.
2. Combivir contains both lamivudine and zidovudine and should not be used with medications containing these components including Retrovir, Trizivir, Epzicom, and Epivir.
3. Unlike other NRTIs, pharmacokinetic studies do not support once-daily dosing of Combivir.
4. Combivir or any medication containing lamivudine has activity against HBV; therefore, it is important to check for HBV because using Combivir or any medication containing lamivudine alone in HBV–infected individuals leads to rapid resistance to lamivudine.

■ LAMIVUDINE PLUS ZIDOVUDINE PLUS ABACAVIR (Trizivir)

BASIC CHARACTERISTICS

Class: Nucleoside reverse transcriptase inhibitors (NRTIs).

Mechanism of Action: Converted by cellular enzymes to its active drugs lamivudine triphosphate (a cytosine analogue), zidovudine triphosphate (a thymidine analogue), and carbavir triphosphate (a guanosine triphosphate). These triphosphate analogues compete with the naturally occurring nucleotides for incorporation in newly forming HIV DNA. Because the triphosphate analogues do not have terminal hydroxyl groups, they halt transcription and replication of the virus.

Mechanisms of Resistance: Zidovudine resistance mutations change the structure of HIV reverse transcriptase, which leads to pyrophosphorolysis of the nucleoside analogues, allowing transcription of DNA to continue. Lamivudine resistance mutations change the structure of HIV reverse transcriptase leading to preferred incorporation of cytosine triphosphate and decreased incorporation of lamivudine triphosphate, which allows transcription of DNA to continue. Abacavir resistance mutations change the structure of HIV reverse transcriptase, leading to preferred incorporation of guanosine triphosphate and decreased incorporation of carbavir triphosphate, which allows transcription of DNA to continue.

Resistance mutations that emerge in those on Trizivir include M184V and the "TAMS": 41L, 67N, 70R, 210W, 215F and 219E.

Metabolic Route: Zidovudine is primarily eliminated by hepatic metabolism. The major metabolite of zidovudine is 3′-azido-3′-deoxy-5′-*O*-β-*D*-glucopyranuronosylthymidine. The majority of lamivudine is eliminated unchanged in urine by active organic cationic secretion. Abacavir is metabolized by alcohol dehydrogenase and glucuronyl transferase into inactive metabolites that are eliminated primarily in the feces.

FDA FDA-APPROVED INDICATIONS

FDA-Approved Indications: Trizivir is approved to be used in combinations with other antiretrovirals or alone for the treatment of HIV infection. However, although it is approved for use alone, its preferred use is in combination with other antiretrovirals.

SIDE EFFECTS/TOXICITY

WARNING: Hypersensitivity to Trizivir or any medication containing abacavir can be fatal. The hypersensitivity syndrome is a multiorgan clinical syndrome with two or more of the following: fever, rash, gastrointestinal symptoms, constitutional

WARNINGS: (cont.)

WARNINGS: (cont.):

symptoms, and respiratory symptoms. Trizivir or any medication containing abacavir should be discontinued immediately if the hypersensitivity syndrome develops, and never restarted. Reintroduction can lead to serious or fatal reactions. Hypersensitivity occurs in up to 8% of patients and usually occurs within the first month of therapy. Determining patient's HLA-B5701 status may screen for the risk of reaction: if HLA-B5701 test is negative, the risk of hypersensitivity is near zero; if positive, the risk is 50%.

Trizivir or any medication containing zidovudine is associated with **hematologic toxicity** including neutropenia and severe anemia, particularly in patients with advanced HIV.

Prolonged use of Trizivir or any medication containing zidovudine has been associated with symptomatic myopathy.

Lactic acidosis and severe hepatomegaly with steatosis, including fatal cases, have been reported with the use of nucleoside analogues alone or in combination, including zidovudine, lamivudine, and abacavir.

Severe acute exacerbations of hepatitis B have been reported in patients who are coinfected with hepatitis B virus (HBV) and HIV and have discontinued Trizivir or any medication containing lamivudine. Hepatic function should be monitored closely with both clinical and laboratory follow-up for at least several months in patients who discontinue Trizivir or any medication containing lamivudine and are coinfected with HIV and HBV. If appropriate, initiation of anti-HBV therapy may be warranted.

Other side effects/toxicities: Immune reconstitution inflammatory syndrome; fat redistribution including central obesity and dorsocervical fat enlargement, peripheral wasting, facial wasting, and breast enlargement; fever; rash; headache; malaise and fatigue; nausea; vomiting; diarrhea, and abnormal dreams/sleep.

DRUG INTERACTIONS/FOOD INTERACTIONS

Trizivir can be taken with or without food and is unaffected by pH.

Trizivir should not be used with stavudine, because zidovudine and stavudine are both thymidine analogues and may be antagonistic.

Trizivir should not be administered with ribavirin because of additive effects on anemia.

Trizivir should not be used with emtricitabine because both lamivudine and emtricitabine are cytosine analogues and may be antagonistic.

Trizivir should not be given with other antiretrovirals containing lamivudine, abacavir, or zidovudine. These include Epivir, Combivir, Ziagen, Epzicom, and Retrovir.

DOSING

Trizivir is administered in a fixed-dose combination of zidovudine 300 mg, lamivudine 150 mg, and abacavir 300 mg. The recommended adult dosage is one tablet twice daily.

SPECIAL POPULATIONS

RENAL IMPAIRMENT: In patients with renal impairment, this formulation should not be used.

HEPATIC DYSFUNCTION: In patients with hepatic dysfunction, this formulation should not be used.

PEDIATRIC PATIENTS: Not recommended for those aged younger than 12 years.

PREGNANCY: Category C.

BREASTFEEDING: It is recommended that HIV-positive mothers not breastfeed their children, to decrease mother-to-child transmission of HIV.

THE ART OF ANTIMICROBIAL THERAPY

Clinical Pearls:

1. Even though Trizivir contains three antiretrovirals, it should be used in combination with other antiretroviral agents because of less efficacy compared with other antiretroviral regimens.
2. Trizivir contains lamivudine, abacavir, and zidovudine and should not be used with other medications containing these components, including Retrovir, Combivir, Epzicom, Ziagen, and Epivir.
3. Unlike other NRTIs, pharmacokinetic studies do not support once-daily dosing of Trizivir.
4. An HLA-B5701 test should be done before starting any medication containing abacavir; if positive, Trizivir or any medication containing abacavir should be avoided.
5. If a person has suspected hypersensitivity, Trizivir and any medication containing abacavir should not be used.
6. Trizivir has activity against HBV; therefore, it is important to check for HBV infection, because using Trizivir or any medication containing lamivudine alone in HBV-infected individuals leads to rapid resistance to lamivudine.

LEVOFLOXACIN (Levaquin)

BASIC CHARACTERISTICS

Class: Fluoroquinolone

Mechanism of Action: Inhibits bacterial topoisomerase IV and DNA gyrase.

Mechanisms of Resistance: Mutations in DNA gyrase and/or topoisomerase IV; or through altered efflux.

Metabolic Route: Levofloxacin is predominantly excreted in the urine.

FDA FDA-APPROVED INDICATIONS

FDA-Approved Indications: Levofloxacin is indicated for the treatment of serious infections caused by susceptible strains of microorganisms in pneumonia (nosocomial and community-acquired), acute bacterial sinusitis, acute bacterial exacerbation of chronic bronchitis, skin and skin structure infections (complicated and uncomplicated), chronic bacterial prostatitis, urinary tract infections (complicated and uncomplicated), acute pyelonephritis, and inhalational anthrax (postexposure).

Also Used for: Treatment of *Mycobacterium tuberculosis* and nontuberculous mycobacteria in combination with other medications, and *Chlamydia trachomatis* infection.

SIDE EFFECTS/TOXICITY

WARNING: Fluoroquinolones, including levofloxacin, are associated with an increased risk of **tendinitis and tendon rupture** in all ages. This risk is further increased in older patients usually aged older than 60 years, in patients taking corticosteroid drugs, and in patients with kidney, heart, or lung transplants.

Levofloxacin is **contraindicated** in persons with a history of hypersensitivity associated with the use of levofloxacin or any quinolone.

Side effects/toxicities include, most commonly, nausea, headache, diarrhea, insomnia, constipation, and dizziness. Also reported are anaphylactic reactions and allergic skin reactions, occasionally fatal, which may occur after the first dose; photosensitivity; renal toxicity; hepatotoxicity, sometimes fatal; central nervous system effects including convulsions, anxiety, confusion, depression, and insomnia (use with caution in patients at risk for seizures); peripheral neuropathy; *Clostridium difficile*–associated colitis; prolongation of the QT interval and torsade de pointes (avoid use in patients with known prolongation of QT, hypokalemia, and with other drugs that prolong the QT interval); agranulocytosis; and thrombocytopenia.

DRUG INTERACTIONS/FOOD INTERACTIONS

Levofloxacin tablets can be administered without regard to food. Levofloxacin oral solution should be taken 1 hour before or 2 hours after eating.

Antacids containing calcium, magnesium, or aluminum; sucralfate; divalent or trivalent cations such as iron; or multivitamins containing zinc should not be taken within the 2-hour period before or within the 2-hour period after taking levofloxacin.

Levofloxacin may enhance the effects of warfarin. However, no dosage adjustments are necessary for concomitantly administered probenecid, cimetidine, digoxin, or cyclosporine.

The concomitant administration of a nonsteroidal antiinflammatory drug with a quinolone may increase the risk of central nervous system stimulation and convulsive seizures.

Disturbances of blood glucose, including hyperglycemia and hypoglycemia, may be seen in patients treated concurrently with antidiabetic agents.

Levofloxacin may produce false-positive urine screening results for opiates.

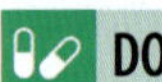

DOSING

Levofloxacin is supplied in 250-mg, 500-mg, and 750-mg tablets and an oral solution containing 25 mg/mL. Levofloxacin is also available for intravenous administration.

Type of Infection	*Dose Every 24 hours (Intravenous or Oral)*	*Duration (Days)*
Nosocomial pneumonia	750 mg	7–14
Community-acquired pneumonia	500 mg	7–14
	750 mg	5
Acute bacterial sinusitis	750 mg	5
	500 mg	10–14
Acute exacerbation of chronic bronchitis	500 mg	7
Complicated skin and skin structure infections	750 mg	7–14
Uncomplicated skin and skin structure infections	500 mg	7–10
Chronic bacterial prostatitis	500 mg	28
Complicated urinary tract infection or acute pyelonephritis	750 mg	5

Type of Infection	*Dose Every 24 hours (Intravenous or Oral)*	*Duration (Days)*
Complicated urinary tract infection or acute pyelonephritis	250 mg	10
Uncomplicated urinary tract infection	250 mg	3
Inhalational anthrax (postexposure)		
Adults and pediatric patients ≥ 50 kg and aged ≥ 6 months	500 mg	60
Pediatric patients < 50 kg and aged ≥ 6 months	8 mg/kg twice a day	60
M tuberculosis	500 mg to 1000 mg	Varies with antituberculosis regimen used

SPECIAL POPULATIONS

RENAL IMPAIRMENT:

Normal Renal Function	*CrCl 20 mL/min to 49 mL/min*	*CrCl 10 mL/min to 19 mL/min*	*Hemodialysis, CAPD, or CRRT*
750 mg daily	750 mg every 48 hours	750 mg, then 500 mg every 48 hours	750 mg, then 500 mg every 48 hours
500 mg daily	500 mg, then 250 mg every 24 hours	500 mg, then 250 mg every 48 hours	500 mg, then 250 mg every 48 hours
250 mg daily	No dosage adjustment	250 mg every 48 hours	No information

Note: CrCl = Creatinine Clearance, CAPD = Chronic Ambulatory Peritoneal Dialysis, CRRT = Continuous Renal Replacement Therapy.

HEPATIC DYSFUNCTION: A maximum dosage of 400 mg of levofloxacin per day should not be exceeded.

PEDIATRIC PATIENTS: Levofloxacin is indicated in pediatric patients for the prophylaxis of inhalational anthrax. Prolonged therapy has not been studied in children.

PREGNANCY: Category C.

BREASTFEEDING: Levofloxacin should not be administered to breastfeeding mothers.

THE ART OF ANTIMICROBIAL THERAPY

Clinical Pearls

1. Levofloxacin should be given 2 hours before or after cations.
2. All fluoroquinolones can lead to tendon rupture, especially in patients aged older than 60 years.
3. All fluoroquinolones can prolong QT intervals and caution should be used when given with medications that affect QT intervals.
4. All fluoroquinolones can cause phototoxicity.
5. All fluoroquinolones can lower the seizure threshold.
6. Levofloxacin should be avoided, if possible, in children, pregnant women, and breastfeeding mothers because of concern for cartilage developmental problems.
7. Levofloxacin has activity against mycobacteria; therefore, levofloxacin monotherapy (e.g., for pneumonia) should be avoided if mycobacterial infection is possible.
8. Treatment of gonorrhea with fluoroquinolones should be undertaken with caution because of rising resistance.

LINEZOLID (Zyvox)

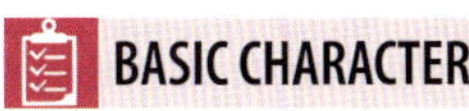

BASIC CHARACTERISTICS

Class: Oxazolidinone

Mechanism of Action: Binds the bacterial 23S ribosomal RNA of the 50S subunit and prevents the formation of a functional 70S initiation complex, which is an essential component of the bacterial translation process.

Mechanisms of Resistance:

1. Mutations in the 23S ribosomal RNA is the major cause of linezolid resistance in vancomycin-resistant enterococci (VRE) and methicillin-resistant *Staphylococcus aureus* (MRSA), and
2. resistance can also be conveyed by the *cfr* rRNA methyltransferase conferring resistance to lincosamides, oxazolidinones, and streptogramins.

Metabolic Route: Linezolid is metabolized by oxidation and excreted in the urine as both linezolid and linezolid metabolites.

FDA-APPROVED INDICATIONS

FDA-Approved Indications: Vancomycin-resistant *Enterococcus faecium* infections; nosocomial pneumonia caused by *S. aureus* or *Streptococcus pneumoniae;* complicated skin and skin structure infections, including diabetic foot infections without concomitant osteomyelitis, caused by *S. aureus, Streptococcus pyogenes*, or *Streptococcus agalactiae;* uncomplicated skin and skin structure infections caused by *S. aureus* or *S. pyogenes;* community-acquired pneumonia caused by *S. pneumoniae* or *S. aureus.*

Also Used For: Resistant *Mycobacterium tuberculosis,* nocardiosis, and atypical mycobacterial infection.

SIDE EFFECTS/TOXICITY

Side effects/toxicities include anaphylaxis, rash including Stevens-Johnson syndrome, myelosuppression (including anemia, leukopenia, pancytopenia, and thrombocytopenia), *Clostridium difficile*–associated diarrhea, lactic acidosis, peripheral and optic neuropathy (primarily in patients treated for longer than the maximum recommended duration of 28 days), nausea, vomiting, diarrhea, headache, tongue and tooth discoloration, taste alteration, oral and vaginal candidiasis, and seizures.

DRUG INTERACTIONS/FOOD INTERACTIONS

Linezolid can be taken without regard to food.

Serotonin syndrome (cognitive dysfunction, fever, hyperreflexia, and incoordination): Unless patients are carefully observed for signs and/or symptoms of serotonin syndrome, linezolid should not be administered to patients with carcinoid syndrome and/or patients taking any of the following medications: selective serotonin reuptake inhibitors (SSRIs), tricyclic antidepressants, serotonin 5-HT1 receptor agonists (triptans), meperidine, or buspirone.

Monoamine oxidase (MAO) inhibition: Linezolid is an inhibitor of MAO and has the potential for interaction with adrenergic and serotonergic agents; it should not be used in patients taking MAO inhibitors (within 2 weeks) and should not be administered to patients with uncontrolled hypertension, pheochromocytoma, thyrotoxicosis, and/or patients taking any of the following types of medications: directly and indirectly acting sympathomimetic agents (e.g., pseudoephedrine or phenylpropanolamine), vasopressive agents (e.g., epinephrine, norepinephrine), or dopaminergic agents (e.g., dopamine, dobutamine). Patients receiving linezolid need to avoid consuming large amounts of foods or beverages with high tyramine content.

DOSING

Linezolid is available in 400-mg and 600-mg tablets, as an oral suspension containing 100 mg/5 mL, and for intravenous administration.

Complicated skin infections: 600 mg oral or IV every 12 hours for 10 to 14 days

Pneumonia: 600 mg oral or IV every 12 hours for 10 to 14 days

VRE infection: 600 mg oral or IV every 12 hours for 14 to 28 days

Uncomplicated skin infections: 400 mg to 600 mg oral every 12 hours for 10 to 14 days

SPECIAL POPULATIONS

RENAL IMPAIRMENT: No dosage adjustment is necessary.

HEPATIC DYSFUNCTION: No dosage adjustment is necessary.

PEDIATRIC PATIENTS (aged up to 11 years; older patients should receive the adult dosage):

Complicated skin infections: 10 mg/kg oral or IV every 8 hours for 10 to 14 days

Pneumonia: 10 mg/kg oral or IV every 8 hours for 10 to 14 days

VRE infection: 10 mg/kg oral or IV every 8 hours for 14 to 28 days

Uncomplicated skin infections: 10 mg oral every 8 to 12 hours for 10 to 14 days

PREGNANCY: Category C.

BREASTFEEDING: Caution should be exercised.

THE ART OF ANTIMICROBIAL THERAPY

Clinical Pearls

1. Linezolid is not approved for and should not be used for the treatment of patients with catheter-related bloodstream infections or catheter-site infections.
2. Linezolid has no clinical activity against gram-negative pathogens and is not indicated for the treatment of gram-negative infections.
3. Use caution when linezolid is administered with SSRIs, MAO inhibitors, or adrenergic agents.
4. Monitor complete blood counts weekly when a patient is using linezolid for more than 2 weeks.
5. Peripheral and optic neuropathy can be seen with prolonged linezolid use; visual function should be monitored.
6. In the chronic treatment of resistant tuberculosis, linezolid (in combination with other drugs) is used at a dosage of 600 mg daily.
7. Many experts add pyridoxine 100 mg for prolonged linezolid administration

■ LOPINAVIR PLUS RITONAVIR (Kaletra)

 BASIC CHARACTERISTICS

Class: Protease inhibitor

Mechanism of Action: Reversibly binds the active site of the enzyme protease. Inhibition of protease prevents cleavage of the *gag* and *gag-pol* polyprotein resulting in the production of immature, noninfectious virus.

Mechanism of Resistance: Development of mutations on the enzyme protease causes a conformational change that prevents lopinavir from binding the active site allowing protease activity to continue. Many protease mutations are required for the virus to become resistant to lopinavir.

Metabolic Route: Lopinavir is metabolized by the liver and excreted in the feces.

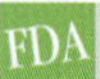 FDA-APPROVED INDICATIONS

FDA-Approved Indication: Treatment of HIV-1 in combinations with other antiretroviral agents.

 SIDE EFFECTS/TOXICITY

> **WARNING:** Coadministration of ritonavir with certain nonsedating antihistamines, sedative hypnotics, antiarrhythmics, or ergot alkaloid preparations may result in potentially serious and/or life-threatening adverse events because of possible effects of ritonavir on the hepatic metabolism of certain drugs.

Side effects/toxicities include new-onset diabetes mellitus, exacerbation of preexisting diabetes mellitus, and hyperglycemia; increased bleeding including spontaneous skin hematomas and hemarthrosis in patients with hemophilia type A or B; redistribution or accumulation of body fat including central obesity, dorsocervical fat enlargement (buffalo hump), peripheral wasting, facial wasting, and breast enlargement; cushingoid appearance; immune reconstitution syndrome; diarrhea; QTc prolongation; torsade de pointes; abdominal pain; headache; anorexia; dyspepsia; epigastric pain; hepatitis; mouth ulceration; vomiting; anemia; leukopenia; thrombocytopenia; increases in alkaline phosphatase, amylase, creatine phosphokinase, lactic dehydrogenase, SGOT, SGPT, and gamma glutamyl transpeptidase; hyperlipemia; hyperuricemia; hypoglycemia; and dehydration.

DRUG INTERACTIONS/FOOD INTERACTIONS

Lopinavir plus ritonavir tablets may be taken with or without food. The tablets should be swallowed whole and not chewed, broken, or crushed. Lopinavir plus ritonavir oral solution must be taken with food.

Drugs that **should not be coadministered** with lopinavir plus ritonavir include amiodarone, quinidine, rifampin, ergot derivatives, Saint-John's-Wort, HMG-CoA reductase inhibitors simvastatin or lovastatin, pimozide, proton pump inhibitors, benzodiazepines, voriconazole, ritonavir, phenobarbitol, phenytoin, carbamazepine, tipranavir, fosamprenavir, darunavir, salmeterol, and sildenafil for pulmonary hypertension.

Lopinavir is an inhibitor of the CYP3A enzyme; coadministration of lopinavir and drugs primarily metabolized by CYP3A may result in increased plasma concentrations of the other drug that could increase or prolong its therapeutic and adverse effects.

Lopinavir is metabolized by CYP3A; coadministration of lopinavir and drugs that induce CYP3A may decrease lopinavir plasma concentrations and reduce its therapeutic effect. Coadministration of lopinavir and drugs that inhibit CYP3A may increase lopinavir plasma concentrations. Because of these metabolic affects, potential drug interactions that may require dosage change or clinical/laboratory monitoring are listed below:

Medication	*Adjustment or Action*
Itraconzole	Do not exceed 200 mg/day; monitor for toxicity
Ketoconazole	Do not exceed 200 mg/day
Hormonal clarithromycin	Reduce clarithromycin dosage in moderate to severe renal impairment
Rifabutin	Decrease rifabutin to 150 mg every other day or 3 times per week
Hormonal contraceptives	Use alternative or additional method
Atorvastatin	Use lowest possible dosage with close monitoring
Methadone	Monitor; may require higher methadone dosage
Sildenafil	25 mg every 48 hours (maximum)
Tadalafil	10 mg in 72 hours (maximum)
Vardenafil	2.5 mg in 72 hours (maximum)
Tenofovir	Monitor for tenofovir toxicity
Efavirenz, nevirapine	Increase lopinavir plus ritonavir to 600 mg/150 mg in treatment-experienced patients receiving efavirenz or nevirapine; no dosage adjustment in treatment-naïve patients
Maraviroc	Maraviroc dosage should be 150 mg twice a day
Cyclosporine, tacrolimus, rapamycin	Monitor concentration of immunosuppressant

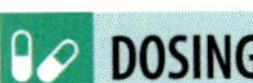

DOSING

Lopinavir plus ritonavir is supplied in 200 mg lopinavir/50 mg ritonavir tablets, 100 mg lopinavir/25 mg ritonavir tablets, and a light yellow to orange–colored liquid containing

80 mg lopinavir/20 mg ritonavir per mL. For therapy-naïve patients, the recommended dosage is lopinavir 400 mg /100 mg (two tablets or 5 mL) twice daily, or 800 mg/200 mg (four tablets or 10 mL) once daily.

For therapy-experienced patients, the recommended dosage is 400 mg/100 mg (two tablets or 5.0 mL) twice daily.

SPECIAL POPULATIONS

RENAL IMPAIRMENT: There is no dosage adjustment needed.

HEPATIC DYSFUNCTION: Administer with caution.

PEDIATRIC PATIENTS: Lopinavir plus ritonavir should not be administered once daily in patients aged younger than 18 years:

- **Age 14 days to 6 months:** the recommended dosage is 16 mg/4 mg per kg or 300 mg/75 mg per m^2 twice daily.
- **Age 6 months to 18 years:** the recommended dosage is 230 mg/57.5 mg per m^2 given twice daily, not to exceed the recommended adult dosage, or the dosage for patients who weigh less than 15 kg is 12 mg/3 mg per kg given twice daily, and the dosage for patients who weigh 15 kg to 40 kg is 10 mg/2.5 mg per kg given twice daily.

PREGNANCY: Category C.

BREASTFEEDING: It is recommended that HIV-positive mothers not breastfeed their children, to decrease mother-to-child transmission of HIV.

THE ART OF ANTIMICROBIAL THERAPY

Clinical Pearls

1. Lopinavir plus ritonavir should always be used in combination with other antiretrovirals.
2. Even though lopinavir plus ritonavir can be administered with or without food, it is likely that gastrointestinal side effects are decreased when it is taken with food.
3. Kaletra contains ritonavir, and all side effects of both lopinavir and ritonavir should be considered when administering it.
4. When assessing for resistance to lopinavir plus ritonavir, a phenotype assay may be helpful.
5. Whenever initiating lopinavir plus ritonavir, review all medications the patient is receiving to limit drug interactions.

 BASIC CHARACTERISTICS

Class: Second-generation cephalosporin

Mechanism of Action: Binds penicillin-binding protein (PBP), disrupting cell wall synthesis.

Mechanisms of Resistance:

1. The PBP can be altered, with reduced affinity,
2. production of a β-lactamase resulting in hydrolysis of the β-lactam ring, and
3. decreased ability of the antibiotic to reach the PBP when bacteria decrease porin production, resulting in a decrease of the drug concentration within the cell.

Metabolic Route: Loracarbef is excreted unchanged in the urine.

 FDA-APPROVED INDICATIONS

FDA-Approved Indications: Treatment of the following infections when caused by susceptible organisms: secondary bacterial infection of acute bronchitis, acute bacterial exacerbations of chronic bronchitis, pneumonia, otitis media, acute maxillary sinusitis, pharyngitis and tonsillitis, skin and skin structure infections, and urinary tract infections.

 SIDE EFFECTS/TOXICITY

Loracarbef is **contraindicated** in patients with allergy to cephalosporins. Loracarbef should be used with caution if hypersensitivity exists to penicillins.

Side effects/toxicities include fever; anaphylaxis; rash including Stevens-Johnson syndrome, erythema multiforme, and toxic epidermal necrolysis; angioedema; flushing; serum sickness–like reactions; encephalopathy; seizures; diarrhea; *Clostridium difficile*–associated diarrhea and pseudomembranous colitis; oral candidiasis; anorexia; nausea; vomiting; stomach cramps; flatulence; hepatitis; renal impairment; genital candidiasis; vaginitis; hemorrhage; prolonged prothrombin time; pancytopenia; hemolytic anemia; positive Coombs' test; and false-positive test for urinary glucose.

 DRUG INTERACTIONS/FOOD INTERACTIONS

Loracarbef is administered orally either at least 1 hour before eating or at least 2 hours after eating.

Probenecid inhibits the renal excretion of loracarbef.

False-positive reaction for ketones in the urine may occur with tests that use nitroprusside, but not with those that use nitroferricyanide. Cephalosporins may cause false-positive urine glucose determinations when one is using cupric sulfate solution

(Benedict's solution, Clinitest). Tests utilizing glucose oxidase (Tes-Tape, Clinistix) are not affected by cephalosporins.

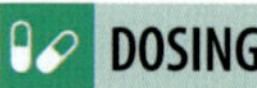

DOSING

Loracarbef is supplied in 200-mg and 400-mg tablets as well as a suspension.

Infection	*Dosage*	*Duration*
Secondary infection of acute bronchitis	200 mg to 400 mg every 12 hours	7 days
Acute exacerbations of chronic bronchitis	400 mg every 12 hours	7 days
Pneumonia	400 mg every 12 hours	14 days
Acute sinusitis	400 mg every 12 hours	10 days
Pharyngitis/tonsillitis	200 mg every 12 hours	10 days
Uncomplicated skin and skin structure infections	200 mg every 12 hours	7 days
Uncomplicated urinary tract infections	200 mg per day	7 days
Pyelonephritis	400 mg every 12 hours	14 days

SPECIAL POPULATIONS

RENAL IMPAIRMENT:

- Creatinine clearance 10 mg/mL to 49 mg/mL: half dose at usual intervals, or full dose at double interval
- Creatinine clearance less than 10 mg/mL: full dose every 3 to 5 days
- Hemodialysis: full dose every 3 to 5 days and 1 dose after hemodialysis

HEPATIC DYSFUNCTION: No dosage adjustment is necessary

PEDIATRIC PATIENTS (aged 6 months to 12 years):

Otitis media: 15 mg/kg every 12 hours for 10 days

Acute maxillary sinusitis: 15 mg/kg every 12 hours for 10 days

Pharyngitis/tonsillitis: 7.5 mg/kg every 12 hours for 10 days

Impetigo: 7.5 mg/kg every 12 hours for 7 days

PREGNANCY: Category B.

BREASTFEEDING: Loracarbef should be used with caution in breastfeeding mothers.

THE ART OF ANTIMICROBIAL THERAPY

Clinical Pearls

1. Loracarbef dosage must be adjusted for patients with renal insufficiency.
2. Cross-allergy with penicillins is less than 10%.

MARAVIROC (Selzentry)

BASIC CHARACTERISTICS

Class: CCR5 co-receptor antagonist

Mechanism of Action: Antagonizes the interaction between human CCR5 and HIV-1 gp120. Blocking this interaction prevents CCR5-tropic HIV-1 entry into cells. **Maraviroc is not active against all HIV strains, only those that use CCR5 solely as the co-receptor for entry.**

Mechanism of Resistance: Two amino acid residue substitutions in the V3-loop region of the HIV-1 envelope glycoprotein, gp160—A316T and I323V—lead to resistance to maraviroc.

Metabolic Route: Maraviroc is principally metabolized by the cytochrome P450 system.

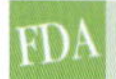

FDA-APPROVED INDICATIONS

FDA-Approved Indications: Treatment of HIV-1 in combinations with other antiretroviral agents for adult patients infected with only CCR5-tropic HIV-1, who have evidence of viral replication and HIV-1 strains resistant to multiple antiretroviral agents. Maraviroc is currently approved for both treatment-experienced and treatment-naïve patients.

SIDE EFFECTS/TOXICITY

WARNING: Hepatotoxicity has been reported with maraviroc use. Evidence of a **systemic allergic reaction** (e.g., pruritic rash, eosinophilia, or elevated IgE) before the development of hepatotoxicity may occur. Patients with signs or symptoms of hepatitis or allergic reaction following use of maraviroc should be evaluated immediately.

Other side effects/toxicities include hypersensitivity, fever, rash, eosinophilia, hepatotoxicity, upper respiratory tract infection, cough, dizziness, diarrhea, edema, sleep disorders, symptomatic postural hypotension, and immune reconstitution syndrome.

Maraviroc antagonizes the CCR5 co-receptor located on some immune cells, and, therefore, could potentially increase the patient's risk of developing infections. Patients should be monitored closely for evidence of infections while they are receiving maraviroc.

Because of maraviroc's mechanism of action it could affect immune surveillance and increase the risk of malignancy. Use with caution in patients at increased risk for cardiovascular events.

 DRUG INTERACTIONS/FOOD INTERACTIONS

Maraviroc can be taken with or without food.

Saint-John's-wort should not be taken with maraviroc.

Because maraviroc is metabolized by CYP3A, coadministration of maraviroc and drugs that induce CYP3A may decrease maraviroc plasma concentrations and reduce its therapeutic effect. Coadministration of maraviroc and drugs that inhibit CYP3A may increase maraviroc plasma concentrations. Because of these metabolic effects, potential drug interactions that may require dosage change or clinical/laboratory monitoring are:

Medication	*Adjustment or Action*
Itraconazole and ketoconazole	Decrease maraviroc to 150 mg twice a day
Voriconazole	Monitor for toxicities
Clarithromycin	Decrease maraviroc to 150 mg twice a day
Rifampin	Increase maraviroc to 600 mg twice a day
Rifabutin	When coadministerd with a protease inhibitor (except tipranavir/ritonavir or fosamprenavir/ritonavir), maraviroc dose should be decreased to 150 mg twice daily. Otherwise, maraviroc dose should be 300 mg twice daily.
Phenobarbital, phenytoin, or carbamazepine	Increase maraviroc to 600 mg twice a day
All protease inhibitors except tipranavir/ritonavir or fosamprenavir/ritonavir	Decrease maraviroc to 150 mg twice a day
Efavirenz	Increase maraviroc to 600 mg twice a day
Tipranavir/ritonavir, fosamprenavir/ritonavir, nevirapine, all NRTIs, and enfuvirtide	300 mg twice a day

 DOSING

Maraviroc is supplied in 150-mg and 300-mg tablets. The normal dosage is 300 mg given twice daily.

SPECIAL POPULATIONS

RENAL IMPAIRMENT: Maraviroc should be used with caution in those with renal impairment.

HEPATIC DYSFUNCTION: Maraviroc should be used with caution in those with hepatic impairment.

PEDIATRIC PATIENTS: Maraviroc has not been studied in pediatric patients and, therefore, should not be used in patients aged younger than 16 years.

PREGNANCY: Category B.

BREASTFEEDING: It is recommended that HIV-positive mothers not breastfeed their children, to decrease mother-to-child transmission of HIV.

THE ART OF ANTIMICROBIAL THERAPY

Clinical Pearls

1. Maraviroc should always be used in combination with other antiretrovirals.
2. A tropism test must be done to see whether the patient has virus that uses only the CCR5 receptor, to ensure that maraviroc's use is appropriate.
3. If the virus uses the CXCR4 coreceptor or is dual-tropic, maraviroc should not be used.
4. Whenever initiating maraviroc, one should make sure to review all medications the patient is receiving to minimize drug interactions.

MEBENDAZOLE (Vermox)

BASIC CHARACTERISTICS

Class: Broad-spectrum anthelminthic

Mechanism of Action: Inhibits tubulin polymerization, resulting in loss of cytoplasmic microtubules.

Metabolic Route: Mebendazole is excreted in the feces.

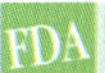

FDA-APPROVED INDICATIONS

FDA-Approved Indications: Treatment of *Enterobius vermicularis* (pinworm), *Trichuris trichiura* (whipworm), *Ascaris lumbricoides* (common roundworm), *Ancylostoma duodenale* (common hookworm), and *Necator americanus* (American hookworm) in single or mixed infections.

Also Used for: Treatment of trichinellosis.

SIDE EFFECTS/TOXICITY

Side effects/toxicities include transient abdominal pain and diarrhea in cases of massive infection, expulsion of worms, rash, urticaria, angioedema, convulsions, hepatitis, neutropenia, and agranulocytosis.

DRUG INTERACTIONS/FOOD INTERACTIONS

Mebendazole can be given with food.

Cimetidine inhibits mebendazole metabolism and may result in an increase in plasma concentrations of mebendazole.

DOSING

Mebendazole is administered as 100-mg chewable tablets. The tablet may be chewed, swallowed, or crushed and mixed with food. The same dosage schedule applies to children and adults.

- **Enterobiasis (pinworm):** one tablet for 1 dose
- **Trichuriasis (whipworm):** one tablet twice a day for 3 days
- **Ascariasis (roundworm):** one tablet twice a day for 3 days
- **Ancylostomiasis (hookworm):** one tablet twice a day for 3 days

SPECIAL POPULATIONS

RENAL IMPAIRMENT: There is no dosage adjustment for patients with renal impairment.

HEPATIC DYSFUNCTION: During therapy, monitoring of liver function tests is suggested if prolonged therapy is given.

PEDIATRIC PATIENTS: Mebendazole has not been studied in children aged younger than 2 years; use if benefit outweighs the risks.

PREGNANCY: Category C.

BREASTFEEDING: Caution should be exercised when mebendazole is given to breastfeeding mothers.

THE ART OF ANTIMICROBIAL THERAPY

Clinical Pearls

1. Complete blood counts and liver function tests should be checked if patient is on prolonged therapy.
2. If patient is not cured 3 weeks after therapy, a repeat course of therapy can be given.

MEFLOQUINE HYDROCHLORIDE (Lariam)

BASIC CHARACTERISTICS

Class: Chiral quinolone methanol

Mechanism of Action: Acts against the schizont (erythrocytic stage) of *Plasmodium* species.

Mechanism of Resistance: Data incomplete.

Metabolic Route: Mefloquine is carboxylated and excreted in the feces.

FDA-APPROVED INDICATIONS

FDA-Approved Indications: Prophylaxis and treatment of malaria caused by *Plasmodium falciparum* and *Plasmodium vivax*, including chloroquine-resistant *P falciparum.*

SIDE EFFECTS/TOXICITY

Side effects/toxicities include hypersensitivity; psychiatric symptoms including anxiety, paranoia, depression, hallucinations, and psychosis; diarrhea, nausea and vomiting; circulatory disturbances such as hypotension, tachycardia, bradycardia, A-V block, or other transient conduction alterations; anemia; leukopenia; and thrombocytopenia.

DRUG INTERACTIONS/FOOD INTERACTIONS

Halofantrine use after mefloquine has been associated with fatal prolongation of the QTc and should be avoided.

Concomitant use of mefloquine and other quinine medications should be avoided because of risk of electrocardiographic abnormalities and increased risk of convulsions.

Mefloquine may lower serum levels of anticonvulsants, which should be monitored during concomitant therapy with mefloquine.

DOSING

For malaria prophylaxis: 250 mg once weekly. It should be started 1 week before arrival in endemic areas and continued for 4 weeks after leaving the endemic area. It should be taken with 8 oz. of water and with food.

For malaria treatment: A total dose of 1250 mg given once should be taken with food and 8 oz of fluid.

SPECIAL POPULATIONS

RENAL IMPAIRMENT: There is no dosage adjustment needed.

HEPATIC DYSFUNCTION: There is no dosage adjustment needed; however, levels may increase in those with hepatic dysfunction.

PEDIATRIC PATIENTS:

For treatment: 20 mg/kg to 25 mg/kg body weight; dose can be split into two doses taken 6 to 8 hours apart. Experience with mefloquine in infants aged younger than 3 months or weighing less than 5 kg is limited. The drug should be taken with ample water or crushed and suspended in water, milk, or other beverage.

For prophylaxis: 5 mg/kg body weight once weekly. One 250-mg mefloquine tablet should be taken once weekly in pediatric patients weighing more than 45 kg. In pediatric patients weighing less than 45 kg, the weekly dosage decreases in proportion to body weight:

- 30 kg to <45 kg: ¾ tablet
- 20 kg to <30 kg: ½ tablet
- 10 kg to <20 kg: ¼ tablet
- 5 kg to <10 kg: ⅛ tablet (exact dose should be prepared by a pharmacist)

PREGNANCY: Category C.

BREASTFEEDING: Mefloquine should be given to breastfeeding mothers only if benefit exceeds potential risk.

THE ART OF ANTIMICROBIAL THERAPY

Clinical Pearls

1. Mefloquine should not be given to those with depression, anxiety disorders, psychosis, or schizophrenia.
2. Mefloquine resistance is seen in Southeast Asia and it therefore should not be used for prophylaxis in this region.
3. Mefloquine does not eliminate hepatic-phase parasites, and patients with acute *P vivax* malaria are at high risk of relapse; to avoid relapse, after initial treatment of the acute infection, patients should subsequently be treated with an 8-aminoquinoline derivative (e.g., primaquine).
4. Mefloquine can induce hemolysis in patients with G6PD deficiency.
5. Because of the long half-life of mefloquine, adverse effects can persist for weeks after discontinuation of therapy.

MEGLUMINE ANTIMONATE (Glucantime)

BASIC CHARACTERISTICS

Class: Organometallic pentavalent antimonial

Mechanism of Action: Inhibits DNA topoisomerase, glycolytic enzymes, and fatty acid oxidation.

Metabolic Route: Meglumine antimonate is eliminated rapidly, mainly via the urine.

FDA-APPROVED INDICATIONS

Not FDA-approved, but used against all *Leishmania* species.

SIDE EFFECTS/TOXICITY

Side effects/toxicities include elevated serum amylase, hepatitis, arthralgias, myalgias, anorexia, thrombophlebitis, headache, abdominal pain, nausea, vomiting, pancreatitis, metallic taste, pruritus, arrhythmias, prolongation of QTc interval, thrombocytopenia, and leukopenia.

DRUG INTERACTIONS/FOOD INTERACTIONS

No interactions are known, but drugs that may impair renal function or prolong the QT interval should be used with caution.

DOSING

The recommended dosage by is 20 mg/kg/day; however, twice-daily or thrice-daily doses of 10 mg/kg have been used. It is given by slow intravenous infusion; intramuscular administration is painful, and oral absorption is inadequate.

Cutaneous leishmaniasis is treated for 20 days.

Visceral leishmaniasis is treated for 28 to 30 days.

Mucocutaneous leishmaniasis is treated for 28 days.

SPECIAL POPULATIONS

RENAL IMPAIRMENT: An alternative drug such as liposomal amphotericin B should be used in patients with renal failure.

HEPATIC DYSFUNCTION: No dosage adjustment is necessary.

PEDIATRIC PATIENTS: 20 mg/kg/day with an upper daily limit of 850 mg.

PREGNANCY: Do not use.

BREASTFEEDING: Should be safe.

THE ART OF ANTIMICROBIAL THERAPY

Clinical Pearls

1. Antimonials are more toxic in HIV-infected patients.
2. Children tolerate antimonials better than adults do.
3. Alcohol should be avoided during therapy.
4. Electrocardiographs should be monitored and treatment interrupted for significant QTc prolongation.
5. Meglumine antimonate is not available commercially in the United States. It may be obtained through compounding pharmacies via the National Association of Compounding Pharmacies (800-687-7850) or the Professional Compounding Centers of America (800-331-2498; http://www.pccarx.com).

BASIC CHARACTERISTICS

Class: Aromatic arsenicals

Mechanisms of Action:

1. Inhibits glycolytic kinases,
2. is a potent inhibitor of trypanothione reductase, and
3. interacts with lipoic acid.

Metabolic Route: Melarsoprol B is oxidized in the liver and is excreted in the urine and feces.

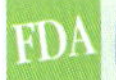

FDA-APPROVED INDICATIONS

Not FDA-approved, but used treatment of African trypanosomiasis in late stages (with central nervous system involvement).

SIDE EFFECTS/TOXICITY

Life threatening encephalopathy may occur in up to 20% of patients receiving melarsoprol. It is more common with Rhodesian than Gambian sleeping sickness and may be an immune-mediated reaction. If this occurs, IV dexamethasone and anticonvulsants may be beneficial and therapy should be switched to eflornithine.

Other side effects/toxicites include fever, rash, polyneuropathy (possibly ameliorated by thiamine), tremors, phlebitis, cellulitis, and abdominal pain.

DRUG INTERACTIONS/FOOD INTERACTIONS

Unknown.

DOSING

Gambian trypanosomiasis: Pentamidine, 4 mg/kg, is given 1 to 3 days before the first injection of melarsoprol (to decrease the possibility of encephalopathy) followed by one of three melarsoprol regimens:

1. 3.6 mg/kg up to 180 mg daily for 3 days then 1 week drug-free, followed by another 3-day series. If the cerebrospinal fluid white-cell count is $\geq 20/mm^3$ the patient should receive a third series.
2. Start with a lower dose, and reach 3.6 mg/kg, up to 180 mg daily after two doses and continue the same total days as described in number 1.
3. 2.2 mg/kg daily for 10 consecutive days.

Rhodesian trypanosomiasis: After two or three doses of suramin as pretreatment (to decrease the possibility of encephalopathy), the following dosing is recommended:

- 0.36 mg/kg on day 1
- 0.72 mg/kg on day 2
- 1.1 mg/kg on day 3
- 1.4 mg/kg on day 10
- 1.8 mg/kg on days 11 and 12
- 2.2 mg/kg on day 19
- 2.9 mg/kg on day 20
- 3.6 mg/kg (up to 180 mg) on days 21, 28, 29, and 30

SPECIAL POPULATIONS

RENAL IMPAIRMENT: There is no dosage adjustment for patients with renal impairment.

HEPATIC DYSFUNCTION: There is no dosage adjustment for patients with hepatic dysfunction.

PEDIATRIC PATIENTS: Dosing is the same as that for adults.

PREGNANCY: May be administered to pregnant women.

BREASTFEEDING: Unknown.

THE ART OF ANTIMICROBIAL THERAPY

Clinical Pearls

1. Melarsoprol can be obtained from the Centers for Disease Control and Prevention Parasitic Diseases Drug Service, 770-488-7775.
2. For late-stage Rhodesian trypanosomiasis, eflornithine is ineffective; thus, melarsoprol is the only option.
3. Prednisolone reduces the risk of encephalopathy by two thirds and mortality by half and should be administered to all patients given melarsoprol as 1 mg/kg daily up to 40 mg, initiated 1 to 2 days before the first dose of melarsoprol, continued at the same dosage until the last injection and then rapidly tapered over 3 days.
4. Pretreatment with suramin or pentamidine may decrease the toxicity of melarsoprol, but its beneficial effect has never been documented.
5. Thiamine may be helpful for the polyneuropathy.

BASIC CHARACTERISTICS

Class: Carbapenem

Mechanism of Action: Binds penicillin-binding protein (PBP), disrupting cell wall synthesis.

Mechanisms of Resistance:

1. The PBP can be altered, with reduced affinity,
2. production of β-lactamases (carbapenemases, metallo-β-lactamases), resulting in hydrolysis of the β-lactam ring,
3. decreased ability of the antibiotic to reach the PBP when bacteria decrease porin production, resulting in a decrease of the drug concentration within the cell, and
4. increased expression of efflux pump components.

Metabolic Route: Meropenem is excreted in the urine.

FDA FDA-APPROVED INDICATIONS

FDA-Approved Indications: Treatment of serious infections caused by susceptible strains of microorganisms in the following conditions: complicated skin and skin structure infections, intraabdominal infections including complicated appendicitis and peritonitis, and bacterial meningitis (patients aged 3 months or older).

SIDE EFFECTS/TOXICITY

Meropenem is **contraindicated** in patients with known hypersensitivity to any component of this product or to other drugs in the same class or in patients who have demonstrated anaphylactic reactions to β-lactams. Before initiation of therapy with meropenem, careful inquiry should be made concerning previous hypersensitivity reactions to penicillins, cephalosporins, other β-lactams, and other allergens, because of the increased possibility of hypersensitivity.

Additional side effects/toxicities include phlebitis; fever; anaphylaxis; rash including Stevens-Johnson syndrome, erythema multiforme, and toxic epidermal necrolysis; angioedema; hypotension; seizures; encephalopathy; hearing loss; diarrhea; *Clostridium difficile*–associated diarrhea and pseudomembranous colitis; oral candidiasis; glossitis; anorexia; nausea; vomiting; stomach cramps; hepatitis; renal impairment; pyuria; hematuria; genital pruritis; dyspnea; polyarthralgia; prolonged prothrombin time; pancytopenia; positive Coombs' test; increased ALT (SGPT), AST (SGOT), alkaline phosphatase, bilirubin, and LDH; decreased serum sodium; and increased potassium and chloride.

DRUG INTERACTIONS/FOOD INTERACTIONS

Meropenem may reduce serum valproic acid concentrations; levels should be monitored.

It is not recommended that probenecid be given with meropenem.

DOSING

The recommended dosage of meropenem is 500 mg IV given every 8 hours for skin and skin structure infections and 1 g given every 8 hours for intraabdominal infections.

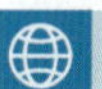

SPECIAL POPULATIONS

RENAL IMPAIRMENT:

CrCl Measurement or Hemodialysis	*Skin and Skin Structure Infections*	*Intraabdominal Infections*
26 mL/min to 50 mL/min	500 mg every 12 hours	1 g every 12 hours
10 mL/min to 25 mL/min	250 mg every 12 hours	500 mg every 12 hours
<10 mL/min	250 mg daily	500 mg daily
After hemodialysis or peritoneal dialysis	500 mg	500 mg
Continuous renal replacement therapy	1 g every 12 hours	1 g every 12 hours

Note: CrCl = Creatinine Clearance.

HEPATIC DYSFUNCTION: No dosage adjustment is necessary.

PEDIATRIC PATIENTS: The safety and effectiveness of meropenem have been established for pediatric patients aged 3 months and older; dosage is as follows:

- **Complicated skin and skin structure infections:** 10 mg/kg (up to 500 mg) every 8 hours
- **Intraabdominal infections:** 20 mg/kg (up to 1 g) every 8 hours
- **Meningitis:** 40 mg/kg (up to 2 g) every 8 hours

PREGNANCY: Category B.

BREASTFEEDING: Meropenem should be used with caution.

THE ART OF ANTIMICROBIAL THERAPY

Clinical Pearls:

1. Dosage of meropenem must be adjusted for patients with renal impairment.

2. Cross-allergy with penicillins is less than 10%.
3. Risk for seizures is greatest in patients with central nervous system disorders or renal dysfunction.
4. Meropenem is active against many organisms that produce extended-spectrum β-lactamases.

BASIC CHARACTERISTICS

Class: Nitroimidazole

Mechanism of Action: After entry into the bacteria, it is reduced into multiple products that are toxic to intracellular targets.

Mechanism of Resistance: Decreased pyruvate:ferredoxin oxidoreductase activity reduces uptake of the drug.

Metabolic Route: The major route of elimination of metronidazole and its metabolites is via the urine (60% to 80% of the dose), with fecal excretion accounting for 6% to 15% of the dose.

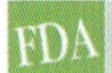

FDA-APPROVED INDICATIONS

FDA-Approved Indications:

Intravenous metronidazole: Treatment of susceptible anaerobic infections, including intraabdominal infections, skin and skin structure infections, gynecological infections, bacterial septicemia, bone and joint infections, central nervous system infections, lower respiratory tract infections, endocarditis, and surgical prophylaxis.

Oral metronidazole: Treatment of symptomatic trichomoniasis, asymptomatic trichomoniasis, treatment of asymptomatic consorts with trichomoniasis, amebiasis, anaerobic bacterial infections (often treated orally after initial IV therapy), intraabdominal infections, skin and skin structure infections, gynecological infections, bacterial septicemia, bone and joint infections, central nervous system infections, lower respiratory tract infections, and endocarditis.

Also Used for: *Clostridium difficile*–associated diarrhea; giardiasis; *Dientamoeba fragilis* infections; in combination with amoxicillin, clarithromycin, and a proton pump inhibitor for *Helicobacter pylori* infections; bacterial vaginosis; and bacterial overgrowth syndromes.

SIDE EFFECTS/TOXICITY

> **WARNING:** Metronidazole has been shown to be carcinogenic in animals.

Contraindicated in patients with a prior history of hypersensitivity to metronidazole or other nitroimidazole derivatives.

Side effects/toxicities include seizures, peripheral neuropathy, fever, thrombophlebitis, pruritus, rash, urticaria, flushing, nasal congestion, anorexia, furry tongue, glossitis, metallic taste, nausea, vomiting, abdominal discomfort, pancreatitis, diarrhea, headache, dizziness, syncope, vertigo, ataxia, confusion, incoordination, dysuria, cystitis, polyuria, incontinence, darkened urine, neutropenia, thrombocytopenia, flattening of the T-wave, and interference with laboratory determinations of AST, ALT, LDH, triglycerides, and glucose.

DRUG INTERACTIONS/FOOD INTERACTIONS

Metronidazole may potentiate the anticoagulant effect of warfarin and other oral coumarin anticoagulants.

Phenytoin or phenobarbital and other drugs that induce hepatic microsomal enzymes may accelerate the elimination of metronidazole.

Drugs that decrease hepatic microsomal enzyme activity, such as cimetidine, may prolong the half-life and decrease plasma clearance of metronidazole.

Alcoholic beverages should not be consumed during metronidazole therapy because abdominal cramps, nausea, vomiting, headaches, and flushing may occur.

Metronidazole should not be given to patients who have taken disulfiram within the past 2 weeks; psychotic reactions have been reported.

DOSING

Metronidazole is administered as 250-mg and 500-mg capsules. It is also administered intravenously.

Intravenous

Treatment of anaerobic infections: The recommended dosage is 15 mg/kg loading dose followed by 7.5 mg/kg every 6 hours, with a maximum of 4 g during a 24-hour period.

Surgical prophylaxis: 15 mg/kg followed by 7.5 mg/kg at 6 hours and 12 hours after the initial dose. The first dose should be administered 30 to 60 minutes before incision.

Oral

Trichomoniasis:

- 1-day treatment: 2 g as a single dose or in two divided doses of 1 g each given in the same day.
- 7-day course of treatment: 250 mg three times daily for 7 consecutive days.

Amebiasis:

- For acute intestinal amebiasis (acute amebic dysentery): 750 mg orally three times daily for 5 to 10 days.
- For amebic liver abscess: 500 mg or 750 mg orally three times daily for 5 to 10 days.

SPECIAL POPULATIONS

RENAL IMPAIRMENT:

CrCl Measurement or Hemodialysis	*Dosage*
≥ 10 mL/min	Usual dosage and intervals

<10 mL/min	Usual dosage every 8 hours (maximum)
Hemodialysis	Administer after dialysis only
Chronic ambulatory peritoneal dialysis	Usual dosage every 8 hours (maximum)
Continuous renal replacement therapy	Usual dosage and intervals

Note: CrCl = Creatinine Clearance.

HEPATIC DYSFUNCTION: Patients with severe hepatic disease metabolize metronidazole slowly, with resultant accumulation of metronidazole and its metabolites in the plasma. Accordingly, for such patients, dosages below those usually recommended should be administered cautiously. Close monitoring of plasma metronidazole levels and toxicity is recommended.

PEDIATRIC PATIENTS: 35 mg/kg to 50 mg/kg every 24 hours, divided into three doses.

PREGNANCY: Category B; should not be used in the first trimester to treat trichomoniasis. Otherwise, metronidazole should be used in pregnancy only if clearly needed.

BREASTFEEDING: Interruption of breastfeeding is recommended.

THE ART OF ANTIMICROBIAL THERAPY

Clinical Pearls

1. Patients should avoid ethanol when they are taking metronidazole.
2. Metronidazole should not be used in the first trimester of pregnancy.
3. Metronidazole has poor activity against anaerobic non–spore-forming gram-positive bacilli, e.g., *Bifidobacterium, Eubacterium, Actinomyces, Propionibacterium*, and *Lactobacillus.*
4. In a mixed aerobic and anaerobic infection, antimicrobials appropriate for the treatment of the aerobic infection and gram-positive anaerobes (see #3) should be used in addition to metronidazole.

BASIC CHARACTERISTICS

Class: Echinocandin

Mechanism of Action: Inhibits synthesis of 1,3-β-D-glucan, an essential component of fungal cell walls.

Mechanism of Resistance: Data incomplete.

Metabolic Route: Micafungin undergoes slow chemical degradation to multiple products with the majority of them excreted in the feces. It is not metabolized by the cytochrome P450 enzymes.

FDA-APPROVED INDICATIONS

FDA-Approved Indications: Treatment of candidemia, intraabdominal candidal infections, and esophageal candidiasis in HIV-infected patients; and prevention of fungal infections in patients undergoing hematopoietic transplantation.

SIDE EFFECTS/TOXICITY

Side effects/toxicities include possible histamine-related syndrome, characterized by rash, urticaria, flushing, and pruritus; injection-site reactions when administered through peripheral lines; fever; rash; erythema multiforme; nausea; vomiting; diarrhea; hepatitis with liver failure; renal failure; arrhythmia; arthralgia; seizure; encephalopathy; hyponatremia; hypokalemia; and pancytopenia.

DRUG INTERACTIONS

Patients receiving sirolimus, nifedipine, or itraconazole with micafungin should be monitored for toxicity attributable to sirolimus, nifedipine, or itraconazole; dosage reductions of these drugs may be necessary.

DOSING

Candidemia or intraabdominal candidiasis: 100 mg IV daily

Esophageal candidiasis: 150 mg IV daily

Prophylaxis for hematopoietic transplant recipients: 50 mg IV daily

SPECIAL POPULATIONS

RENAL IMPAIRMENT: There is no dosage adjustment needed.

HEPATIC IMPAIRMENT: No dosage adjustment is needed.

PEDIATRIC PATIENTS: Safety and dosing have not been studied in children.

PREGNANCY: Category C.

BREASTFEEDING: It is not known whether micafungin is secreted in human milk.

THE ART OF ANTIMICROBIAL THERAPY

Clinical Pearls

1. Echinocandins have activity only against *Candida* species and *Aspergillus* species.
2. Micafungin is active against all pathogenic *Candida* species, including those resistant to fluconazole.

MILTEFOSINE (Impavido and Miltex)

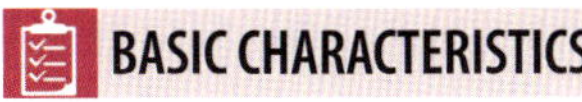

BASIC CHARACTERISTICS

Class: Alkylphospholipid

Mechanism of Action: Inhibits phosphocholine cytidylyl transferase resulting in interference of cellular membranes and cellular apoptosis.

Mechanism of Resistance: A single point mutation has been identified.

Metabolic Route: Unknown.

FDA-APPROVED INDICATIONS

Not FDA-approved, but used for treatment of visceral, cutaneous, and mucosal leishmaniasis.

SIDE EFFECTS/TOXICITY

Contraindications: pregnancy, lactation, and concurrent radiation therapy.

The main side effects/toxicities reported with miltefosine treatment are nausea and vomiting.

Also seen: hepatotoxicity, nephrotoxicity, QTc prolongation, leukocytosis, thrombocytosis, and retinal degeneration.

DRUG INTERACTIONS/FOOD INTERACTIONS

None known.

DOSING

Miltefosine is administered as 50-mg and 10-mg tablets. The usual dosage for leishmaniasis is 2.5 mg/kg in two divided doses daily for 28 days.

SPECIAL POPULATIONS

RENAL IMPAIRMENT: No dosage adjustment is needed.

HEPATIC DYSFUNCTION: No dosage adjustment is needed.

PEDIATRIC PATIENTS: The drug is not to be used in children aged younger than 2 years. In children aged 2 years and older, the dosage is 2.5 mg/kg divided in two doses daily.

PREGNANCY: Miltefosine should not be used in pregnancy.

BREASTFEEDING: Unknown.

THE ART OF ANTIMICROBIAL THERAPY

Clinical Pearls

1. Miltefosine is not available in the United States. It is available in Brazil, South America, India, Pakistan, and Afghanistan.
2. A negative pregnancy test before drug initiation and effective contraception during and for 2 months after treatment is recommended.

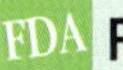 BASIC CHARACTERISTICS

Class: Tetracycline

Mechanism of Action: Reversibly bind the 30s ribosomal subunit preventing the addition of new amino acids into the growing peptide chain.

Mechanisms of Resistance: Decreased entry into the cell or increased excretion of the drug. Rarely, the tetracyclines are inactivated.

Metabolic Route: Minocycline is metabolized in the liver.

FDA FDA-APPROVED INDICATIONS

FDA-Approved Indications: Treatment of serious infections caused by susceptible strains of microorganisms in the following conditions: respiratory tract and skin and skin structure infections; Rocky Mountain spotted fever; typhus fever and the typhus group; Q fever, rickettsialpox, and tick fevers caused by *Rickettsiae*; *Mycoplasma pneumonia;* lymphogranuloma venereum; psittacosis; trachoma; inclusion conjunctivitis; nongonococcal urethritis; relapsing fever; chancroid; plague; tularemia; cholera; infections caused by *Campylobacter fetus;* brucellosis; bartonellosis; granuloma inguinale; syphilis; yaws; listeriosis; anthrax; actinomycosis; Vincent's infection; intestinal amebiasis; *Clostridium* infections; acne; gonococcal infections; syphilis; *Mycobacterium marinum;* and asymptomatic carriers of *Neisseria meningitidis.*

Also Used for: Treatment of community-acquired methicillin-resistant *Staphylococcus aureus,* nocardiosis, and rapidly-growing mycobacteria.

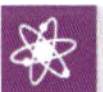 SIDE EFFECTS/TOXICITY

Minocycline is **contraindicated** in persons who have shown hypersensitivity to any of the tetracyclines.

Tetracyclines should not be used during pregnancy or in children under 8 years of age unless absolutely necessary and no reasonable alternative exists.

Side effects/toxicities include hypersensitivity reactions, including rash, anaphylaxis, and urticaria; angioneurotic edema; serum sickness; photosensitivity; lupuslike syndrome; nausea; vomiting; diarrhea; glossitis; esophagitis; hepatotoxicity; pseudomembranous colitis; renal failure; bulging fontanels in infants and benign intracranial hypertension in adults; vertigo; pseudotumor cerebri; tinnitus and decreased hearing; dosage-related rise in BUN; hemolytic anemia; thrombocytopenia; neutropenia; and eosinophilia.

 DRUG INTERACTIONS/FOOD INTERACTIONS

Minocycline hydrochloride tablets should be taken at least 1 hour before meals or 2 hours after meals.

Concurrent use of minocycline may render oral contraceptives less effective.

Patients who are on anticoagulant therapy may require downward adjustment of their anticoagulant dosage.

It is advisable to avoid giving tetracycline-class drugs in conjunction with penicillin.

Absorption of oral tetracyclines is impaired by antacids containing aluminum, calcium, or magnesium, and iron-containing preparations.

The concurrent use of minocycline and methoxyflurane has been reported to result in fatal renal toxicity.

Administration of isotretinoin should be avoided shortly before, during, and shortly after minocycline therapy. Each drug alone has been associated with pseudotumor cerebri.

DOSING

Minocycline is administered as 50-mg, 75-mg, and 100-mg tablets and capsules.

Usual dosage of minocycline is 200 mg initially followed by 100 mg every 12 hours.

Gonococcal urethritis: 100 mg every 12 hours for 5 days

Other gonococcal infections: 200 mg initially, followed by 100 mg every 12 hours for 4 days

Syphilis: usual dosage, over 10 to 15 days

Meningococcal carrier state: 100 mg every 12 hours for 5 days

***M marinum* infections:** 100 mg every 12 hours for 6 to 8 weeks

Chlamydial genitourinary infection: 100 mg every 12 hours for 7 days

SPECIAL POPULATIONS

RENAL IMPAIRMENT: No dosage adjustment is necessary.

HEPATIC DYSFUNCTION: Data insufficient.

PEDIATRIC PATIENTS: Above 8 years of age, 4 mg/kg initially followed by 2 mg/kg every 12 hours.

PREGNANCY: Category D.

BREASTFEEDING: Do not administer to breastfeeding mothers.

THE ART OF ANTIMICROBIAL THERAPY

Clinical Pearls

1. To reduce the risk of esophageal irritation and ulceration, tetracyclines should be taken with adequate amounts of fluid and should not be taken immediately before going to bed.

2. Minocycline can cause fetal harm when administered to a pregnant woman.
3. The use of drugs of the tetracycline class during tooth development (last half of pregnancy, infancy, and childhood to the age of 8 years) may cause permanent discoloration of the teeth (yellow-gray-brown).
4. Minocycline should not be administered with calcium or other cations.
5. Central nervous system side effects including light-headedness, dizziness, or vertigo have been reported with minocycline therapy. Patients who experience these symptoms should be cautioned about driving vehicles or using hazardous machinery while on minocycline therapy. These symptoms may disappear during therapy and usually disappear rapidly when the drug is discontinued.

MOXIFLOXACIN (Avelox)

BASIC CHARACTERISTICS

Class: Fluoroquinolone

Mechanism of Action: Inhibits bacterial topoisomerase IV and DNA gyrase.

Mechanisms of Resistance: Mutations in DNA gyrase and/or topoisomerase IV, or through altered efflux.

Metabolic Route: Moxifloxacin is metabolized via glucuronide and sulfate conjugation by the liver and the metabolites are excreted in the feces and urine.

FDA-APPROVED INDICATIONS

FDA-Approved Indications: Treatment of serious infections caused by susceptible strains of microorganisms in the following conditions: acute bacterial sinusitis, acute bacterial exacerbation of chronic bronchitis, community-acquired pneumonia, uncomplicated skin and skin structure infections, complicated intraabdominal infections, and complicated skin and skin structure infections.

Also Used for: Treatment of tuberculosis.

SIDE EFFECTS/TOXICITY

> **WARNING:** Fluoroquinolones, including moxifloxacin, are associated with an increased risk of **tendinitis and tendon rupture** in all ages. This risk is further increased in older patients usually aged older than 60 years, in patients taking corticosteroid drugs, and in patients with kidney, heart, or lung transplants.

Moxifloxacin is **contraindicated** in persons with a history of hypersensitivity associated with the use of moxifloxacin or any quinolone.

Other side effects/toxicities include anaphylactic reactions and allergic skin reactions including toxic epidermal necrolysis and Stevens-Johnson syndrome; photosensitivity; renal toxicity; hepatotoxicity (sometimes fatal); central nervous system effects including headache, dizziness, seizures, anxiety, confusion, depression, and insomnia (use with caution in patients at risk of seizures); peripheral neuropathy; nausea; diarrhea; constipation; *Clostridium difficile*–associated colitis; prolongation of the QT interval and torsade de pointes (avoid use in patients with known prolongation of QT, hypokalemia, and with other drugs that prolong the QT interval); and pancytopenia.

DRUG INTERACTIONS/FOOD INTERACTIONS

Moxifloxacin should be taken 4 hours before or 8 hours after antacids containing calcium, magnesium, or aluminum; sucralfate; divalent or trivalent cations such as iron; or multivitamins containing zinc.

The concomitant administration of a nonsteroidal antiinflammatory drug with a quinolone may increase the risk of central nervous system stimulation and seizures.

Disturbances of blood glucose, including hyperglycemia and hypoglycemia, may be seen in patients treated concurrently with antidiabetic agents.

DOSING

Moxifloxacin can be administered as 400-mg tablets or via intravenous injection.

Infection	*Dosage*	*Duration*
Acute bacterial sinusitis	400 mg every 24 hours	10 days
Acute exacerbation of chronic bronchitis	400 mg every 24 hours	5 days
Community-acquired pneumonia	400 mg every 24 hours	7 to 14 days
Uncomplicated skin and skin structure infections	400 mg every 24 hours	7 days
Complicated skin and skin structure infections	400 mg every 24 hours	7 to 21 days
Complicated intraabdominal infections[a]	400 mg every 24 hours	5 to 14 days

[a]For complicated intraabdominal infections, therapy should usually be initiated with the intravenous formulation.

SPECIAL POPULATIONS

RENAL IMPAIRMENT: No dosage adjustment is necessary.

HEPATIC DYSFUNCTION: No dosage adjustment is necessary.

PEDIATRIC PATIENTS: Safety and efficacy in patients aged younger than 18 years have not been established.

PREGNANCY: Category C.

BREASTFEEDING: Moxifloxacin should not be administered to breastfeeding mothers.

THE ART OF ANTIMICROBIAL THERAPY

Clinical Pearls

1. Moxifloxacin should be given at least 4 hours before or 8 hours after ingestion of cations.
2. All fluoroquinolones can cause tendon rupture, especially in patients aged older than 60 years.

3. Caution should be used when moxifloxacin is given with medications that affect QT intervals.
4. All fluoroquinolones can cause phototoxicity.
5. All fluoroquinolones can cause seizures.
6. Moxifloxacin should be avoided if possible in children, pregnant women, and breastfeeding mothers because of concerns for cartilage developmental problems.
7. Moxifloxacin has activity against mycobacteria; therefore, moxifloxacin monotherapy (e.g., for community-acquired pneumonia) should be avoided if mycobacterial infection is possible.
8. Treatment of gonorrhea with fluoroquinolones should be undertaken with caution because of rising resistance.
9. Moxifloxacin is not indicated for urinary tract infections.
10. Unlike the other fluoroquinolones, moxifloxacin has significant activity against gram-negative anaerobes.

 BASIC CHARACTERISTICS

Class: Semisynthetic penicillin

Mechanism of Action: Binds penicillin-binding protein (PBP), disrupting cell wall synthesis.

Mechanisms of Resistance:

1. The PBP can be altered, with reduced affinity,
2. production of a β-lactamase resulting in hydrolysis of the β-lactam ring, and
3. decreased ability of the antibiotic to reach the PBP when bacteria decrease porin production, resulting in a decrease of the drug concentration within the cell.

Metabolic Route: The majority of nafcillin is inactivated by the liver and excreted in the bile. The remaining 30% is excreted unchanged in the urine.

FDA-APPROVED INDICATIONS

FDA-Approved Indications: Treatment of infections caused by susceptible penicillinase-producing staphylococci.

 SIDE EFFECTS/TOXICITY

A history of allergic reaction to any of the penicillins is a **contraindication.**

Side effects/toxicities include *Clostridium difficile*–associated diarrhea; interstitial nephritis including rash, fever, eosinophilia, hematuria, proteinuria, and renal insufficiency; thrombophlebitis; hypersensitivity reactions including rash, erythema multiforme, and Stevens-Johnson syndrome; hepatitis; nausea; vomiting; diarrhea; stomatitis; black or hairy tongue; hyperactivity and seizures; anemia; thrombocytopenia; neutropenia; and eosinophilia.

DRUG INTERACTIONS/FOOD INTERACTIONS

Chloramphenicol, macrolides, sulfonamides, and tetracyclines may interfere with the bactericidal effects of penicillins.

When nafcillin and warfarin are used concomitantly, the prothrombin time should be closely monitored.

When cyclosporine and nafcillin are used concomitantly in organ transplant patients, the cyclosporine levels should be monitored.

High urine concentrations of nafcillin may result in false-positive reactions when one is testing for the presence of glucose in urine with Clinitest. It is recommended that glucose tests based on enzymatic glucose oxidase reactions (such as Clinistix) be used instead. Nafcillin may cause false-positive urine reaction for protein.

DOSING

The usual intravenous dosage for adults is 500 mg every 4 hours.

For severe infections, 1 g every 4 hours is recommended.

SPECIAL POPULATIONS

RENAL IMPAIRMENT: No dosage adjustment is necessary.

HEPATIC DYSFUNCTION: No dosage adjustment is necessary.

COMBINED RENAL AND HEPATIC INSUFFICIENCY: Measurement of nafcillin serum levels should be performed and dosage adjusted accordingly.

PEDIATRIC PATIENTS: Safety and effectiveness in pediatric patients have not been established.

PREGNANCY: Category B.

BREASTFEEDING: Nafcillin should be used only with caution in breastfeeding mothers.

THE ART OF ANTIMICROBIAL THERAPY

Clinical Pearls

1. Nafcillin does not need dosage adjustment for patients with renal dysfunction.
2. Occasional skin sloughing at the injection site has been reported.
3. Nafcillin should be used with caution in patients with both renal and hepatic insufficiency.

NELFINAVIR (Viracept)

BASIC CHARACTERISTICS

Class: Protease inhibitor

Mechanism of Action: Reversibly binds the active site of the enzyme protease. Inhibition of protease prevents cleavage of the *gag* and *gag-pol* polyprotein resulting in the production of immature, noninfectious virus.

Mechanism of Resistance: Development of mutations on the enzyme protease causes a conformational change that prevents nelfinavir from binding the active site, allowing protease activity to continue. The most frequent resistance mutations include D30N and L90M.

Metabolic Route: Numerous oxidative metabolites and unchanged nelfinavir are excreted in the feces.

FDA-APPROVED INDICATIONS

FDA-Approved Indications: Treatment of HIV-1 in combinations with other antiretroviral agents

SIDE EFFECTS/TOXICITY

The most common side effect is diarrhea. Additional side effects/toxicities include new-onset diabetes mellitus; exacerbation of preexisting diabetes mellitus; hyperglycemia; increased bleeding, including spontaneous skin hematomas and hemarthrosis, in patients with hemophilia type A or B; redistribution/accumulation of body fat including central obesity, dorsocervical fat enlargement (buffalo hump), peripheral wasting, facial wasting, and breast enlargement; cushingoid appearance; immune reconstitution syndrome; QTc prolongation; torsade de pointes; abdominal pain; headache; anorexia; dyspepsia; epigastric pain; hepatitis; mouth ulceration; pancreatitis; vomiting; anemia; leukopenia; thrombocytopenia; increases in alkaline phosphatase, amylase, creatine phosphokinase, lactic dehydrogenase, SGOT, SGPT, and gamma glutamyl transpeptidase; hyperlipemia; hyperuricemia; hypoglycemia; and dehydration.

DRUG INTERACTIONS/FOOD INTERACTIONS

Nelfinavir should be taken with a meal.

Patients with phenylketonuria: nelfinavir oral powder contains 11.2 mg phenylalanine per gram of powder.

Drugs that **should not be coadministered** with nelfinavir include amiodarone, quinidine, rifampin, ergot derivatives, Saint-John's-wort, pimozide, proton pump inhibitors, benzodiazepines, and simvastatin or lovastatin.

Nelfinavir is an inhibitor of the CYP3A enzyme; coadministration of nelfinavir and drugs primarily metabolized by CYP3A may result in increased plasma concentrations of the other drug that could increase or prolong its therapeutic and adverse effects.

Nelfinavir is metabolized by CYP3A and CYP2C19; coadministration of nelfinavir and drugs that induce CYP3A or CYP2C19 may decrease nelfinavir plasma concentrations and reduce its therapeutic effect. Coadministration of nelfinavir and drugs that inhibit CYP3A or CYP2C19 may increase nelfinavir plasma concentrations. Because of these metabolic affects, potential drug interactions that may require dosage change or clinical/laboratory monitoring are listed:

Medication	*Adjustment or Action*
Itraconazole	Monitor for toxicity
Voriconazole	Monitor for toxicity
Rifabutin	Decrease rifabutin to 150 mg every other day or 300 mg three times per week
Hormonal contraceptives	Use alternative or additional method
Atorvastatin	Use lowest possible dosage with close monitoring
Phenobarbital, phenytoin, or carbamazepine	Monitor anticonvulsant level; consider alternative
Methadone	Monitor; may require higher methadone dosage
Sildenafil	25 mg every 48 hours
Tadalafil	5 mg, no more than 10 mg in 72 hours
Vardenafil	No more than 2.5 mg in 24 hours

DOSING

The recommended dosage is 1250 mg (five 250-mg tablets or two 625-mg tablets) twice daily or 750 mg (three 250-mg tablets) three times daily. Patients unable to swallow the 250-mg or 625-mg tablets may dissolve the tablets in a small amount of water. Once the tablets are dissolved, patients should mix the cloudy liquid well, and consume it immediately. The glass should be rinsed with water and the rinse swallowed to ensure that the entire dose is consumed.

SPECIAL POPULATIONS

RENAL IMPAIRMENT: There is no dosage adjustment needed.

HEPATIC DYSFUNCTION: In patients with known or suspected history of hepatitis B or C infection and in patients treated with other medications associated with liver toxicity, monitoring of liver enzymes is recommended.

PEDIATRIC PATIENTS: In children aged 2 years and older, the recommended oral dose of nelfinavir is 45 mg/kg to 55 mg/kg twice daily or 25 mg/kg to 35 mg/kg three times daily. All doses should be taken with a meal.

PREGNANCY: Category B.

BREASTFEEDING: It is recommended that HIV-positive mothers not breastfeed their children, to decrease mother-to-child transmission of HIV.

THE ART OF ANTIMICROBIAL THERAPY

Clinical Pearls

1. Nelfinavir should always be used in combination with other antiretrovirals.
2. Nelfinavir should be taken with food to increase absorption and to decrease diarrhea.
3. Whenever initiating nelfinavir, one should make sure to review all medications the patient is receiving to make sure drug interactions are limited.

NEOMYCIN (Neo-Fradin)

BASIC CHARACTERISTICS

Class: Poorly absorbed oral aminoglycoside

Mechanism of Action: Inhibits the synthesis of protein in susceptible bacterial cells.

Metabolic Route: Neomycin is poorly absorbed and is excreted in the feces.

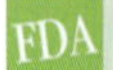

FDA-APPROVED INDICATIONS

FDA-Approved Indications: Treatment of hepatic coma.

Also Used for: Suppression of intestinal bacteria in preoperative bowel preparation.

SIDE EFFECTS/TOXICITY

Warning: Systemic absorption of neomycin occurs following oral administration, and toxic reactions may occur, including **neurotoxicity, ototoxicity,** and **nephrotoxicity.** Serial vestibular and audiometric tests, as well as tests of renal function, should be performed.

The risk of toxicity is greater in patients with impaired renal function, advanced age, and dehydration. **Neuromuscular blockade** and respiratory paralysis have been reported, especially in patients receiving anesthetics, neuromuscular blocking agents such as tubocurarine, succinylcholine, decamethonium, or in patients receiving massive transfusions of citrate anticoagulated blood. If blockage occurs, calcium salts may reverse these phenomena, but mechanical respiratory assistance may be necessary.

Concurrent and/or sequential systemic, oral, or topical use of other aminoglycosides including paromomycin and other potentially nephrotoxic and/or neurotoxic drugs such as bacitracin, cisplatin, vancomycin, amphotericin B, polymyxin B, colistin, and viomycin should be avoided because the toxicity may be additive.

The concurrent use of neomycin with potent diuretics such as ethacrynic acid or furosemide should be avoided since certain diuretics by themselves may cause ototoxicity. In addition, when administered intravenously, diuretics may enhance neomycin toxicity by altering the antibiotic concentration in serum and tissue.

Contraindicated

1. in the presence of intestinal obstruction.
2. in individuals with a history of hypersensitivity to the drug.
3. in patients with a history of hypersensitivity to other aminoglycosides, and
4. in patients with inflammatory or ulcerative gastrointestinal disease.

Side effects/toxicities include: numbness, skin tingling, muscle twitching, convulsions, nausea, vomiting, diarrhea, nephrotoxicity, ototoxicity, neuromuscular blockade, and malabsorption.

DRUG INTERACTIONS/FOOD INTERACTIONS

Caution should be taken in concurrent or serial use of other neurotoxic and/or nephrotoxic drugs including aminoglycosides and polymyxins.

Oral neomycin inhibits the gastrointestinal absorption of penicillin V, oral vitamin B12, methotrexate, 5-fluorouracil, and digoxin.

Oral neomycin sulfate may enhance the effect of coumarin anticoagulants by decreasing vitamin K availability.

DOSING

Neomycin sulfate is supplied as 500-mg tablets or as an oral solution (Neo-Fradin) containing 125 mg/mL.

Hepatic coma: the recommended dosage is 4 g to 12 g per day given in divided doses

Preoperative prophylaxis for elective colorectal surgery: Neomycin sulfate 1 g and erythromycin base 1 g orally three times the day before surgery

SPECIAL POPULATIONS

RENAL IMPAIRMENT: No dosage adjustment is necessary.

HEPATIC DYSFUNCTION: No dosage adjustment is necessary.

PEDIATRIC PATIENTS: The safety and efficacy of oral neomycin sulfate in patients aged younger than 18 years have not been established. If treatment of a patient aged younger than 18 years is necessary, neomycin should be used with caution and the period of treatment should not exceed 2 weeks because of absorption from the gastrointestinal tract.

PREGNANCY: Category D.

BREASTFEEDING : A decision should be made whether to discontinue breastfeeding or to discontinue the drug, taking into account the importance of the drug to the mother.

THE ART OF ANTIMICROBIAL THERAPY

Clinical Pearls

1. Small amounts of orally administered neomycin are absorbed through intact intestinal mucosa.
2. Neomycin irrigation of absorptive surfaces (e.g., pleura) has resulted in systemic absorption and neurotoxicity.

NEVIRAPINE (Viramune)

BASIC CHARACTERISTICS

Class: Nonnucleoside reverse transcriptase inhibitor

Mechanism of Action: Inhibits reverse transcriptase activity by binding the enzyme.

Mechanism of Resistance: Changes in the structure of reverse transcriptase lead to the inability of nevirapine to bind the enzyme and allow transcription to continue. The most frequent resistance mutations include K103N and Y181C.

Metabolic Route: Nevirapine is metabolized by the cytochrome P450 system to hydroxylated metabolites.

FDA-APPROVED INDICATIONS

FDA-Approved Indications: Treatment of HIV-1 in combinations with other antiretroviral agents.

SIDE EFFECTS/TOXICITY

WARNING: Severe, life-threatening, and in some cases fatal **hepatotoxicity,** particularly in the first 18 weeks, has been reported in patients treated with nevirapine. These events are often associated with rash. Women with CD4 counts greater than 250 cells/mm^3, including pregnant women, are at the greatest risk. However, hepatotoxicity associated with nevirapine use can occur in both genders, all CD4 counts, and at any time during treatment. Patients with signs or symptoms of hepatitis, or with increased transaminases combined with rash or other systemic symptoms, must discontinue nevirapine and seek medical evaluation immediately. Severe, life-threatening **skin reactions**, including fatal cases, have occurred in patients treated with nevirapine. These have included cases of Stevens-Johnson syndrome, toxic epidermal necrolysis, and hypersensitivity reactions characterized by rash, constitutional findings, and organ dysfunction. Patients developing signs or symptoms of severe skin reactions or hypersensitivity reactions must discontinue nevirapine and seek medical evaluation immediately. Transaminase levels should be checked immediately for all patients who develop a rash in the first 18 weeks of treatment. Patients must be monitored intensively during the first 18 weeks of therapy with nevirapine to detect potentially life-threatening hepatotoxicity or skin reactions. Extra vigilance is warranted during the first 6 weeks of therapy, which is the period of greatest risk of these events. Do not restart nevirapine following severe hepatic, skin, or hypersensitivity reactions. In some cases, hepatic injury has progressed despite discontinuation of treatment.

Other **side effects/toxicities** include elevated cholesterol, fat redistribution, immune reconstitution syndrome, fever, anemia, neutropenia, rhabdomyolysis, and paresthesias.

 DRUG INTERACTIONS/FOOD INTERACTIONS

Food has no significant effect on nevirapine.

Nevirapine should not be administered concurrently with astemizole, bepridil, cisapride, midazolam, pimozide, triazolam, ketoconazole, ergot derivatives, Saint-John's-wort, atazanavir, or etravirine.

Nevirapine is principally metabolized by the liver via the cytochrome P450 isoenzymes, 3A4 and 2B6. Nevirapine causes hepatic enzyme induction of CYP3A4; coadministration of nevirapine with drugs primarily metabolized by 3A4 and 2B6 isozymes may result in altered plasma concentrations of the coadministered drug; Drugs that induce CYP3A4 activity would be expected to increase the clearance of nevirapine resulting in lowered plasma concentrations. Because of these metabolic activities, the following drug interactions warrant consideration of dosage adjustment and monitoring of clinical effects and serum levels of affected drugs:

Medication	*Adjustment or Action*
Fluconazole	Risk of hepatotoxicity; monitor for toxicity
Voriconazole	Monitor for toxicity
Clarithromycin	Consider alternative agent to clarithromycin
Rifampin	Use rifabutin and monitor for rifabutin toxicity
Hormonal contraceptives	Use alternative or additional method
Methadone	Opiate withdrawal common; titrate methadone
Indinavir	Indinavir 1000 mg every 8 hours plus ritonavir 100 mg twice a day
Lopinavir/ritonavir	Use 600 mg/ 150 mg lopinavir/ritonavir twice a day
Warfarin	Monitor warfarin effect

In addition, **potential** drug interactions warrant monitoring for decreased effects of the following when given with nevirapine: antiarrhythmics, anticonvulsants, calcium channel blockers, immunosuppressants, and cancer chemotherapeutic agents.

 DOSING

Nevirapine is administered in 200-mg tablets and a white oral suspension containing 50 mg nevirapine in each 5 mL. The recommended dosage for nevirapine is one 200-mg tablet daily for the first 14 days, followed by one 200-mg tablet twice daily, in combination with other antiretroviral agents.

SPECIAL POPULATIONS

RENAL IMPAIRMENT: There is no dosage adjustment needed.

HEPATIC DYSFUNCTION: Nevirapine is contraindicated in patients with moderate or severe (Child Pugh class B or C, respectively) hepatic impairment.

PEDIATRIC PATIENTS : The recommended oral dosage for patients aged 15 days and older is 150 mg/m^2 once daily for 14 days followed by 150 mg/m^2 twice daily thereafter. The total daily dose should not exceed 400 mg for any patient. Body surface area may be calculated with the Mosteller formula.

PREGNANCY: Category B.

BREASTFEEDING: It is recommended that HIV-positive mothers not breastfeed their children, to decrease mother-to-child transmission of HIV.

THE ART OF ANTIMICROBIAL THERAPY

Clinical Pearls

1. Nevirapine should always be used in combination with other antiretrovirals.
2. Nevirapine should not be initiated in women with CD4 counts greater than 250 cells/mm^3 or men with CD4 counts greater than 400 cells/mm^3.
3. Patients must be monitored intensively during the first 18 weeks of therapy with nevirapine to detect potentially life-threatening hepatotoxicity or skin reactions.
4. Nevirapine has a very long half-life. If a patient is stopping an antiretroviral regimen, to decrease resistance, the other medications should be continued for at least another 48 hours.
5. Whenever initiating nevirapine, one should make sure to review all medications the patient is receiving, to limit drug interactions.

BASIC CHARACTERISTICS

Class: Salicylanilide

Mechanism of Action: Blocks the uptake of glucose by intestinal tapeworms resulting in the tapeworms' death.

Metabolic Route: Minimal absorption occurs.

FDA-APPROVED INDICATIONS

Not FDA-approved, but effective against intestinal tapeworms including *Taenia saginata, Taenia solium, Diphyllobothrium latum*, and *Hymenolepis nana.*

SIDE EFFECTS/TOXICITY

Side effects/toxicities include nausea, vomiting, diarrhea, light-headedness, malaise, and pruritus.

DRUG INTERACTIONS/FOOD INTERACTIONS

Alcohol should be avoided when one is taking this drug—it increases niclosamide absorption, increasing the risk of side effects.

DOSING

***Taenia* and *Diphyllobothrium* infections**: A single 2-gram dose should be used. The tablets should be thoroughly chewed and washed down with a small amount of water.

H nana: 2 grams on first day followed by 1 gram daily for 6 days.

SPECIAL POPULATIONS

RENAL IMPAIRMENT: No data available.

HEPATIC DYSFUNCTION: No data available.

PEDIATRIC PATIENTS: Children weighing 10 kg to 35 kg are given a single dose of 1 g orally. Those weighing less than 10 kg are given a single dose of 0.5 g orally. The tablet should be crushed and then mixed with water.

PREGNANCY: Niclosamide may be used in pregnancy.

BREASTFEEDING: Unknown.

THE ART OF ANTIMICROBIAL THERAPY

Clinical Pearls

1. Niclosamide is not available commercially in the United States. It may be obtained from a compounding pharmacy through the National Association of

Compounding Pharmacies (800-687-7850) or Professional Compounding Centers of America: http://www.pccarx.com.

2. Niclosamide is not active against the larval form of *T solium* (cysticercosis), because it is poorly absorbed.
3. Niclosamide should be chewed thoroughly before swallowing.
4. For children, the pill should be crushed and mixed with water.

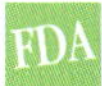

BASIC CHARACTERISTICS

Class: Nitrofuran derivative

Mechanism of Action: Forms nitro anion radicals resulting in decreased protein and nucleic acid synthesis, breakage of DNA, and inhibition of growth of the parasite.

Metabolic Route: Data incomplete.

FDA-APPROVED INDICATIONS

Not FDA-approved, but used for treatment of *Trypanosoma cruzi* infections.

SIDE EFFECTS/TOXICITY

Side effects/toxicities include nausea, vomiting, abdominal pain, anorexia, insomnia, twitching, paresthesias, disorientation, seizures, and rash.

DRUG INTERACTIONS/FOOD INTERACTIONS

Unknown.

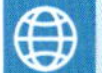

DOSING

Administered as 30 mg and 120-mg tablets.

Treatment is 8 mg/kg to 10 mg/kg daily in four divided doses for 90 to 120 days.

SPECIAL POPULATIONS

RENAL IMPAIRMENT: Should not be administered.

HEPATIC DYSFUNCTION: Should not be administered.

PEDIATRIC PATIENTS: For children aged 1 to 10 years, the dosage is 15 mg/kg to 20 mg/kg per day in four divided doses for 90 to 120 days.

For adolescents, the daily dosage is 12.5 mg/kg to 15 mg/kg daily in four divided doses for 90 to 120 days.

PREGNANCY: Should not be administered.

BREASTFEEDING: Should not be administered.

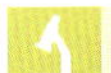

THE ART OF ANTIMICROBIAL THERAPY

Clinical Pearls

1. Nifurtimox may be obtained in the United States from the Centers for Disease Control and Prevention Parasitic Diseases Drug Service, 770-488-7775.
2. The clinical efficacy of nifurtimox is limited, especially with chronic *T. cruzi* infection, which has only a 20% parasitologic cure rate.

NITAZOXANIDE (Alinia)

BASIC CHARACTERISTICS

Class: Nitrothiazolyl-salicylamide

Mechanism of Action: Inhibits pyruvate ferredoxin oxidoreductase in protozoa.

Metabolic Route: One third of the administered dose is excreted in the urine and two thirds in the feces.

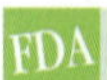

FDA-APPROVED INDICATIONS

FDA-Approved Indications: Nitazoxanide for oral suspension (patients aged 1 year and older) and tablets (patients aged 12 years and older) are indicated for the treatment of diarrhea caused by *Giardia lamblia* or *Cryptosporidium parvum.*

Also Used for: *Entamoeba histolytica, Cyclospora cayetanensis, Trichomonas vaginalis, Encephalitozoon intestinalis, Isospora belli, Blastocystis hominis, Balantidium coli, Enterocytozoon bieneusi, Ascaris lumbricoides, Trichuris trichiura, Taenia saginata, Hymenolepis nana,* and *Fasciola hepatica.*

SIDE EFFECTS/TOXICITY

Side effects/toxicities include nausea, vomiting, diarrhea, and abdominal pain.

DRUG INTERACTIONS/FOOD INTERACTIONS

Food will increase the absorption of nitazoxanide.

DOSING

Treatment with nitazoxanide of diarrhea caused by *G lamblia* or *C parvum:*

Age of Patient	*Dosage*	*Duration*
1 to 3 years	5 mL (100 mg) every 12 hours with food	3 days
4 to 11 years	10 mL (200 mg) every 12 hours with food	3 days
≥ 12 years	1 tablet (500 mg) every 12 hours with food or 25 mL (500 mg) every 12 hours with food	3 days

SPECIAL POPULATIONS

RENAL IMPAIRMENT: No dosage adjustment is necessary.

HEPATIC DYSFUNCTION: No dosage adjustment is necessary.

PEDIATRIC PATIENTS: See table in "Dosing" section.

PREGNANCY: This drug has not been studied in pregnant women so caution is advised.

BREASTFEEDING: It is not known whether nitazoxanide passes into breastmilk.

THE ART OF ANTIMICROBIAL THERAPY

Clinical Pearl

Nitazoxanide has not been shown to be superior to placebo for the treatment of diarrhea caused by *C. parvum* in HIV-infected or immunodeficient patients.

NITROFURANTOIN (Furadantin, Macrobid, Macrodantin)

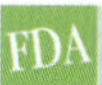

BASIC CHARACTERISTICS

Class: Imidazolidinedione

Mechanism of Action: Nitrofurantoin is reduced by bacterial flavoproteins to reactive intermediates that inactivate or alter bacterial ribosomal proteins and other macromolecules.

Mechanism of Resistance: Development of resistance to nitrofurantoin has not been a significant problem.

Metabolic Route: Nitrofurantoin is excreted in the urine.

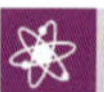

FDA-APPROVED INDICATIONS

FDA-Approved Indications: Treatment of urinary tract infections (not pyelonephritis) caused by susceptible bacteria.

SIDE EFFECTS/TOXICITY

Contraindications: hypersensitivity to nitrofurantoin, history of hepatotoxicity from nitrofurantoin, anuria, oliguria, creatinine clearance less than 60 mL/min, pregnancy at term, and in neonates aged younger than 1 month.

Side effects/toxicities include hypersensitivity with fever and rash; exfoliative dermatitis and erythema multiforme; acute, subacute, or chronic pulmonary reactions with consolidation, pleural effusion, diffuse interstitial pneumonitis, or pulmonary fibrosis; nausea; vomiting; hepatitis; jaundice; pancreatitis; *Clostridium difficile*–associated diarrhea; changes in electrocardiograms; peripheral neuropathy; optic neuritis; vertigo; nystagmus; headache; benign intracranial hypertension (pseudotumor cerebri); confusion; depression; psychosis; sialadenitis; lupuslike syndrome; leukopenia; thrombocytopenia; megaloblastic anemia; hemolytic anemia in G6PDH-deficient patients; and cyanosis secondary to methemoglobinemia.

DRUG INTERACTIONS/FOOD INTERACTIONS

Nitrofurantoin should be given with food to improve absorption.

Antacids containing magnesium trisilicate should not be administered with nitrofurantoin.

Probenecid and sulfinpyrazone can inhibit secretion of nitrofurantoin.

A false-positive reaction for glucose in the urine may occur with Benedict's and Fehling's solutions but not with the glucose enzymatic test.

DOSING

Furadantin is available in a 25 mg/5 mL liquid suspension and the usual dosage is 50 mg to 100 mg four times a day for 7 days.

Macrobid is available as 100-mg capsules and the usual dosage is 100 mg every 12 hours for 7 days.

Macrodantin is available in 25-mg, 50-mg, and 100-mg capsules and the usual dosage is 50 mg to 100 mg four times a day for 7 days.

SPECIAL POPULATIONS

RENAL IMPAIRMENT: Do not administer if creatinine clearance is less than 60 mL/min.

HEPATIC DYSFUNCTION: Monitor liver function tests.

PEDIATRIC PATIENTS: Safety and effectiveness of nitrofurantoin in neonates aged younger than 1 month have not been established.

The usual dosage of **furadantin** and **macrodantin** is 5 mg/kg to 7 mg/kg of body weight per 24 hours, given in four divided doses for 7 days.

Macrobid is indicated in patients older than 12 years and the dosage is similar to that for adults: 100 mg twice daily for 7 days.

PREGNANCY: Category B.

BREASTFEEDING: Nitrofurantoin should not be administered to the breastfeeding mother.

THE ART OF ANTIMICROBIAL THERAPY

Clinical Pearls

1. Nitrofurantoin is most consistently active against *Escherichia coli*; it is not active against most strains of *Proteus* or *Serratia* species and has no activity against *Pseudomonas* species.
2. Antagonism has been demonstrated in vitro between nitrofurantoin and quinolone antimicrobial agents.
3. Nitrofurantoin is not indicated for the treatment of pyelonephritis or any systemic infections.
4. Nitrofurantoin can cause pulmonary fibrosis, especially if given for long durations of time.
5. Nitrofurantoin should be administered with food.
6. The different formulations of nitrofurantoin have different dosage recommendations and are absorbed differently; therefore, they are not interchangeable.

NORFLOXACIN (Noroxin)

BASIC CHARACTERISTICS

Class: Fluoroquinolone

Mechanism of Action: Inhibits bacterial topoisomerase IV and DNA gyrase.

Mechanisms of Resistance: Mutations in DNA gyrase and/or topoisomerase IV; or through altered efflux.

Metabolic Route: Norfloxacin is eliminated through metabolism, biliary excretion, and renal excretion.

FDA-APPROVED INDICATIONS

FDA-Approved Indications: Treatment of serious infections caused by susceptible strains of microorganisms in urinary tract infections, uncomplicated urethral and cervical gonorrhea, and prostatitis.

SIDE EFFECTS/TOXICITY

> **WARNING:** Fluoroquinolones, including norfloxacin, are associated with an increased risk of **tendinitis and tendon rupture** in all ages. This risk is further increased in older patients, usually aged older than 60 years, in patients taking corticosteroid drugs, and in patients with kidney, heart, or lung transplants.

Contraindicated in persons with a history of hypersensitivity, tendinitis, or tendon rupture associated with the use of norfloxacin or any of the quinolones.

Other side effects/toxicities include anaphylactic reactions with cardiovascular collapse; angioedema; allergic skin reactions including toxic epidermal necrolysis and Stevens-Johnson syndrome; photosensitivity; renal toxicity; hepatotoxicity (sometimes fatal); central nervous system effects including headache, dizziness, seizures, anxiety, confusion, depression, and insomnia (use with caution in patients at risk of seizures); peripheral neuropathy; nausea; diarrhea; onstipation; *Clostridium difficile*–associated colitis; prolongation of the QT interval and torsade de pointes (avoid use in patients with known prolongation of QT, hypokalemia, and with other drugs that prolong the QT interval); pancytopenia; hemolysis in patients with G6PD deficiency; and exacerbations of myasthenia gravis.

DRUG INTERACTIONS/FOOD INTERACTIONS

Antacids containing calcium, magnesium, or aluminum; sucralfate; divalent or trivalent cations such as iron; or multivitamins containing zinc should not be taken within the 2-hour period before or within the 2-hour period after taking norfloxacin.

Cimetidine results in significant increases in half-life of some quinolones.

Most quinolone antimicrobial drugs inhibit cytochrome P450 enzyme activity to varying degrees. Because of this inhibition, norfloxacin may produce increased drug concentrations of concomitantly administered caffeine, clozapine, ropinirole, tacrine, theophylline, tizanidine, cyclosporine, and warfarin.

The concomitant administration of a nonsteroidal antiinflammatory drug with a quinolone may increase the risk of central nervous system stimulation and convulsive seizures.

The concomitant use of probenecid with quinolones decreases renal tubular secretion.

Disturbances of blood glucose may be seen, including hyperglycemia and hypoglycemia, in patients treated concurrently with quinolones and antidiabetic agents.

Concomitant administration of nitrofurantoin may antagonize the effect of norfloxacin in the urinary tract.

DOSING

Norfloxacin is administered as 400-mg capsules.

Infection	*Dosage*	*Duration*
Cystitis	400 mg every 12 hours	3 days
Uncomplicated urinary tract infections	400 mg every12 hours	7 to 10 days
Complicated urinary tract infections	400 mg every 12 hours	10 to 21 days
Uncomplicated gonorrhea	800 mg for one dose	1 day
Acute or chronic prostatitis	400 mg every 12 hours	28 days

SPECIAL POPULATIONS

RENAL IMPAIRMENT: If creatinine clearance is less than 30 mL/min, 400 mg daily should be administered.

HEPATIC DYSFUNCTION: A maximum dosage of 400 mg of norfloxacin per day should not be exceeded.

PEDIATRIC PATIENTS: Safety and efficacy in patients aged younger than 18 years have not yet been established.

PREGNANCY: Category C.

BREASTFEEDING: Norfloxacin should not be administered to breastfeeding mothers.

THE ART OF ANTIMICROBIAL THERAPY

Clinical Pearls

1. Norfloxacin should be given at least 2 hours separately from cations.
2. All fluoroquinolones can lead to tendon rupture, especially patients aged older than 60 years.
3. All fluoroquinolones can prolong QT intervals and caution should be used when they are given with medications that affect QT intervals.
4. All fluoroquinolones can cause phototoxicity
5. All fluoroquinolones can lower seizure threshold.
6. Fluoroquinolones should be avoided in children, pregnant women, and nursing mothers because of possible disturbance in cartilage development.
7. Treatment of gonorrhea with fluoroquinolones should be undertaken with caution because of rising resistance.

OFLOXACIN (Floxin)

BASIC CHARACTERISTICS

Class: Fluoroquinolone

Mechanism of Action: Inhibits bacterial topoisomerase IV and DNA gyrase.

Mechanisms of Resistance: Mutations in DNA gyrase and/or topoisomerase IV, or through altered efflux.

Metabolic Route: Ofloxacin is predominantly excreted in the urine.

FDA-APPROVED INDICATIONS

FDA-Approved Indications: Treatment of the following serious infections caused by susceptible strains of microorganisms: acute bacterial exacerbations of chronic bronchitis, community-acquired pneumonia, uncomplicated skin and skin structure infections, acute uncomplicated urethral and cervical gonorrhea, nongonococcal urethritis and cervicitis, mixed infections of the urethra and cervix, acute pelvic inflammatory disease, uncomplicated cystitis, complicated urinary tract infections, and prostatitis.

SIDE EFFECTS/TOXICITY

Although ofloxacin does not have a boxed warning, other fluoroquinolones are associated with an increased risk of **tendinitis and tendon rupture** in all ages. This risk is further increased in older patients, usually aged older than 60 years, in patients taking corticosteroid drugs, and in patients with kidney, heart, or lung transplants.

Ofloxacin is **contraindicated** in persons with a history of hypersensitivity associated with the use of ofloxacin or any quinolone.

Other side effects/toxicities include anaphylactic reactions and allergic skin reactions including toxic epidermal necrolysis and Stevens-Johnson syndrome; photosensitivity; renal toxicity; hepatotoxicity (sometimes fatal); central nervous system effects including headache, dizziness, seizures, anxiety, confusion, depression, and insomnia (use with caution in patients at risk of seizures); peripheral neuropathy; nausea; diarrhea; constipation; *Clostridium difficile*–associated colitis; prolongation of the QT interval and torsade de pointes (avoid use in patients with known prolongation of QT, hypokalemia, and with other drugs that prolong the QT interval), and pancytopenia.

DRUG INTERACTIONS/FOOD INTERACTIONS

Antacids containing calcium, magnesium, or aluminum; sucralfate; divalent or trivalent cations such as iron; or multivitamins containing zinc should not be taken within the 2-hour period before or after taking ofloxacin.

Cimetidine results in significant increases in half-life of some quinolones, possibly including ofloxacin.

Ofloxacin may enhance the effect of theophylline, cyclosporine, and warfarin, via inhibition of P450 enzyme activity.

The concomitant administration of a nonsteroidal antiinflammatory drug with a quinolone may increase the risk of central nervous system stimulation and convulsive seizures.

The concomitant use of probenecid with quinolones decreases renal tubular secretion.

Disturbances of blood glucose have been seen, including hyperglycemia and hypoglycemia, in patients treated concurrently with quinolones and antidiabetic agents.

Ofloxacin may produce false-positive urine screening results for opiates.

DOSING

Ofloxacin is supplied as 200-mg, 300-mg, and 400-mg tablets.

The usual dosage of ofloxacin is 200 mg to 400 mg orally every 12 hours.

Infection	*Dosage*	*Duration*
Acute exacerbation of chronic bronchitis	400 mg every 12 hours	10 days
Community-acquired pneumonia	400 mg every 12 hours	10 days
Uncomplicated skin and skin structure infections	400 mg every 12 hours	10 days
Acute urethral and cervical gonorrhea	400 mg, single dose	1 day
Nongonococcal cervicitis/urethritis	300 mg every 12 hours	7 days
Infection of the urethra and cervix	300 mg every 12 hours	7 days
Acute pelvic inflammatory disease	400 mg every 12 hours	10 to 14 days
Cystitis	200 mg every 12 hours	3 days
Uncomplicated urinary tract infection	200 mg every 12 hours	7 days
Complicated urinary tract infection	200 mg every 12 hours	10 days
Prostatitis	300 mg every 12 hours	6 weeks

SPECIAL POPULATIONS

RENAL IMPAIRMENT:

CrCl Measurement or Hemodialysis	*Maintenance Dosage*	*Frequency*
20 mL/min to 50 mL/min	The usual recommended unit dose	Every 24 hours
<20 mL/min	½ the usual recommended unit dose	Every 24 hours
Hemodialysis	½ the usual recommended unit dose	Every 12 hours
Chronic ambulatory peritoneal dialysis	½ the usual recommended unit dose	Every 24 hours
Continuous renal replacement therapy	300 mg	Every 24 hours

Note: CrCl = Creatinine Clearance.

HEPATIC DYSFUNCTION: A maximum dosage of 400 mg of ofloxacin per day should not be exceeded.

PEDIATRIC PATIENTS: Safety and efficacy in patients aged younger than 18 years have not yet been established.

PREGNANCY: Category C.

BREASTFEEDING: Ofloxacin should not be administered to breastfeeding mothers.

THE ART OF ANTIMICROBIAL THERAPY

Clinical Pearls

1. Ofloxacin should be given at least 2 hours separately from cations.
2. All fluoroquinolones can lead to tendon rupture, especially patients aged older than 60 years.
3. All fluoroquinolones can prolong QT intervals and caution should be used when they are given with other medications that affect QT intervals.
4. All fluoroquinolones can cause phototoxicity.
5. All fluoroquinolones can lower the seizure threshold.
6. Fluoroquinolones should be avoided if possible in children, pregnant women, and breastfeeding mothers, because of possible disturbance in cartilage development.
7. Treatment of gonorrhea with fluoroquinolones should be undertaken with caution because of rising resistance.

OSELTAMIVIR (Tamiflu)

BASIC CHARACTERISTICS

Class: Neuraminidase inhibitor

Mechanism of Action: Inhibits influenza virus neuraminidase affecting release of viral particles.

Mechanisms of Resistance: Mutations in the viral neuraminidase or viral hemagglutinin (or both).

Metabolic Route: Oseltamivir phosphate is an ethyl ester prodrug requiring ester hydrolysis for conversion to the active form, oseltamivir carboxylate. It is excreted unchanged in the urine.

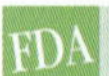

FDA-APPROVED INDICATIONS

FDA-Approved Indications: Prophylaxis and treatment of influenza A and B in patients aged 1 year and older.

SIDE EFFECTS/TOXICITY

Side effects/toxicities include nausea, vomiting, bronchitis, insomnia, vertigo, rash including Stevens-Johnson syndrome, delirium, and seizure.

DRUG INTERACTIONS/FOOD INTERACTIONS

Oseltamivir is well absorbed orally, with or without food.

No pharmacokinetic interactions have been observed.

DOSING

Oseltamivir phosphate is available as 30-mg, 45-mg, or 75-mg capsules and as a powder for oral suspension, which, when constituted with water as directed, contains 12 mg/mL oseltamivir base.

Dosage for treatment in those aged 13 years and older is 75 mg twice daily for 5 days.

Dosage for prophylaxis in those aged 13 years and older is 75 mg once daily for at least 10 days.

SPECIAL POPULATIONS

RENAL IMPAIRMENT:

- For patients with creatinine clearance between 10 mL/min and 30 mL/min: 75 mg once daily for treatment and 75 mg every other day or 30 mg every day for prophylaxis

- For patients on hemodialysis: 30 mg on nondialysis days
- For patients on chronic ambulatory peritoneal dialysis: 30 mg one or two times per week

HEPATIC DYSFUNCTION: No dosage adjustment is recommended for patients with mild or moderate hepatic impairment. Oseltamivir should not be administered to those with severe hepatic impairment.

PEDIATRIC PATIENTS: Oseltamivir is not indicated for treatment of influenza in patients aged younger than 1 year.

Weight	*Treatment*	*Prophylaxis*
> 15 kg	30 mg twice daily	30 mg once daily
> 15 kg to 23 kg	45 mg twice daily	45 mg once daily
> 23 kg to 40 kg	60 mg twice daily	60 mg once daily
> 40 kg	75 mg twice daily	75 mg once daily

PREGNANCY: Category C.

BREASTFEEDING: Oseltamivir should only be used if the potential benefit for the lactating mother justifies the potential risk to the breastfed infant.

THE ART OF ANTIMICROBIAL THERAPY

Clinical Pearls

1. Oseltamivir has activity against both influenza A and B.
2. Oseltamivir is active against avian H5N1 and novel H1N1 influenza.
3. An increased incidence of resistance to oseltamivir has been described.
4. Resistance to oseltamivir may not lead to resistance to zanamivir.
5. Seasonal H1N1 (2008–2009) was resistant to oseltamivir.
6. Delerium and abnormal behavior have been seen in pediatric patients while they were taking oseltamivir.

OXACILLIN SODIUM (Bactocil)

BASIC CHARACTERISTICS

Class: Semisynthetic penicillin

Mechanism of Action: Binds penicillin binding protein (PBP), disrupting cell wall synthesis.

Mechanisms of Resistance:

1. The PBP can be altered, with reduced affinity,
2. production of a β-lactamase resulting in hydrolysis of the β-lactam ring, and
3. decreased ability of the antibiotic to reach the PBP when bacteria decrease porin production, resulting in reduced drug concentration within the cell.

Metabolic Route: Oxacillin is excreted unchanged in the urine.

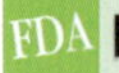

FDA-APPROVED INDICATIONS

FDA-Approved Indications: Treatment of infections caused by susceptible penicillinase-producing staphylococci.

SIDE EFFECTS/TOXICITY

A history of allergic reaction to any of the penicillins is a **contraindication**.

Side effects/toxicities include *Clostridium difficile*–associated diarrhea; thrombophlebitis; hypersensitivity reactions including rash, erythema multiforme, and Stevens-Johnson syndrome; interstitial nephritis; hepatitis; nausea; vomiting; diarrhea; stomatitis; black or hairy tongue; hyperactivity and seizures; anemia; thrombocytopenia; neutropenia; and eosinophilia.

DRUG INTERACTIONS/FOOD INTERACTIONS

Chloramphenicol, macrolides, sulfonamides, and tetracyclines may interfere with the bactericidal effects of penicillins.

When oxacillin and warfarin are used concomitantly, the prothrombin time should be closely monitored.

High urine concentrations of oxacillin may result in false-positive reactions when one is testing for the presence of glucose in urine with Clinitest. It is recommended that glucose tests based on enzymatic glucose oxidase reactions (such as Clinistix) be used instead.

DOSING

The usual intravenous dosage for adults is 250 mg to 500 mg every 4 to 6 hours.

For severe infections, 1 g every 4 to 6 hours is recommended.

SPECIAL POPULATIONS

RENAL IMPAIRMENT: No dosage adjustment is necessary.

HEPATIC DYSFUNCTION: No dosage adjustment is necessary.

COMBINED RENAL AND HEPATIC INSUFFICIENCY: Measurement of oxacillin serum levels should be performed and dosage adjusted accordingly.

PEDIATRIC PATIENTS: Safety and effectiveness in pediatric patients have not been established.

PREGNANCY: Category B.

BREASTFEEDING: Oxacillin should be used only with caution in breastfeeding mothers.

THE ART OF ANTIMICROBIAL THERAPY

Clinical Pearls

1. The dosage of oxacillin does not need to be adjusted for patients with renal impairment.
2. Oxacillin should be used with caution in patients with both renal and hepatic insufficiency.

BASIC CHARACTERISTICS

Class: Hydroquinoline

Mechanism of Action: Unknown.

Metabolic Route: Oxamniquine is oxidized in the liver and excreted in the urine.

FDA-APPROVED INDICATIONS

Not FDA-approved, but used for treatment of *Schistosoma mansoni* infections.

Not active against: *Schistosoma haematobium* or *Schistosoma japonicum.*

SIDE EFFECTS/TOXICITY

Side effects/toxicities include abdominal pain, nausea, vomiting, diarrhea, fever, elevations of ALT and AST, seizures, dizziness, drowsiness, severe headaches, hallucinations, syncope, amnesia, disorientation and confusion, and orange to red discoloration of the urine.

DRUG INTERACTIONS/FOOD INTERACTIONS

Oxamniquine should not be taken with food because food delays its absorption.

DOSING

15 mg/kg to 40 mg/kg as a single or divided dose over 1 to 3 days.

SPECIAL POPULATIONS

RENAL IMPAIRMENT: There is no dosage adjustment.

HEPATIC DYSFUNCTION: There is no dosage adjustment.

PEDIATRIC PATIENTS: As given in adults.

PREGNANCY: Category C.

BREASTFEEDING: Breastfeeding should be withheld for at least 4 hours following administration of oxamniquine.

THE ART OF ANTIMICROBIAL THERAPY

Clinical Pearls

1. Oxamniquine is not available commercially in the United States. It may be obtained from a compounding pharmacy through the National Association of compounding pharmacies (800-687-7850) or Professional Compounding Centers of America: http://www.pccarx.com.
2. Oxamniquine is only active against *S. mansoni,* not against *S. haematobium* or *S. japonicum.*

PARA-AMINOSALICYLATE SODIUM (PAS)

BASIC CHARACTERISTICS

Class: Salicylic acid

Mechanism of Action: Inhibits metabolism of para-aminobenzoic acid in mycobacteria.

Mechanisms of Resistance: Incompletely understood.

Metabolic Route: Acetylated in the liver and excreted in the urine.

FDA-APPROVED INDICATIONS

FDA-Approved Indications: Treatment of active tuberculosis in combination with other antimycobacterials.

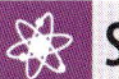

SIDE EFFECTS/TOXICITY

Side effects/toxicities include nausea, vomiting, diarrhea, hepatotoxicity, coagulopathy, hypothyroidism, hypersensitivity, rash, leukopenia, thrombocytopenia, optic neuritis, and crystalluria.

DRUG INTERACTIONS/FOOD INTERACTIONS

Drug should be sprinkled over applesauce or yogurt or mixed with acidic juices (e.g., tomato, apple, or orange). The granules should not be chewed.

Decreases levels of digoxin, warfarin, and orally administered B12.

DOSING

PAS is packaged as granules, with 4 g per packet. The usual dosage is 8 g to 12 g per day divided into two or three times per day.

SPECIAL POPULATIONS

RENAL IMPAIRMENT: No dosage adjustment, but use with caution. It is recommended that PAS be avoided in patients with severe renal failure, but some authorities suggest its cautious use in this situation, if benefit outweighs risk.

HEPATIC DYSFUNCTION: No dosage adjustment, but use with caution.

PEDIATRIC PATIENTS: 200 mg/kg/day to 300 mg/kg/day divided into two to four times daily.

PREGNANCY: Category C.

BREASTFEEDING: PAS is secreted in breastmilk. Use if benefits outweigh risk.

THE ART OF ANTIMICROBIAL THERAPY

Clinical Pearls

1. PAS should never be used alone in the treatment of active tuberculosis.
2. PAS should be refrigerated.
3. PAS should be taken with acidic food to minimize gastrointestinal discomfort.
4. Shells of the PAS granules may be seen in stool.
5. Patients should drink plenty of fluids to limit crystalluria.
6. Monitor thyroid-stimulating hormone levels and liver function tests while patients are on PAS.
7. Patients tolerate PAS best if the dosage is gradually escalated, for example, beginning with 2 g twice a day for a few days, then 2 g in the morning and 4 g at bedtime for a few days, and then 4 g twice a day.
8. Hypothyroidism is more common when PAS is coadministered with ethionamide.

PEGINTERFERON α-2A (Pegasys)

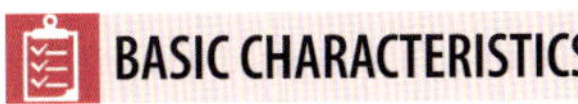

BASIC CHARACTERISTICS

Class: Pegylated alpha interferon

Mechanism of Action: After the drug binds to the cell-surface receptor, production of several interferon-stimulated gene products lead to antiviral, antiproliferative, and immunomodulatory effects; regulation of cell surface major histocompatibility antigen (HLA class I and class II) expression; and regulation of cytokine expression.

Mechanism of Resistance: Unknown.

Metabolic Route: Peginterferon α-2a is metabolized into amino acids.

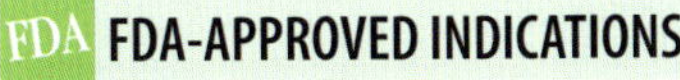

FDA-APPROVED INDICATIONS

FDA-Approved Indications: Peginterferon α-2a, alone or in combination with ribavirin, is indicated for the treatment of adults with chronic hepatitis C virus infection who have compensated liver disease and have not been previously treated with interferon α.

Peginterferon α-2a is also indicated for the treatment of adult patients with HBeAg-positive and HBeAg-negative chronic hepatitis B who have compensated liver disease and evidence of viral replication and liver inflammation.

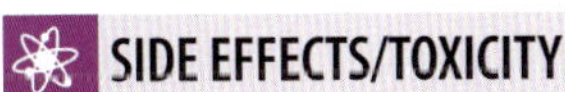

SIDE EFFECTS/TOXICITY

> **WARNING:** Alpha interferons, including peginterferon α-2a, may cause or aggravate fatal or life-threatening neuropsychiatric, autoimmune, ischemic, and infectious disorders. When used with ribavirin: ribavirin may cause birth defects and/or death of the fetus. Extreme care must be taken to avoid pregnancy in female patients and in female partners of male patients. Ribavirin causes hemolytic anemia, which may result in a worsening of cardiac disease. Ribavirin is genotoxic and mutagenic and should be considered a potential carcinogen.

Peginterferon α-2a is **contraindicated** in patients with known hypersensitivity to α interferons or to any component of the product, decompensated hepatic disease (cirrhosis with Child-Pugh score > 6), or autoimmune hepatitis, and in neonates and infants.

Side effects/toxicities include fever; hypersensitivity; neuropsychiatric disorders including depression, suicide, psychosis, aggressive behavior, nervousness, anxiety, emotional lability, abnormal thinking, agitation, apathy, and relapse of drug addiction; infections; bone marrow suppression; cardiovascular disorders including hypertension, tachycardia, palpitation, tachyarrhythmias, supraventricular arrhythmias, chest pain, and myocardial infarction; hypersensitivity; endocrine disorders including hyperthyroidism, hypothyroidism, hyperglycemia, diabetes mellitus, and elevated serum triglycerides; autoimmune disorders including autoimmune thrombocytopenia, idiopathic thrombocytopenic purpura, psoriasis, systemic lupus erythematosus, thyroiditis, and rheumatoid arthritis; pneumonia; interstitial pneumonitis; hemorrhagic/ischemic, ulcerative colitis; pancreatitis; hepatic decompensation; ophthalmologic disorders including decrease or loss of vision, macular edema, retinal artery or vein thrombosis, retinal hemorrhages, cotton wool spots, optic neuritis, and papilledema; and ischemic and hemorrhagic cerebrovascular events.

DRUG INTERACTIONS/FOOD INTERACTIONS

Theophylline serum levels should be monitored.

Patients on methadone should be monitored for the signs and symptoms of methadone toxicity.

DOSING

Chronic hepatitis C: 180 μg (1.0-mL vial or 0.5-mL prefilled syringe) once weekly (for 24 weeks for Hepatitis C genotype 2 or 3 and for 48 weeks for genotype 1 or 4) by subcutaneous administration in the abdomen or thigh.

Chronic hepatitis B: 180 μg (1.0-mL vial or 0.5-mL prefilled syringe) once weekly for 48 weeks by subcutaneous administration in the abdomen or thigh.

SPECIAL POPULATIONS

RENAL IMPAIRMENT: For patients with end-stage renal disease requiring hemodialysis: 135 μg once weekly.

HEPATIC DYSFUNCTION: Peginterferon α-2a should not be administered to those with decompensated liver disease (cirrhosis with Child-Pugh > 6). Liver function tests should be monitored closely:

- In patients with chronic hepatitis C who have ALT increases above baseline values, reduce peginterferon α-2a dose to 135 μg; prior dose can be resumed after ALT flares subside.
- In patients with chronic hepatitis B who have elevations in ALT (> 5 × ULN), reduce the dose of peginterferon α-2a to 135 μg or temporarily discontinue treatment. Therapy can be resumed after ALT flares subside. If flares are severe and persistent (ALT > 10 times above the upper limit of normal) consider discontinuing treatment.

PEDIATRIC PATIENTS: Not recommended for those aged younger than 18 years.
PREGNANCY: Category C.
BREASTFEEDING: Should not be administered to breastfeeding mothers.
DEPRESSION: Reduce dosage to 135 μg.
HEMATOLOGIC DYSFUNCTION:

- ANC < 750/mm: reduce dosage to 135 μg.
- Platelet count < 50,000: reduce dosage to 90 μg.

THE ART OF ANTIMICROBIAL THERAPY

Clinical Pearls

1. Before initiating peginterferon α-2a, one should evaluate for psychiatric issues including depression.
2. Hepatitis C genotypes 2 and 3 respond better to therapy compared with types 1 and 4.
3. It is current standard of care to administer peginterferon α-2a in combination with ribavirin for hepatitis C.
4. If a 2-log drop of hepatitis C RNA is not noticed by 12 weeks, treatment can be stopped because the patient is most likely going to be a nonresponder.
5. Monitor complete blood counts during therapy. Discontinue in patients who develop severe decreases in neutrophil ($< 0.5 \times 10^9$/L) or platelet counts ($< 50 \times 10^9$/L).
6. Hepatic function should be closely monitored, and interferon treatment should be immediately discontinued if symptoms of hepatic decompensation, such as jaundice, ascites, coagulopathy, or decreased serum albumin, are observed.
7. All patients should receive an eye examination at baseline. Patients with preexisting ophthalmologic disorders (e.g., diabetic or hypertensive retinopathy) should receive periodic ophthalmologic examinations during interferon α treatment. Any patient who develops ocular symptoms should receive a prompt and complete eye examination.
8. **If HIV co-infected:** duration of therapy is 48 weeks regardless of hepatitis C genotype.

PEGINTERFERON α-2B (Pegintron)

 BASIC CHARACTERISTICS

Class: Pegylated alpha interferon

Mechanism of Action: After the drug binds to the cell-surface receptor, production of several interferon-stimulated gene products leads to antiviral, antiproliferative, and immunomodulatory effects; regulation of cell surface major histocompatibility antigen (HLA class I and class II) expression; and regulation of cytokine expression.

Mechanism of Resistance: Unknown.

Metabolic Route: Peginterferon α-2b is metabolized into amino acids.

FDA FDA-APPROVED INDICATIONS

FDA-Approved Indications: Peginterferon α-2b in combination with ribavirin is indicated for the treatment of adults with chronic hepatitis C virus infection who have compensated liver disease and have not been previously treated with interferon α.

 SIDE EFFECTS/TOXICITY

> **WARNING:** May cause or aggravate fatal or life-threatening neuropsychiatric, autoimmune, ischemic, and infectious disorders.
> When used with ribavirin: ribavirin may cause birth defects and fetal death; avoid pregnancy in female patients and female partners of male patients. Ribavirin is a potential carcinogen.

Peginterferon α-2b is **contraindicated** in patients with known hypersensitivity to α interferons or to any component of the product, decompensated hepatic disease (cirrhosis with Child-Pugh class > 6), autoimmune hepatitis, neonates, and infants.

Side effects/toxicities include fever; hypersensitivity; neuropsychiatric disorders including depression, suicide, psychosis, aggressive behavior, nervousness, anxiety, emotional lability, abnormal thinking, agitation, apathy, and relapse of drug addiction; infections, bone marrow suppression; cardiovascular disorders including hypertension, tachycardia, palpitation, tachyarrhythmias, supraventricular arrhythmias, chest pain, and myocardial infarction; hypersensitivity; endocrine disorders including hyperthyroidism, hypothyroidism, hyperglycemia, diabetes mellitus, and elevated serum triglycerides; autoimmune disorders including autoimmune thrombocytopenia, idiopathic thrombocytopenic purpura, psoriasis, systemic lupus erythematosus, thyroiditis, and rheumatoid arthritis; pneumonia; interstitial pneumonitis; hemorrhagic/ischemic, ulcerative colitis; pancreatitis; hepatic decompensation; ophthalmologic disorders including decrease or loss of vision, macular edema, retinal artery or vein thrombosis, retinal hemorrhages, cotton wool spots, optic neuritis, and papilledema; and ischemic and hemorrhagic cerebrovascular events.

DRUG INTERACTIONS/FOOD INTERACTIONS

Patients on methadone should be monitored for the signs and symptoms of methadone toxicity.

Theophylline serum levels should be monitored.

DOSING

1.5 μg/kg/week subcutaneously in combination with 800 mg to 1400 mg of ribavirin orally based on patient body weight. The treatment duration for patients with genotype 1 or 4 is 48 weeks. Patients with genotype 2 or 3 should be treated for 24 weeks.

If one is using peginterferon α-2b monotherapy, the dosage is 1 μg/kg/week for 48 weeks.

SPECIAL POPULATIONS

RENAL IMPAIRMENT:

- Creatinine clearance 30 mL/min to 50mL/min: dosage reduction of 25%
- Creatinine clearance 10 mL/min to 29 mL/min, or hemodialysis: dosage reduction of 50%.

HEPATIC DYSFUNCTION: Peginterferon α-2b should not be administered to those with decompensated liver disease (cirrhosis with Child-Pugh class > 6). Liver function tests should be monitored closely.

PEDIATRIC PATIENTS: The recommended dosage is 60 μg/m^2/week subcutaneously.

PREGNANCY: Category C.

BREASTFEEDING: Peginterferon α-2b should not be administered to breastfeeding mothers.

THE ART OF ANTIMICROBIAL THERAPY

Clinical Pearls

1. Before initiating peginterferon α-2b, one should evaluate for psychiatric issues including depression.
2. Hepatitis C genotypes 2 and 3 respond better to therapy compared with types 1 and 4.
3. It is current standard of care to administer peginterferon α-2b in combination with ribavirin for hepatitis C.

4. If a 2-log drop of hepatitis C RNA is not noticed by 12 weeks, treatment can be stopped because the patient is most likely going to be a nonresponder.
5. Monitor complete blood counts during therapy. Discontinue peginterferon α-2b in patients who develop severe decreases in neutrophil ($< 0.5 \times 10^9$/L) or platelet counts ($< 50 \times 10^9$/L).
6. Hepatic function should be closely monitored, and interferon treatment should be immediately discontinued if symptoms of hepatic decompensation, such as jaundice, ascites, coagulopathy, or decreased serum albumin, are observed.
7. All patients should receive an eye examination at baseline. Patients with preexisting ophthalmologic disorders (e.g., diabetic or hypertensive retinopathy) should receive periodic ophthalmologic examinations during interferon α treatment. Any patient who develops ocular symptoms should receive a prompt and complete eye examination.
8. **If HIV co-infected:** duration of therapy is 48 weeks regardless of hepatitis C genotype.

PENICILLIN [Penicillin G, Penicillin V, Penicillin G procaine, Penicillin G benzathine (Bicillin L-A, Permapen)]

BASIC CHARACTERISTICS

Class: Penicillin

Mechanism of Action: Binds penicillin-binding protein (PBP), disrupting cell wall synthesis.

Mechanisms of Resistance:

1. The PBP can be altered, with reduced affinity,
2. production of a β-lactamase resulting in hydrolysis of the β-lactam ring, and
3. decreased ability of the antibiotic to reach the PBP when bacteria decrease porin production, resulting in a decrease of the drug concentration within the cell.

Metabolic Route: Penicillin is excreted unchanged in the urine.

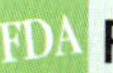

FDA-APPROVED INDICATIONS

FDA-Approved Indications:

- **Penicillin G potassium** injection is indicated in the treatment of susceptible strains of microorganisms causing septicemia, empyema, pneumonia, pericarditis, endocarditis, and meningitis. It is also indicated for pneumococcal infection, fusospirochetosis, anthrax, actinomycosis, clostridial infections, *Erysipelothrix*, spirochetal infections, listeriosis, *Pasteurella multocida*, rat-bite fever, syphilis, susceptible gonococcal and meningococcal infection, and prevention of rheumatic fever.
- **Penicillin V** is indicated for **mild-to-moderate** infections caused by susceptible organisms including streptococcal infections (without bacteremia) of the upper respiratory tract, scarlet fever, and mild erysipelas; pneumococcal infections; fusospirochetosis; and prevention of rheumatic fever. Severe pneumonia, empyema, bacteremia, pericarditis, meningitis, and arthritis should not be treated with penicillin V during the acute stage.
- **Penicillin G procaine** is indicated in the treatment of **moderately severe** infections susceptible to low serum levels of penicillin G, including upper respiratory tract infections, skin and skin structure infections, scarlet fever, erysipelas, fusospirochetosis, pneumococcal infection, syphilis, yaws, bejel, pinta, an adjunct to antitoxin for prevention of the carrier stage of diphtheria, anthrax, rat-bite fever, *Erysipelothrix rhusiopathiae*, and subacute bacterial endocarditis caused by group A streptococci.
- **Penicillin G benzathine** is indicated in the treatment of infections that are susceptible to low and prolonged serum levels: upper respiratory tract streptococcal infection, syphilis, yaws, bejel, and pinta, and prevention of rheumatic fever.

 SIDE EFFECTS/TOXICITY

A history of allergic reaction to any of the penicillins is a **contraindication**.

Side effects/toxicities include hypersensitivity, including rashes, ranging from maculopapular eruptions to exfoliative dermatitis; urticaria; serum sickness–like reactions, including chills, fever, edema, arthralgia, and prostration; anaphylaxis; *Clostridium difficile*–associated diarrhea; mucocutaneous candidiasis; nausea; vomiting; diarrhea; black hairy tongue; rise in AST (SGOT) and/or ALT (SGPT), crystalluria, interstitial nephritis, anemia, thrombocytopenia, eosinophilia, leukopenia, hyperactivity, and convulsions.

Procaine side effects/toxicities include anxiety, confusion, agitation, depression, weakness, seizures, hallucinations, combativeness, and expressed "fear of impending death."

Procaine and benzathine penicillin injection side effects/toxicities: inadvertent intravascular administration has resulted in severe neurovascular damage, transverse myelitis, gangrene, and necrosis. Other side effects/toxicities include pallor, mottling, or cyanosis of the extremity; severe edema quadriceps femoris fibrosis; and atrophy.

 DRUG INTERACTIONS/FOOD INTERACTIONS

Penicillin tablets and oral suspensions may be given without regard to meals.

Concurrent use of penicillin and probenecid may result in increased and prolonged blood levels of penicillin.

Chloramphenicol, macrolides, sulfonamides, and tetracyclines may interfere with the bactericidal effects of penicillin.

 DOSING

Penicillin G Potassium Injection

Clinical Indication	*Dosage*
Septicemia, empyema, pneumonia, pericarditis, endocarditis, and meningitis	12 million to 24 million units/day in equally divided doses every 4 to 6 hours
Anthrax	8 million units/day in divided doses every 6 hours.
Actinomycosis	
Cervicofacial disease	1 million to 6 million units/day
Thoracic and abdominal disease	10 million to 20 million units/day
Clostridial infections	20 million units/day

Clinical Indication	*Dosage*
Diphtheria	2 million to 3 million units/day in divided doses
Erysipelothrix endocarditis	12 million to 20 million units/day
Fusospirochetosis	5 million to 10 million units/day
Listeria infections	
Meningitis	15 million to 20 million units/day
Endocarditis	15 million to 20 million units/day
Pasteurella infections	4 million to 6 million units/day
Rat-bite fever	12 million to 20 million units/day
Disseminated gonococcal infections	10 million units/day
Syphilis (neurosyphilis)	12 million to 24 million units/day, as 2 to 4 million units every 4 hours
Meningococcal meningitis and/or septicemia	24 million units/day as 2 million units every 2 hours

Penicillin V: Penicillin V potassium is administered as 250-mg (400,000 units) or 500-mg (800,000 units) tablets and an oral solution containing 125 mg (200,000 units) per 5 mL and 250 mg (400,000 units) per 5 mL.

- **Streptococcal infections:** 125 mg to 250 mg every 6 to 8 hours for 10 days
- **Pneumococcal infections, fusospirochetosis, or staphylococcal infections:** 250 mg to 500 mg every 6 hours
- For the **prevention of recurrence following rheumatic fever and/or chorea**: 125 mg to 250 mg twice daily on a continuing basis

Penicillin G Procaine: Should be administered by intramuscular injection in the upper, outer quadrant of the buttock. It is supplied in 600,000-unit and 1,200,000-unit injections.

- **Pneumonia, streptococcal infections, staphylococcal infections, bacterial endocarditis, cutaneous anthrax, fusospirochetosis, erysipeloid, and rat-bite fever:** 600,000 units to 1,000,000 units daily
- **Primary, secondary, and latent syphilis:** 600,000 units daily for total 4,800,000 units
- **Late (tertiary, neurosyphilis, and latent) syphilis** with positive spinal fluid examination or no spinal fluid examination): 600,000 units daily for 10 to 15 days for a total of 6 million to 9 million units

- **Diphtheria adjunctive therapy** with antitoxin: 300,000 units to 600,000 units daily
- **Diphtheria carrier state:** 300,000 units daily for 10 days
- **Anthrax-inhalational** (post-exposure): 1,200,000 units every 12 hours

Benzathine Penicillin: Should be administered by intramuscular injection in the upper, outer quadrant of the buttock. It comes in 600,000 units, 1,200,000 units, and 2,400,000 units per syringe.

- **Upper respiratory infections:** a single injection of 1,200,000 units
- **Primary, secondary, and early latent syphilis:** 2,400,000 units for one dose
- **Late syphilis:** 2,400,000 units at 7-day intervals for three doses
- **Yaws, bejel, and pinta:** 1,200,000 units in one dose.
- **Prophylaxis of rheumatic fever:** 1,200,000 units once a month or 600,000 units every 2 weeks

 SPECIAL POPULATIONS

RENAL IMPAIRMENT:

Penicillin G

CrCl Measurement or Hemodialysis	*Dosage*
10 mL/min to 50 mL/min	1 million to 2 million units every 4 hours
<10 mL/min	1 million units every 6 hours
Hemodialysis	2 million units after dialysis
Chronic ambulatory peritoneal dialysis	1 million units every 6 hours
Continuous renal replacement therapy	1 million to 2 million units every 4 hours

Note: CrCl = Creatinine Clearance.

Penicillin V

CrCl or Hemodialysis	*Dosage*
10 mL/min to 50 mL/min	No change
<10 mL/min	250 mg to 500 mg every 8 hours
Hemodialysis	250 mg after dialysis
Chronic ambulatory peritoneal dialysis	250 mg to 500 mg after dialysis
Continuous renal replacement therapy	Correct dose unknown

Note: CrCl = Creatinine Clearance.

HEPATIC DYSFUNCTION: No dosage adjustment is necessary.

PEDIATRIC PATIENTS:

Penicillin G

Clinical Indication	*Dosage*
Serious infections	150,000 to 300,000 units/kg/day divided in equal doses every 4 to 6 hours
Meningitis	250,000 units/kg/day divided in equal doses every 4 hours
Disseminated gonococcal infections	Weight less than 45 kg:
Arthritis	100,000 units/kg/day in four equally divided doses
Meningitis	250,000 units/kg/day in equal doses every 4 hours
Endocarditis	250,000 units/kg/day in equal doses every 4 hours
Arthritis, meningitis, endocarditis	Weight 45 kg or greater: 10 million units/day in four doses
Syphilis (congenital and neurosyphilis) after the newborn period	200,000 to 300,000 units/kg/day (administered as 50,000 units/kg every 4 to 6 hours)
Diphtheria	150,000 to 250,000 units/kg/day in equal doses every 6 hours
Rat-bite fever	150,000 to 250,000 units/kg/day in equal doses every 4 hours

Penicillin G Procaine: In neonates, infants, and small children, the midlateral aspect of the thigh may be preferable. When doses are repeated, vary the injection site.

In pneumonia, streptococcal infections, and staphylococcal infections in pediatric patients who weigh less than 60 lbs: 300,000 units daily.

Congenital syphilis infections in pediatric patients who weigh less than 70 lbs: 50,000 units/kg/day for 10 days.

Anthrax-inhalational (post-exposure): 25,000 units per kilogram of body weight (maximum 1,200,000 units) every 12 hours in children.

Benzathine Penicillin:

Upper respiratory infections in older pediatric patients: a single injection of 900,000 units

Upper respiratory infections in infants and pediatric patients who weigh less than 60 lbs: 300,000 units to 600,000 units

Congenital syphilis in patients who are aged younger than 2 years: 50,000 units/kg/body weight

Congenital syphilis in patients who are aged 2 to 12 years: adjust dosage based on adult dosage schedule.

PREGNANCY: Category B.

BREASTFEEDING: Caution should be exercised when penicillin is administered to a breastfeeding mother.

THE ART OF ANTIMICROBIAL THERAPY

Clinical Pearls

1. Dosage of penicillin needs to be adjusted for patients with renal dysfunction.
2. The Jarisch-Herxheimer reaction can occur following treatment of syphilis as well as other spirochetal infections.
3. Penicillin G potassium, USP (1 million units contains 1.68 mEq of potassium ion) may cause serious and even fatal electrolyte disturbances, such as hyperkalemia, when given intravenously in large doses, especially in patients with renal failure.
4. Chloramphenicol, macrolides, sulfonamides, and tetracyclines may interfere with the bactericidal effects of penicillins.

PENTAMIDINE (Pentam, NebuPent)

BASIC CHARACTERISTICS

Class: Aromatic diamidine

Mechanism of Action: Inhibits putrescine and spermidine uptake competitively.

Metabolic Route: Pentamidine is hydroxylated by the liver and subsequently excreted.

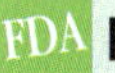

FDA-APPROVED INDICATIONS

FDA-Approved Indications:

IV pentamidine is a third-line drug for the treatment of *Pneumocystis jiroveci* infections.

Inhaled pentamidine is indicated for prophylaxis of *P jiroveci* pneumonia in patients with AIDS who have a history of *P jiroveci* infection and CD4 count less than 200.

Also Used for:

Inhaled pentamidine is also used for treatment of mild infection caused by *P jiroveci.*

IV pentamidine is used for early-stage *Trypanosoma gambiense.*

IV pentamidine is a second-line agent for visceral leishmaniasis.

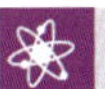

SIDE EFFECTS/TOXICITY

Intravenous pentamadine can cause hypotension, especially if given in less than 1 hour, renal failure, hypocalcemia, hypomagnesemia, hyperkalemia, hyponatremia, hypoglycemia, fatal pancreatitis, diabetes, neutropenia, anemia, thrombocytopenia, nausea, vomiting, abnormal liver function tests, and ventricular arrhythmias as well as QT interval prolongation and changes in ST segment and T waves.

IM pentamidine may also result in sterile abscesses.

Aerosolized pentamidine can cause coughing and bronchospasm.

DRUG INTERACTIONS/FOOD INTERACTIONS

Data incomplete.

DOSING

Should be given IV if possible, because of pain and abscess formation from IM administration.

PENTAMIDINE (Pentam, NebuPent)

Disease	*Dosage and Duration*
P. jiroveci pneumonia in AIDS patients	4 mg/kg daily for 21 days
P. jiroveci pneumonia non–HIV-infected patients	4 mg/kg daily for 14 days
P. jiroveci pneumonia prophylaxis	300 mg inhaled once a month
T. gambiense trypanosomiasis	Seven daily injections of 4 mg/kg
Visceral leishmaniasis	2 mg/kg to 4 mg/kg daily for up to 15 days or 4 mg/kg three times a week until negative splenic aspirates are obtained

SPECIAL POPULATIONS

RENAL IMPAIRMENT: No dosage adjustment is necessary for renal impairment; however, if creatinine increases by 1 mg/dL or more, the daily dosage should be decreased to 2 mg/kg to 3 mg/kg.

HEPATIC DYSFUNCTION: No dosage adjustment is necessary.

PEDIATRIC PATIENTS: The same dosage as in adults; however, for pediatric cases of African trypanosomiasis a daily dose of 5 mg/kg should be administered.

PREGNANCY: If possible, pentamidine should be avoided during the first trimester of pregnancy.

BREASTFEEDING: Unknown.

THE ART OF ANTIMICROBIAL THERAPY

Clinical Pearls

1. Although inhaled pentamidine is used for mild *P. jiroveci* pneumonia, other agents are preferable (e.g., trimethoprim plus sulfamethoxazole, clindamycin plus primaquine).
2. Although inhaled pentamidine is recommended for prophylaxis for *P. jiroveci* pneumonia, other agents are more effective (e.g., trimethoprim plus sulfamethoxazole, dapsone, atovaquone).
3. Severe complications may occur in patients receiving pentamidine including hypotension, hypoglycemia, pancreatitis, and renal failure. Close monitoring is necessary.
4. Pentamidine is administered to patients with Gambian trypanosomiasis because of severe encephalopathy with melarsoprol.

BASIC CHARACTERISTICS

Class: Ureidopenicillin

Mechanism of Action: Binds penicillin-binding protein (PBP), disrupting cell wall synthesis.

Mechanisms of Resistance:

1. The PBP can be altered, with reduced affinity,
2. production of a β-lactamase resulting in hydrolysis of the β-lactam ring, and
3. decreased ability of the antibiotic to reach the PBP when bacteria decrease porin production, resulting in a decrease of the drug concentration within the cell.

Metabolic Route: Piperacillin is excreted by both biliary and renal routes.

FDA FDA-APPROVED INDICATIONS

FDA-Approved Indications: Treatment of infections caused by susceptible (only β-lactamase–negative) strains of microorganisms in the following conditions: intraabdominal infections, urinary tract infections, gynecologic infections, septicemia, lower respiratory tract infections, skin and skin structure infections, bone and joint infections, uncomplicated gonococcal urethritis, and prophylaxis for surgery.

SIDE EFFECTS/TOXICITY

Contraindicated in patients with a history of allergic reactions to any of the penicillins or cephalosporins.

Side effects/toxicities include *Clostridium difficile*–associated diarrhea, hypersensitivity reactions including anaphylaxis, rash including erythema multiforme and Stevens-Johnson syndrome, mucocutaneous candidiasis, nausea, vomiting, diarrhea, constipation, black hairy tongue, headache, arrhythmias, hyperactivity and seizures, confusion, hepatitis, renal dysfunction, crystalluria, anemia, thrombocytopenia, eosinophilia, leukopenia, and abnormalities of coagulation.

DRUG INTERACTIONS/FOOD INTERACTIONS

Concurrent use of piperacillin and probenecid may result in increased and prolonged blood levels of piperacillin. Neuromuscular blockade produced by any of the nondepolarizing muscle relaxants could be prolonged in the presence of piperacillin. The clearance of methotrexate may be reduced.

Chloramphenicol, macrolides, sulfonamides, and tetracyclines may interfere with the bactericidal effects of penicillins.

High urine concentrations of piperacillin may result in false-positive reactions when one is testing for the presence of glucose in urine with Clinitest. It is recommended that glucose tests based on enzymatic glucose oxidase reactions (such as Clinistix) be used instead.

DOSING

Piperacillin may be administered intramuscularly or intravenously.

Condition	*Dosage*[a]
Sepsis	12 g to 18 g IV daily divided every 4 to 6 hours
Nosocomial pneumonia	12 g to 18 g IV daily divided every 4 to 6 hours
Intraabdominal infections	12 g to 18 g IV daily divided every 4 to 6 hours
Gynecological infections	12 g to 18 g IV daily divided every 4 to 6 hours
Skin and skin structure infections	12 g to 18 g IV daily divided every 4 to 6 hours
Complicated urinary tract infections	8 g to 16 g IV daily divided every 6 to 8 hours
Uncomplicated urinary tract infections	6 g to 8 g IM or IV daily divided every 6 to 12 hours
Uncomplicated gonococcal infections	2 g IM with 1 g of probenecid 30 minutes earlier
Prophylaxis for surgery	2 g 20 to 30 minutes before anesthesia

[a]Maximum dosage for serious infection: 24 g/day.

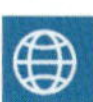

SPECIAL POPULATIONS

RENAL IMPAIRMENT:

CrCl Measurement or Hemodialysis	*Uncomplicated UTI*	*Complicated UTI*	*Serious Infections*
20 mL/min to 40 mL/min	6 g to 8 g IM or IV divided every 6 to 12 hours	3 g every 8 hours	4 g every 8 hours
<20 mL/min	3 g IM or IV every 12 hours	3 g every 12 hours	4 g every 12 hours
Hemodialysis	Maximum daily dosage is 2 g every 8 hours and 1 g after dialysis		
Chronic ambulatory peritoneal dialysis	Maximum daily dosage is 2 g every 8 hours and 2 g after dialysis		
Continuous renal replacement therapy	3 g IM or IV every 8 hours		

Note: CrCl = Creatinine Clearance; UTI = urinary tract infection.

HEPATIC DYSFUNCTION: No dosage adjustment is necessary.

RENAL AND HEPATIC FAILURE: Should measure levels of piperacillin.

PEDIATRIC PATIENTS: Dosages in patients aged younger than 12 years have not been studied in adequate and well-controlled clinical trials.

PREGNANCY: Category B.

BREASTFEEDING: Piperacillin should be used only with caution in breastfeeding mothers.

THE ART OF ANTIMICROBIAL THERAPY

Clinical Pearls

1. Dosage of piperacillin needs to be adjusted for patients with renal dysfunction.
2. Piperacillin is a monosodium salt containing 1.85 mEq of Na+ per g (42.5 mg of Na+ per g). This should be considered when one is treating patients requiring restricted salt intake.
3. Neuromuscular blockade produced by any of the nondepolarizing muscle relaxants could be prolonged in the presence of piperacillin.
4. As with other semisynthetic penicillins, piperacillin therapy has been associated with an increased incidence of fever and rash in patients with cystic fibrosis.
5. When one is treating *Pseudomonas* infections, piperacillin dosage should be 24 g/day IM or IV, in four divided doses.

PIPERACILLIN PLUS TAZOBACTAM (Zosyn)

BASIC CHARACTERISTICS

Class: Ureidopenicillin and β-lactamase inhibitor combination

Mechanism of Action: Binds penicillin-binding protein (PBP), disrupting cell wall synthesis.

Mechanisms of Resistance:

1. The PBP can be altered, with reduced affinity,
2. production of a β-lactamase resulting in hydrolysis of the β-lactam ring, and
3. decreased ability of the antibiotic to reach the PBP when bacteria decrease porin production, resulting in reduced drug concentration within the cell.

Metabolic Route: Piperacillin is excreted unchanged in the urine. Tazobactam and its metabolite are excreted in the urine.

FDA-APPROVED INDICATIONS

FDA-Approved Indications: Treatment of infections caused by susceptible strains of microorganisms in the following conditions: appendicitis, uncomplicated and complicated skin and skin structure infections, postpartum endometritis or pelvic inflammatory disease, community-acquired pneumonia (moderate severity only), and nosocomial pneumonia (moderate to severe).

SIDE EFFECTS/TOXICITY

Contraindicated in patients with a history of allergic reactions to any of the penicillins, cephalosporins, or β-lactamase inhibitors.

Side effects/toxicities include *Clostridium difficile*–associated diarrhea, hypersensitivity reactions including anaphylaxis, rash including erythema multiforme and Stevens-Johnson syndrome, mucocutaneous candidiasis, nausea, vomiting, diarrhea, constipation, black hairy tongue, headache, arrhythmias, hyperactivity and seizures, confusion, hepatitis, renal dysfunction, crystalluria, anemia, thrombocytopenia, eosinophilia, leukopenia, abnormalities of coagulation, false-positive reaction for urinary glucose, and hypokalemia.

DRUG INTERACTIONS/FOOD INTERACTIONS

Concurrent use of piperacillin plus tazobactam and probenecid may result in increased and prolonged blood levels of piperacillin plus tazobactam. Neuromuscular blockade produced by any of the nondepolarizing muscle relaxants could be prolonged in the presence of piperacillin. The clearance of methotrexate may be reduced.

Chloramphenicol, macrolides, sulfonamides, and tetracyclines may interfere with the bactericidal effects of penicillin.

High urine concentrations of piperacillin may result in false-positive reactions when one is testing for the presence of glucose in urine with Clinitest. It is recommended that glucose tests based on enzymatic glucose oxidase reactions (such as Clinistix) be used instead.

 DOSING

The usual dosage is 3.375 g IV every 6 hours.

For nosocomial pneumonia, the dosage should be 4.5 g every 6 hours IV along with an aminoglycoside.

 SPECIAL POPULATIONS

RENAL IMPAIRMENT:

CrCl Measurement or Hemodialysis	*Usual Dosage*	*Nosocomial Pneumonia*
20 mL/min to 40 mL/min	2.25 g every 6 hours	3.375 g every 6 hours
<20 mL/min	2.25 g every 8 hours	2.25 g every 6 hours
Hemodialysis	2.25 g every 12 hours	2.25 g every 8 hours; an additional 0.75 g should be administered following each dialysis
Chronic ambulatory peritoneal dialysis	2.25 g every 8 hours	2.25 g every 6 hours
Continuous renal replacement therapy	2.25 g every 12 hours	2.25 g every 8 hours

Note: CrCl = Creatinine Clearance.

HEPATIC DYSFUNCTION: No dosage adjustment is necessary.

PEDIATRIC PATIENTS: For patients aged 9 months and older, the recommended dosage is 100 mg piperacillin/12.5 mg tazobactam/kg every 8 hours.

For patients aged between 2 months and 9 months, the recommended dosage is 80 mg piperacillin/10 mg tazobactam/kg every 8 hours.

PREGNANCY: Category B.

BREASTFEEDING: Piperacillin plus tazobactam should be used only with caution in breastfeeding mothers.

THE ART OF ANTIMICROBIAL THERAPY

Clinical Pearls

1. Dosage of piperacillin plus tazobactam needs to be adjusted for patients with renal dysfunction.
2. Piperacillin plus tazobactam is a monosodium salt of piperacillin and a monosodium salt of tazobactam and contains a total of 2.79 mEq (64 mg) of Na+ per gram of piperacillin in the combination product. This should be considered when one is treating patients requiring restricted salt intake.
3. As with other semisynthetic penicillins, piperacillin therapy has been associated with an increased incidence of fever and rash in patients with cystic fibrosis.
4. Nosocomial pneumonia caused by *Pseudomonas aeruginosa* should be treated in combination with an aminoglycoside.
5. Neuromuscular blockade produced by any of the nondepolarizing muscle relaxants could be prolonged in the presence of piperacillin.

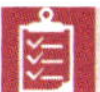

BASIC CHARACTERISTICS

Class: Cyclic secondary amine

Mechanism of Action: Inhibits extrasynaptic γ-aminobutyric acid. (GABA) receptors, causing an influx of Cl^- ions in the nematode.

Metabolic Route: Piperazine citrate is excreted unchanged in the urine.

FDA-APPROVED INDICATIONS

Not FDA-approved, but used for treatment of *Ascaris lumbricoides* and *Enterobius vermicularis.*

SIDE EFFECTS/TOXICITY

Contraindicated in patients with seizure disorders.

Side effects/toxicities include nausea, vomiting, diarrhea, abdominal pain, headache, visual disturbances, ataxia, and hypotonia.

DRUG INTERACTIONS/FOOD INTERACTIONS

Data incomplete.

DOSING

75 mg/kg/day for 2 days.

SPECIAL POPULATIONS

RENAL IMPAIRMENT: Contraindicated.

HEPATIC DYSFUNCTION: Contraindicated.

PEDIATRICS: Same dosage as adults.

PREGNANCY: Should not be used in pregnant women.

BREASTFEEDING: Unknown.

THE ART OF ANTIMICROBIAL THERAPY

Clinical Pearls

1. Piperazine should not be used in patients with seizure disorders.
2. Piperazine is used when less toxic anthelminthics (e.g., mebendazole or albendazole) are unavailable or can not be administered.
3. Piperazine is not available in the United States; however, it is available in Canada.

 BASIC CHARACTERISTICS

Class: Triazole

Mechanism of Action: Inhibits lanosterol 14-α-demethylase, which is involved in the synthesis of ergosterol, an essential component of fungal cell membranes.

Mechanisms of Resistance:

1. Point mutations in the gene (*ERG11*) encoding for the target enzyme lead to an altered target with decreased affinity for azoles,
2. overexpression of *ERG11* results in the production of high concentrations of the target enzyme, creating the need for higher intracellular drug concentrations to inhibit all of the enzyme molecules in the cell, and
3. active efflux of posaconazole out of the cell through the activation of two types of multidrug efflux transporters.

Metabolic Route: Posaconazole is predominantly eliminated unchanged in the feces.

FDA FDA-APPROVED INDICATIONS

FDA-Approved Indications: Prophylaxis of invasive *Aspergillus* and *Candida* infections in patients aged 13 years and older who are at high risk of developing these infections because of being severely immunocompromised, such as hematopoietic stem cell transplant (HSCT) recipients with graft-versus-host disease (GVHD) or those with hematologic malignancies with prolonged neutropenia from chemotherapy; and treatment of oropharyngeal candidiasis, including oropharyngeal candidiasis refractory to itraconazole and/or fluconazole.

Also Used for: Posaconazole has activity against *Zygomycetes* species.

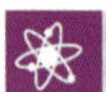 SIDE EFFECTS/TOXICITY

Caution should be used when one is prescribing posaconazole to patients with hypersensitivity to other azoles.

Posaconazole should be administered with caution to patients with potentially proarrhythmic conditions and should not be administered with drugs that are known to prolong the QTc interval and are metabolized through CYP3A4.

Other side effects/toxicities include fever, neutropenia, thrombocytopenia, abdominal pain, hepatotoxicity, nausea, vomiting, diarrhea, rash, adrenal insufficiency, thrombocytopenia, and hypokalemia.

 DRUG INTERACTIONS/ADMINISTRATION

Administer posaconazole with food or a nutritional supplement.

Because posaconazole is a strong inhibitor of CYP3A4, plasma concentrations of drugs predominantly metabolized by CYP3A4 may be increased by posaconazole. The following drug interactions may be seen and may require dosage adjustment when appropriate:

Drug	*Adjustment or Action*
Astemizole	**Contraindicated**
Benzodiazepines	May see increased levels of benzodiazepines
Calcium channel blockers	May increase levels of calcium channel blockers
Cimetidine	May lower levels of posaconazole
Cisapride	**Contraindicated**
Cyclosporine	Reduce cyclosporine dosage to approximately three fourths of the original dosage and monitor cyclosporine levels
Digoxin	May increase levels of digoxin
Efavirenz	May lower levels of posaconazole
Ergot alkaloids	**Contraindicated**
Halofantrine	**Contraindicated**
HMG-CoA reductase inhibitors (statins)	May increase concentrations of statins
Phenytoin	May lower levels of posaconazole; levels of phenytoin may increase
Pimozide	**Contraindicated**
Protease inhibitors	May increase levels of protease inhibitors
Quinidine	Contraindicated
Rifabutin	May lower levels of posaconazole; also, levels of rifabutin may increase
Sirolimus	**Contraindicated**
Tacrolimus	Reduce tacrolimus dosage to approximately one third of the original dosage and monitor tacrolimus levels
Terfenadine	**Contraindicated**
Vinca alkaloids	May increase levels of vinca alkaloids

DOSING

Posaconazole is available in a solution for oral administration containing 40 mg/mL.

- **Prophylaxis:** 200 mg three times a day; duration is based on recovery from neutropenia or immunosuppression
- **Oropharyngeal candidiasis:** 100 mg twice a day on day one, then 100 mg daily for 13 days
- **Refractory oropharyngeal candidiasis:** 400 mg twice a day; duration per clinical response

SPECIAL POPULATIONS

RENAL IMPAIRMENT: No dosage adjustment needed.

HEPATIC IMPAIRMENT: Caution should be used. Liver function tests should be monitored.

PEDIATRIC PATIENTS: Safety and effectiveness of posaconazole in patients aged younger than 13 years have not been established. For pediatric patients 13 years and older, adult dosage should be used.

PREGNANCY: Category C.

BREASTFEEDING: The expected benefits of posaconazole therapy for the mother should be weighed against the potential risk from exposure of posaconazole to the infant.

THE ART OF ANTIMICROBIAL THERAPY

Clinical Pearls

1. Posaconazole should be administered with food.
2. Posaconazole has activity against *Zygomycetes* and has been used in cases refractory to amphotericin.
3. Posaconazole is an inhibitor of cytochrome P450 and can enhance the activity of many commonly used drugs.
4. Liver function tests should be evaluated at the start of and during the course of posaconazole therapy.

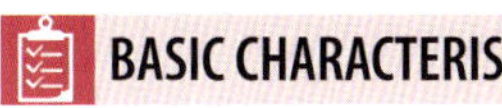

BASIC CHARACTERISTICS

Class: Heterocyclic prazino-isoquinoline derivative

Mechanism of Action: Induces a rapid contraction of schistosomes and causes vacuolization and disintegration of the schistosome tegument.

Metabolic Route: Praziquantel is metabolized by the liver and excreted in the urine.

FDA-APPROVED INDICATIONS

FDA-Approved Indications: Indicated for the treatment of ***Schistosoma*** (e.g., *Schistosoma mekongi, Schistosoma japonicum, Schistosoma mansoni,* and *Schistosoma haematobium*), and infections caused by the **liver flukes**, *Clonorchis sinensis or Opisthorchis viverrini.*

Also Used for: Intestinal tapeworms (*Taenia saginata, Taenia solium, Diphyllobothrium latum, Dipylidium caninum, Hymenolepsis nana,* and *Cysticercus cellulosae*) and for hydatid cyst disease preoperatively or in case of spillage of cyst contents during surgery; and **lung flukes** (*Paragonimus westermani*).

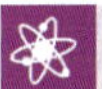

SIDE EFFECTS/TOXICITY

Praziquantel must not be given to patients who previously have shown hypersensitivity to the drug. Because parasite destruction within the eye may cause irreparable lesions, ocular cysticercosis should not be treated with this compound.

Common side effects/toxicities include abdominal pain, nausea, diarrhea, malaise, headache, and dizziness; also reported are hypersensitivity, polyserositis, arrhythmia (including bradycardia, ectopic rhythms, ventricular fibrillation, and AV blocks), seizures, myalgia, somnolence, and vertigo.

DRUG INTERACTIONS/FOOD INTERACTIONS

Praziquantel should be taken with food.

Because praziquantel is metabolized by the liver cytochrome P450 system, concomitant administration of drugs that increase the activity of these enzymes may reduce plasma levels of praziquantel, such as antiepileptic drugs (e.g., phenytoin, phenobarbital, and carbamazepine), dexamethasone, and rifampin. In addition, chloroquine may lower concentrations of praziquantel in blood (mechanism is unclear).

Concomitant administration of drugs that decrease the activity of drug-metabolizing liver enzymes (cytochrome P450), may increase plasma levels of praziquantel (e.g., cimetidine, ketoconazole, itraconazole, and erythromycin); grapefruit juice may also increase plasma levels of praziquantel.

DOSING

Praziquantel is supplied as 600-mg tablets. The tablets should be washed down unchewed with water during meals.

- **Treatment of schistosomiasis:** 20 mg/kg three times a day as a 1-day treatment, at intervals of not less than 4 hours and not more than 6 hours
- **Treatment of clonorchiasis and opisthorchiasis:** 25 mg/kg bodyweight three times a day as a 1-day treatment, at intervals of not less than 4 hours and not more than 6 hours
- **Intestinal tapeworms:** 5 mg/kg to 10 mg/kg once (for *H nana*: 25 mg/kg once)
- ***C cellulosae:*** 100 mg/kg/day in three doses for 1 day, then 50 mg/kg/day in three doses for 29 days
- ***P westermani:*** 75 mg/kg/day in three doses for 2 days

SPECIAL POPULATIONS

RENAL IMPAIRMENT: There is no dosage adjustment for patients with renal insufficiency.

HEPATIC DYSFUNCTION: Caution should be exercised in the administration to patients with moderate to severe liver impairment.

PEDIATRIC PATIENTS: Not studied in children aged younger than 4 years.

PREGNANCY: Category B.

BREASTFEEDING: Mothers should not breastfeed on the day of treatment with praziquantel.

THE ART OF ANTIMICROBIAL THERAPY

Clinical Pearls

1. Although praziquantel is indicated only for the treatment of schistosomiasis and liver flukes, it is the treatment of choice for intestinal tapeworms and lung flukes.
2. Unlike the situation with other liver flukes, praziquantel is **not recommended** for the treatment of ***Fasciola hepatica.***
3. Praziquantel tablets should be washed down unchewed with water during meals to avoid choking.
4. Strong inducers of cytochrome P450 enzymes, such as rifampin, may result in subtherapeutic levels of praziquantel and should be avoided if possible.

PRIMAQUINE PHOSPHATE (Primaquine)

BASIC CHARACTERISTICS

Class: 8-aminoquinoline

Mechanism of Action: Primaquine phosphate is an 8-amino-quinoline compound that eliminates tissue (exoerythrocytic) malarial infection. Thereby, it prevents the development of the blood (erythrocytic) forms of the parasites that are responsible for relapses in vivax malaria. Primaquine phosphate is also active against gametocytes of *Plasmodium falciparum*.

Metabolic Route: Data incomplete.

FDA-APPROVED INDICATIONS

FDA-Approved Indications: Primaquine phosphate is indicated for the radical cure (prevention of relapse) of vivax malaria.

Also Used for: Radical cure of *Plasmodium ovale* and prophylaxis of chloroquine-resistant *P. falciparum*, and for the treatment of *P. jiroveci* with clindamycin.

SIDE EFFECTS/TOXICITY

Hemolytic reactions—leukopenia, hemolytic anemia, and methemoglobinemia—may occur in individuals with glucose-6-phosphate dehydrogenase (G6PD) or nicotinamide adenine dinucleotide (NADH) deficiency or history of favism. Other side effects/toxicities include nausea, vomiting, epigastric distress, and abdominal cramps.

DRUG INTERACTIONS/FOOD INTERACTIONS

Insufficient data to make recommendations. Taking with food may minimize gastrointestinal toxicity.

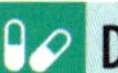

DOSING

Primaquine phosphate is supplied in tablets of 26.3 mg (= 15-mg base). Dosage is one tablet (equivalent to 15-mg base) daily for 14 days.

SPECIAL POPULATIONS

RENAL IMPAIRMENT: There is no dosage adjustment needed.

HEPATIC DYSFUNCTION: There is no dosage adjustment needed.

PEDIATRIC PATIENTS: 0.6 mg/kg/day.

PREGNANCY: Category C.

BREASTFEEDING: Should be given to breastfeeding mothers only if benefit exceeds potential risk.

THE ART OF ANTIMICROBIAL THERAPY

Clinical Pearls

1. Primaquine is used in combination with chloroquine to eradicate the liver (nonerythrocytic) phase of *Plasmodium vivax.*
2. Patients should be screened for G6PD deficiency before administration of primaquine.
3. Complete blood counts should be monitored during therapy.

PYRANTEL PAMOATE (Antiminth)

BASIC CHARACTERISTICS

Class: Tetrahydropyrimidine

Mechanism of Action: Depolarizes the neuromuscular junction of the nematode causing muscular contraction followed by paralysis.

Metabolic Route: Pyrantel pamoate is poorly absorbed from the gastrointestinal tract, and is predominantly eliminated unchanged in the feces.

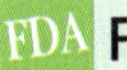

FDA-APPROVED INDICATIONS

Not FDA-approved, but used for treatment of *Ascaris lumbricoides (roundworms), Enterobius vermicularis (pinworms), Trichostrongylus orientalis, Ancylostoma duodenale,* and *Necator americanus (hookworm).*

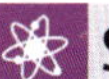

SIDE EFFECTS/TOXICITY

Side effects/toxicities include abdominal cramps, nausea, vomiting, diarrhea, anorexia, headache, dizziness, pruritus, and insomnia.

DRUG INTERACTIONS/FOOD INTERACTIONS

Pyrantel is antagonistic with piperazine and should not be coadministered.

DOSING

11-mg base/kg given once orally with a maximum of 1 g. For the treatment of enterobiasis, the dose should be repeated after 2 weeks.

SPECIAL POPULATIONS

RENAL IMPAIRMENT: There is no dosage adjustment.

HEPATIC DYSFUNCTION: There is no dosage adjustment.

PEDIATRIC PATIENTS: Safety in children aged younger than 2 years has not been established.

PREGNANCY: Unknown.

BREASTFEEDING: Unknown.

THE ART OF ANTIMICROBIAL THERAPY

Clinical Pearls

1. Pyrantel is not available commercially in the United States. It may be obtained through compounding pharmacies via the National Association of Compounding Pharmacies (800-687-7850) or the Professional Compounding Centers of America (800-331-2498, http://www.pccarx.com).
2. Pyrantel is not effective against *Trichuris trichiura.*

BASIC CHARACTERISTICS

Class: Pyrazine analogue of nicotinamide

Mechanisms of Action: Unknown.

Mechanisms of Resistance: Point mutations in the pyrazinamidase gene.

Metabolic Route: Pyrazinamide is hydrolyzed in the liver and excreted in the urine.

FDA FDA-APPROVED INDICATIONS

FDA-Approved Indication: Treatment of active tuberculosis in combination with other antimycobacterials.

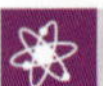

SIDE EFFECTS/TOXICITY

Pyrazinamide inhibits renal excretion of urates, leading to hyperuricemea or gout; more commonly, it produces nongouty polyarthralgias.

Other side effects/toxicities include fever, hypersensitivity, anorexia, nausea, vomiting, diarrhea, hepatitis, cutaneous flushing, porphyria, dysuria, thrombocytopenia, and sideroblastic anemia.

DRUG INTERACTIONS/FOOD INTERACTIONS

Interferes with Ketostix and Acetest—produces a brown color.

Food impairs absorption slightly, but this is of minimal clinical significance and improves gastrointestinal tolerance.

DOSING

Dose should never be divided, but should be given a single dose.

- Daily dosage: 15 mg/kg to 30 mg/kg orally once daily, with a maximum of 2 g per day.
- Twice-weekly dosage: 40 kg to 55 kg: 2000 mg; 56 kg to 75 kg: 3000 mg; 76 kg to 90 kg: 4000 mg (maximum)
- Thrice-weekly dosage: 40 kg to 55 kg: 1500 mg; 56 kg to 75 kg: 2500 mg; 76 kg to 90 kg: 3000 mg (maximum)

SPECIAL POPULATIONS

RENAL IMPAIRMENT: 25 mg/kg to 35 mg/kg, three times per week (not daily).

HEPATIC DYSFUNCTION: No dosage adjustment, but use with caution.

PEDIATRIC PATIENTS: Pyrazinamide is administered orally 15 mg/kg to 30 mg/kg once daily, with a maximum of 2 g per day. Twice-weekly dosage: 50 mg/kg, maximum 4 g.

PREGNANCY: Category C.

BREASTFEEDING: Pyrazinamide should be used with caution in breastfeeding mothers.

THE ART OF ANTIMICROBIAL THERAPY

Clinical Pearls

1. Pyrazinamide should never be used alone in the treatment of active tuberculosis.
2. The regimen of pyrazinamide plus rifampin for prophylaxis is no longer indicated, because of hepatotoxicity.
3. Patients with acute gout should not receive pyrazinamide.
4. Pyrazinamide should be used with caution in patients with liver disease and avoided if possible in patients with severe liver damage.
5. Hepatic and hematologic function should be monitored at least monthly in all patients who are taking pyrazinamide.

PYRIMETHAMINE (Daraprim)

BASIC CHARACTERISTICS

Class: Diaminopyrimidine

Mechanism of Action: Antagonizes folic acid.

Metabolic Route: Data incomplete.

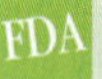

FDA-APPROVED INDICATIONS

FDA-Approved Indications: Treatment of toxoplasmosis when used conjointly with a sulfonamide; alternative treatment of acute malaria with a sulfonamide; and chemoprophylaxis of malaria caused by susceptible strains of *Plasmodia.*

Also Used for: Prophylaxis of toxoplasmosis (with dapsone) in patients with HIV who cannot tolerate trimethoprim plus sulfamethoxazole.

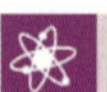

SIDE EFFECTS/TOXICITY

Contraindicated in patients with known hypersensitivity to pyrimethamine or in patients with documented megaloblastic anemia caused by folate deficiency.

Side effects/toxicities include hypersensitivity reactions, occasionally severe (such as Stevens-Johnson syndrome, toxic epidermal necrolysis, erythema multiforme, and anaphylaxis), hyperphenylalaninemia, anorexia, vomiting, atrophic glossitis, hematuria, arrhythmias, pulmonary eosinophilia, megaloblastic anemia, leukopenia, thrombocytopenia, and pancytopenia.

DRUG INTERACTIONS/FOOD INTERACTIONS

Pyrimethamine should be taken with food to decrease side effects.

The concomitant use of other antifolic drugs including sulfonamides or trimethoprim plus sulfamethoxazole combinations, proguanil, zidovudine, or cytostatic agents (e.g., methotrexate) may increase the risk of bone marrow suppression.

DOSING

For treatment of toxoplasmosis: Starting dosage is 50 mg to 75 mg of the drug daily for 1 to 3 weeks. Then half the dose previously given and continued for an additional 4 to 5 weeks.

For treatment of acute malaria: 25 mg daily for 2 days with a sulfonamide will initiate transmission control and suppression of non-*falciparum* malaria.

Should circumstances arise wherein pyrimethamine must be used alone in semi-immune persons, the adult dosage for acute malaria is 50 mg for 2 days.

For chemoprophylaxis of malaria: 25 mg (1 tablet) once weekly.

SPECIAL POPULATIONS

RENAL IMPAIRMENT: Use with caution.

HEPATIC DYSFUNCTION: Use with caution.

PEDIATRIC PATIENTS:

For toxoplasmosis: 1 mg/kg/day divided into two equal daily doses; after 2 to 4 days this dosage may be reduced to one half and continued for approximately 1 month.

For chemoprophylaxis of malaria:

- Pediatric patients aged older than 10 years: 25 mg (1 tablet) once weekly
- Children aged 4 through 10 years: 12.5 mg (½ tablet) once weekly
- Infants and children aged younger than 4 years: 6.25 mg (¼ tablet) once weekly

PREGNANCY: Category C.

BREASTFEEDING: Mothers should discontinue breastfeeding if they are taking pyrimethamine.

THE ART OF ANTIMICROBIAL THERAPY

Clinical Pearls

1. The action of pyrimethamine is enhanced when it is used with sulfa compounds.
2. Most *Plasmodia* around the world are resistant to pyrimethamine.
3. Folinic acid (leucovorin) should be administered in a dosage of 5 mg to 15 mg daily (orally, IV, or IM) to all patients receiving pyrimethamine.

QUINACRINE HYDROCHLORIDE (Atabrine)

BASIC CHARACTERISTICS

Class: Acridine derivative

Mechanism of Action: Unknown.

Metabolic Route: Quinacrine hydrochloride is excreted in the urine.

FDA FDA-APPROVED INDICATIONS

Not FDA-approved, but used for treatment of *Giardia lamblia* infections; it is no longer used for malaria or tapeworm infections because of its toxicity.

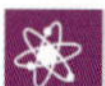

SIDE EFFECTS/TOXICITY

Quinacrine should not be given to patients with a history of psychosis or to patients with psoriasis because of possible exacerbations.

Side effects/toxicities include dizziness, abdominal pain, nausea, vomiting, diarrhea, headache, and yellow discoloration of the skin and urine.

DRUG INTERACTIONS/FOOD INTERACTIONS

Quinacrine should not be administered with primaquine because it increases the plasma concentration of primaquine.

DOSING

100 mg three times a day for 5 to 7 days.

SPECIAL POPULATIONS

RENAL IMPAIRMENT: Unknown.

HEPATIC DYSFUNCTION: Unknown.

PEDIATRIC PATIENTS: 2 mg/kg three times a day for 5 to 7 days.

PREGNANCY: Unknown.

BREASTFEEDING: Unknown.

THE ART OF ANTIMICROBIAL THERAPY

Clinical Pearls

1. Quinacrine should not be used for malaria or tapeworm infections.
2. Quinacrine should not be given to patients with a history of psychosis or psoriasis.
3. Quinacrine is not available in United States or Canada.

BASIC CHARACTERISTICS

Class: Arylaminoalcohol

Mechanism of Action: Acts primarily as an intraerythrocytic schizonticide, with little effect upon sporozoites or upon preerythrocytic parasites. Quinidine is gametocidal to *Plasmodium vivax* and *Plasmodium malariae*, but not to *Plasmodium falciparum*.

Metabolic Route: Most quinidine is metabolized by the liver's cytochrome P450 system.

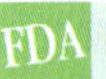

FDA-APPROVED INDICATIONS

FDA-Approved Indications: Treatment of life-threatening *P. falciparum* malaria and for the conversion of atrial fibrillation/flutter and the treatment of ventricular arrhythmias.

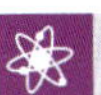

SIDE EFFECTS/TOXICITY

Quinidine is **contraindicated:**

1. in patients who are known to be allergic to it, or who have developed thrombocytopenic purpura during prior therapy with quinidine or quinine,
2. in the absence of a functioning artificial pacemaker, quinidine is also contraindicated in any patient whose cardiac rhythm is dependent upon a junctional or idioventricular pacemaker, including patients in complete atrioventricular block, and
3. in those with myasthenia gravis and others who might be adversely affected by an anticholinergic agent.

Other side effects/toxicities include fever, angioedema rash, cinchonism (a syndrome that may also include tinnitus, reversible high-frequency hearing loss, deafness, vertigo, blurred vision, diplopia, photophobia, headache, confusion, and delirium), prolongation of QTc interval leading to torsade de pointes, other ventricular arrhythmias, paradoxical increase in ventricular rate in atrial flutter/fibrillation, bradycardia in patients with sick sinus syndrome, hepatotoxicity, bronchospasm, pneumonitis, lymphadenopathy, uveitis, visual disturbances, the sicca syndrome, arthralgia, myalgia, vasculitis, a lupuslike syndrome, psychosis, seizures, ataxia, elevation in serum levels of skeletal muscle enzymes, hemolytic anemia, thrombocytopenic purpura, and agranulocytosis.

DRUG INTERACTIONS/FOOD INTERACTIONS

Quinidine levels may be **increased** by drugs that alkalinize the urine (carbonic–anhydrase inhibitors, sodium bicarbonate, thiazide diuretics), amiodarone or cimetidine, ketoconazole, and diltiazem.

Quinidine levels may be **decreased** by nifedipine, phenobarbital, phenytoin, rifampin, and verapamil.

Quinidine may result in **increased levels** or potentiated effects of digoxin, warfarin, drugs metabolized by cytochrome P450 IID6 (e.g., phenothiazines, polycyclic antidepressants, codeine, hydrocodone), procainamide, verapamil, haloperidol, calcium channel blockers, and depolarizing neuromuscular blocking agents.

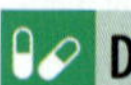

DOSING

Treatment of *P. falciparum* malaria: loading dose of 24 mg/kg of quinidine gluconate (15 mg/kg of quinidine base) infused over 4 hours. Thereafter a maintenance regimen of 12 mg/kg quinidine gluconate (7.5 mg/kg base) infused over 4 hours every 8 hours, starting 8 hours after the beginning of the loading dose. Continue for 7 days. (In patients able to swallow, the maintenance infusions can be discontinued, and approximately the same daily doses of quinidine can be given orally, with 300-mg tablets of quinidine sulfate).

SPECIAL POPULATIONS

RENAL IMPAIRMENT: Quinidine levels may increase, so dosage reduction is recommended.

HEPATIC DYSFUNCTION: Quinidine levels may increase, so dosage reduction is recommended.

PEDIATRIC PATIENTS: Same dosage as adults.

PREGNANCY: Category C.

BREASTFEEDING: Administration of quinidine should (if possible) be avoided in lactating women who continue to breastfeed.

THE ART OF ANTIMICROBIAL THERAPY

Clinical Pearls

1. Overly rapid infusion of quinidine may cause peripheral vascular collapse and severe hypotension.
2. Patients should be monitored for the side effects/toxicities listed previously, particularly for hypoglycemia and electrocardiographic abnormalities (e.g., QTc prolongation).
3. Quinidine has many drug–drug interactions, which affect the levels of coadministered drugs as well as the levels of quinidine.

QUININE SULFATE (Qualaquin)

Note: Quinine sulfate is available as Qualaquin for oral administration; quinine can also be administered intravenously or intramuscularly.

BASIC CHARACTERISTICS

Class: Arylaminoalcohol

Mechanism of Action: Quinine inhibits nucleic acid synthesis, protein synthesis, and glycolysis in *Plasmodium falciparum* and can bind with hemazoin in parasitized erythrocytes.

Metabolic Route: Quinine is metabolized by the liver and excreted partially in the urine.

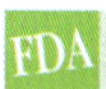

FDA-APPROVED INDICATIONS

FDA-Approved Indications: Oral quinine sulfate is indicated only for treatment of uncomplicated *P. falciparum* malaria.

Also Used for: Administered IV or IM for severe malaria.

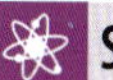

SIDE EFFECTS/TOXICITY

Quinine is **contraindicated** in patients with a prolonged QT interval, G6PD deficiency, myasthenia gravis, optic neuritis, or known hypersensitivity to quinine, mefloquine, or quinidine.

Side effects/toxicities: "cinchonism" occurs to some degree in almost all patients taking quinine. Symptoms include headache, vasodilation and sweating, nausea, tinnitus, hearing impairment, vertigo or dizziness, blurred vision, and disturbance in color perception. More severe symptoms of cinchonism are vomiting, diarrhea, abdominal pain, deafness, blindness, and disturbances in cardiac rhythm or conduction. Most symptoms of cinchonism are reversible and resolve with discontinuation of quinine.

Other side effects/toxicites include fever, chills, sweating, flushing, asthenia, lupuslike syndrome, hypersensitivity reactions, agranulocytosis, hypoprothrombinemia, thrombocytopenia, disseminated intravascular coagulation, hemolytic anemia, hemolytic uremic syndrome, thrombotic thrombocytopenic purpura, coagulopathy, lupus anticoagulant, headache, diplopia, confusion, seizures, coma, tremors, ataxia, acute dystonic reaction, aphasia, suicide, rashes, pruritus, erythema multiforme, Stevens-Johnson syndrome, toxic epidermal necrolysis, photosensitivity reactions, acral necrosis, cutaneous vasculitis, chest pain, vasodilatation, hypotension, postural hypotension, tachycardia, bradycardia, palpitations, syncope, atrioventricular block, atrial fibrillation, irregular heart rhythm, unifocal premature ventricular contractions, nodal escape beats, U waves, QT prolongation, ventricular fibrillation, ventricular tachycardia, torsade de pointes, cardiac arrest, nausea, vomiting, diarrhea, abdominal pain, gastric irritation, esophagitis, hepatitis, asthma, dyspnea, pulmonary edema, hypoglycemia, myalgias and muscle weakness, hemoglobinuria, renal failure, acute interstitial nephritis, visual disturbances, optic neuritis, blindness, vertigo, tinnitus, hearing impairment, and deafness.

 DRUG INTERACTIONS/FOOD INTERACTIONS

Quinine should be taken with food to minimize gastrointestinal discomfort.

The concomitant administration of the following should be **avoided**: antacids, rifampin, troleandomycin, erythromycin, astemizole, cisapride, terfenadine, halofantrine, imozide, mefloquine, and quinidine.

Concomitant administration of the following may result in changes in the level of quinine and/or the coadministered drug, and monitoring is recommended:

Coadministered Drug	*Effect*
Aminophylline	Aminophylline levels decreased
Carbamazepine	Decreased levels of quinine, increased levels of carbamazepine
CYP2D6 substrates (e.g., desipramine, flecainide, debrisoquine, dextromethorphan, metoprolol, or paroxetine)	Increased level of the CYP2D6 substrate
Digoxin	Increased levels of digoxin
Erythromycin	Increased levels of quinine
Histamine H2-receptor blockers	Increased levels of quinine
HMG-CoA reductase (statins)	Levels of statins increased
Ketoconazole	Increased levels of quinine
Neuromuscular blocking agents (succinylcholine and tubocurarine)	Increased levels of neuromuscular blocking agents
Phenobarbital	Decreased levels of quinine, increased levels of phenobarbital
Phenytoin	Decreased levels of quinine
Tetracycline	Increased levels of quinine
Theophylline	Decreased levels of theophylline
Warfarin	Increased levels of warfarin

Quinine may produce an elevated value for urinary 17-ketogenic steroids when the Zimmerman method is used.

 DOSING

For treatment of **uncomplicated** ***P. falciparum*** **malaria** in adults, oral dosage of quinine sulfate is 648 mg (two capsules) every 8 hours for 3 to 7 days.

For severe illness, quinine is given intravenously, as follows:

Loading dose of 20 mg/kg (salt; 1 mg salt = 0.83 mg base) in 300 mL of normal saline IV over 2 to 4 hours; maintenance dosage: 10 mg/kg every 8 hours.

Parenteral administration of quinine can also be achieved by the intramuscular route, in the same dosages as the intravenous regimens.

SPECIAL POPULATIONS

RENAL IMPAIRMENT: In patients with acute uncomplicated malaria and severe chronic renal failure, the following modified dosage regimen is recommended: one loading dose of 648 mg followed 12 hours later by maintenance doses of 324 mg every 12 hours.

The effects of mild and moderate renal impairment on the pharmacokinetics and safety of quinine sulfate are not known.

HEPATIC DYSFUNCTION: Patients with mild to moderate hepatic impairment (Child-Pugh class A and Child-Pugh class B, respectively), should be monitored closely for adverse reactions; dosage reduction is not warranted.

The effects of severe hepatic impairment (Child-Pugh class C) on the safety and pharmacokinetics of quinine sulfate are not known.

PEDIATRIC PATIENTS: Not studied in those aged younger than 16 years.

Oral dosage for pediatric patients aged 16 years and older: 10 mg/kg for 3 to 7 days.

IV dosage: same as for adults.

PREGNANCY: Category C.

BREASTFEEDING: Risk and benefit to mother and infant should be considered before administration.

THE ART OF ANTIMICROBIAL THERAPY

Clinical Pearls

1. Quinine is not approved for patients with severe or complicated *P. falciparum* malaria or the prophylaxis of malaria.
2. Quinine is not recommended for the treatment of leg cramps.
3. Serologic testing for quinine-specific antibody may be useful for identifying the specific cause of thrombocytopenia in individual cases.
4. Patient should be monitored for the adverse events listed previously, particularly for electrocardiographic abnormalities (e.g., QTc prolongation) and hypoglycemia.

QUINUPRISTIN PLUS DALFOPRISTIN (Synercid)

BASIC CHARACTERISTICS

Class: Streptogramin

Mechanism of Action: Inhibits protein synthesis by irreversibly binding the 50S ribosomal subunit. Quinupristin inhibits peptide chain elongation whereas dalfopristin interferes with peptidyl transferase.

Mechanisms of Resistance: Resistance can occur to macrolides, licosamides, and streptogramins by methylation of their binding site. Resistance may also be mediated by efflux pumps.

Metabolic Route: The majority of quinupristin plus dalfopristin is excreted in the feces.

FDA-APPROVED INDICATIONS

FDA-Approved Indications: Serious or life-threatening infections associated with vancomycin-resistant *Enterococcus faecium* (VREF) bacteremia, and complicated skin and skin structure infections caused by *Staphylococcus aureus* (methicillin-susceptible) or *Streptococcus pyogenes.*

SIDE EFFECTS/TOXICITY

Quinupristin plus dalfopristin is **contraindicated** in patients with known hypersensitivity to other streptogramins (e.g., pristinamycin or virginiamycin).

Side effects/toxicities include venous irritation; arthralgias/myalgias; hypersensitivity; rash, pain, and edema at infusion site; phlebitis; chest pain; palpitation; dyspnea; pleural effusion; stomatitis dyspepsia; oral candidiasis; abdominal pain; constipation; pancreatitis; pseudomembranous enterocolitis; gout; peripheral edema; anxiety; confusion; dizziness; hypertonia; insomnia; leg cramps; paresthesia; vasodilation; vaginitis; hematuria; and hyperbilirubinemia.

DRUG INTERACTIONS/FOOD INTERACTIONS

Because of inhibition of cytochrome P450 3A4, coadministration of quinupristin plus dalfopristin with drugs that are cytochrome P450 3A4 substrates and possess a narrow therapeutic window requires caution and monitoring of these drugs (e.g., cyclosporine) whenever possible. Concomitant medications metabolized by the cytochrome P450 3A4 enzyme system that may prolong the QTc interval should be avoided.

Selected **drugs whose serum levels may be increased** by quinupristin plus dalfopristin include astemizole, terfenadine, delavirdine, nevirapine, indinavir, ritonavir, vinca alkaloids, docetaxel, paclitaxel, midazolam, diazepam, nifedipine, verapamil, diltiazem, HMG-CoA reductase inhibitors (e.g., lovastatin), cisapride, cyclosporine, tacrolimus, methylprednisolone, carbamazepine, quinidine, lidocaine, and disopyramide.

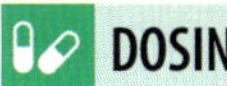

DOSING

Quinupristin plus dalfopristin should be administered by intravenous infusion. The recommended dosage is 7.5 mg/kg, every 8 hours for VREF and every 12 hours for complicated skin and skin structure infections.

SPECIAL POPULATIONS

RENAL IMPAIRMENT: No dosage adjustment is necessary.

HEPATIC DYSFUNCTION: No dosage adjustment is necessary.

PEDIATRIC PATIENTS: Quinupristin plus dalfopristin has been used in a limited number of pediatric patients under emergency-use conditions at a dosage of 7.5 mg/kg every 8 hours or every 12 hours. However, the safety and effectiveness of quinupristin plus dalfopristin in patients aged younger than 16 years have not been established.

PREGNANCY: Category B.

BREASTFEEDING: Caution should be used when one is administering quinupristin plus dalfopristin to breastfeeding mothers.

THE ART OF ANTIMICROBIAL THERAPY

Clinical Pearls

1. Quinupristin plus dalfopristin is not active against *Enterococci* other than *E. faecium.*
2. If severe venous irritation occurs, quinupristin plus dalfopristin can be administered by peripherally inserted central catheter (PICC) or a central venous catheter.
3. If a patient develops severe myalgias, reduction of either the dose or the frequency may alleviate symptoms.

RALTEGRAVIR (Isentress)

BASIC CHARACTERISTICS

Class: Integrase inhibitor

Mechanism of Action: Inhibits the catalytic activity of HIV-1 integrase, which terminates integration of HIV DNA into the host genome.

Mechanism of Resistance: Development of mutations on the enzyme integrase leads to the inability of raltegravir to bind the active site of the enzyme and allows integrase activity to continue. Mutations that lead to resistance to raltegravir include Q148H/K/R and N155H.

Metabolic Route: Raltegravir is glucuronidated by the enzyme UGT1A1 in the liver and then excreted.

FDA FDA-APPROVED INDICATIONS

FDA-Approved Indications: Treatment of HIV-1 in combinations with other antiretroviral agents in adult patients who have evidence of viral replication and HIV-1 strains resistant to multiple antiretroviral agents. Raltegravir is currently approved for both treatment-experienced and treatment-naïve patients.

SIDE EFFECTS/TOXICITY

Side effects/toxicities include immune reconstitution syndrome, fever, headaches, dizziness, hypersensitivity, diarrhea, nausea, myopathy and rhabdomyolysis, abdominal pain, gastritis, hepatitis, genital herpes, herpes zoster, and renal failure.

DRUG INTERACTIONS/FOOD INTERACTIONS

Raltegravir can be taken with or without food.

Raltegravir is not a substrate, inhibitor, or inducer of the CYP3A4 enzymes. Raltegravir is metabolized by UGT1A1. Caution should be used when one is coadministering raltegravir with inducers or inhibitors of UGT1A1 (e.g., rifampin) because of reduced concentration of raltegravir; however, there are no contraindications.

DOSING

400 mg orally, twice daily.

SPECIAL POPULATIONS

RENAL IMPAIRMENT: There is no dosage adjustment needed.

HEPATIC DYSFUNCTION: There is no dosage adjustment needed.

PEDIATRIC PATIENTS: Not indicated for those aged younger than 16 years.

PREGNANCY: Category C.

BREASTFEEDING: It is recommended that HIV-positive mothers not breastfeed their children, to decrease mother-to-child transmission of HIV.

THE ART OF ANTIMICROBIAL THERAPY

Clinical Pearls

1. Raltegravir should always be used in combination with other antiretrovirals.
2. Raltegravir should be given twice daily.
3. Raltegravir is not a substrate, inducer, or inhibitor of the CYP3A4 enzymes.

■ RIBAVIRIN (Rebetol, Copegus, Ribasphere [oral], and Virazole [inhaled])

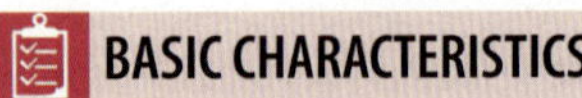

BASIC CHARACTERISTICS

Class: Nucleoside analogue

Mechanism of Action: Not known.

Mechanism of Resistance: Not known.

Metabolic Route: Ribavirin is metabolized by phosphorylation or deribosylation/hydrolysis to yield a triazole carboxylic acid metabolite and is excreted renally.

FDA FDA-APPROVED INDICATIONS

FDA-Approved Indications: Treatment of hepatitis C virus (HCV) and respiratory syncytial virus (RSV) as follows:

Adult use:

- **Copegus** in combination with peginterferon α-2a is indicated for the treatment of adults with chronic HCV infection who have compensated liver disease and have not been previously treated with interferon α.
- **Rebetol** and **Ribasphere** are indicated in combination with interferon α-2b, recombinant α-2b and peginterferon α-2b for the treatment of chronic HCV in patients aged 18 years and older with compensated liver disease previously untreated with α interferon and in patients aged 18 years and older who have relapsed following α interferon therapy.

Pediatric use:

- **Rebetol** is indicated in combination with interferon α-2b for injection for the treatment of chronic HCV in patients aged 5 years and older (capsules) and in patients aged 3 years and older (oral solution) with compensated liver disease previously untreated with α interferon and in patients who have relapsed following α interferon therapy.
- **Virazole** (inhaled ribavirin) is indicated for the treatment of hospitalized infants and young children with severe lower respiratory tract infections caused by RSV. Treatment early in the course of severe lower respiratory tract infection may be necessary to achieve efficacy.

Also Used for: Some authorities recommend consideration of ribavirin therapy for any patient with viral hemorrhagic fever caused by arenavirus (Lassa fever, New World hemorrhagic fevers) or bunyavirus (Hantavirus, Rift Valley fever, Crimean-Congo hemorrhagic fever), or for suspected viral hemorrhagic fever if the etiology is unknown.

SIDE EFFECTS/TOXICITY

WARNING: Ribavirin monotherapy is not effective for the treatment of chronic HCV infection and should not be used alone for this indication. The primary clinical toxicity of ribavirin is hemolytic anemia. The anemia associated with ribavirin therapy may result in worsening of cardiac disease that has led to fatal and nonfatal myocardial infarctions. Patients with a history of significant or unstable cardiac disease should not be treated with ribavirin.

Significant teratogenic and/or embryocidal effects have been demonstrated in all animal species exposed to ribavirin. In addition, ribavirin has a multiple dose half-life of 12 days, and it may persist in nonplasma compartments for as long as 6 months. Ribavirin therapy is **contraindicated** in women who are pregnant and in the male partners of women who are pregnant. Extreme care must be taken to avoid pregnancy during therapy and for 6 months after completion of therapy in both female patients and in female partners of male patients who are taking ribavirin therapy. At least two reliable forms of effective contraception must be utilized during treatment and during the 6-month posttreatment follow-up period.

Ribavirin is **contraindicated** in patients with a history of hypersensitivity, autoimmune hepatitis, and hemoglobinopathies (e.g., thalassemia major, sickle-cell anemia).

Other side effects/toxicities include hemolytic anemia, which may result in worsening of cardiac disease and myocardial infarctions. Also seen are pancreatitis, pneumonia, and dental and periodontal disorders.

Aerosolized ribavirin: Sudden deterioration of respiratory function has been associated with initiation of aerosolized ribavirin use in infants. Respiratory function should be carefully monitored during treatment. If sudden deterioration of respiratory function is noted, treatment should be stopped and reinstituted only with extreme caution, continuous monitoring, and consideration of concomitant administration of bronchodilators. Use of aerosolized ribavirin in patients requiring mechanical ventilator assistance should be undertaken only by physicians and support staff familiar with this mode of administration and the specific ventilator being used. Strict attention must be paid to procedures that have been shown to minimize the accumulation of drug precipitate, which can result in mechanical ventilator dysfunction and associated increased pulmonary pressures.

DRUG INTERACTIONS/FOOD INTERACTIONS

It is recommended to take ribavirin with food.

Coadministration of ribavirin capsules or solution and didanosine is not recommended. Use of ribavirin with zidovudine or stavudine should be undertaken with caution.

DOSING

Ribavirin is supplied in 200-mg capsules; tablets of 200 mg, 400 mg, and 600 mg; and a clear, colorless to pale or light yellow bubble gum–flavored liquid (40 mg/mL).

The recommended daily dosage is based on body weight as follows:

≥ 75 kg: 600 mg twice daily

< 75 kg: 400 mg in the am and 600 mg in the pm

Ribavirin for inhalation is supplied in 100-mL glass vials with 6 g of sterile, lyophilized drug, which is to be reconstituted with 300 mL of sterile water and administered only by a small-particle aerosol generator (SPAG-2). The recommended treatment regimen is 20 mg/mL with continuous aerosol administration for 12 to 18 hours per day for 3 to 7 days.

SPECIAL POPULATIONS

RENAL IMPAIRMENT: Patients with creatinine clearance less than 50 mL/min should not be treated with ribavirin.

HEPATIC DYSFUNCTION: Caution should be used when ribavirin is administered to patients with hepatic impairment.

PEDIATRIC PATIENTS: The recommended dosage is based on body weight as follows:

25 kg to 36 kg: 200 mg twice daily

37 kg to 49 kg: 200 mg in am and 400 mg in pm

50 kg to 61 kg: 400 mg twice daily

> 61 kg: adult dosage

PREGNANCY: Category X.

BREASTFEEDING: The use of ribavirin is not recommended for breastfeeding mothers.

THE ART OF ANTIMICROBIAL THERAPY

Clinical Pearls

1. Treatment early with inhaled ribavirin in infants and young children for severe lower respiratory tract infection may be necessary to achieve efficacy.
2. Ribavirin pills should always be combined with an interferon α product.

3. Ribavirin is pregnancy category X; women should use two barriers of protection for birth control. This caution extends to **when the male sexual partner is taking ribavirin as well**.
4. Routine monitoring during therapy should include complete blood count, liver function tests and thyroid-stimulating hormone, pregnancy tests, and electrocardiography.

RIFABUTIN (Mycobutin)

BASIC CHARACTERISTICS

Class: Rifamycin

Mechanism of Action: Inhibits DNA-dependent RNA polymerase activity in susceptible cells.

Mechanism of Resistance: Resistance occurs as single-step mutations of the DNA-dependent RNA polymerase.

Metabolic Route: Rifabutin is metabolized in the liver into five products that are excreted in the feces and urine.

FDA-APPROVED INDICATIONS

FDA-Approved Indications: Prevention of disseminated *Mycobacterium avium* complex (MAC) disease in patients with advanced HIV infection.

Also Used for: Treatment of MAC in combination with other medications in both HIV-infected and HIV-noninfected patients.

Rifabutin is commonly substituted for rifampin in the treatment of tuberculosis because it interacts with other medications less than rifampin does (approximately 40% less).

SIDE EFFECTS/TOXICITY

Rifabutin is **contraindicated** in patients with a history of hypersensitivity to any of the rifamycins.

Side effects/toxicities include anterior uveitis; liver dysfunction, both hepatocellular damage and jaundice; porphyria; reddish coloration of the urine, sweat, sputum, and tears; "flu syndrome" (fever, chills, and malaise) when used intermittently; anaphylaxis; rash; flushing; epigastric distress; anorexia; nausea; vomiting; flatulence; *Clostridium difficile*–associated diarrhea; disseminated intravascular coagulation; visual disturbances; adrenal insufficiency; renal insufficiency; confusion; elevations in serum uric acid; thrombocytopenia; leukopenia; and hemolytic anemia.

DRUG INTERACTIONS/FOOD INTERACTIONS

Absorption of rifabutin is reduced when the drug is ingested with food, but absorption is usually adequate, and ingestion with food reduces gastrointestinal intolerance.

Rifabutin is known to induce certain cytochrome P450 enzymes. Administration of rifabutin with drugs that undergo biotransformation through these metabolic pathways may accelerate elimination and decrease the therapeutic effect of these coadministered drugs, many of which require monitoring and possible adjustment during and following coadministration with rifabutin. The list of drugs so affected includes the following drugs/classes: antiarrhythmics, oral anticoagulants, anticonvulsants, antifungals, barbiturates, β-blockers, calcium channel blockers, cardiac glycoside preparations, CCR5 inhibitors, chloramphenicol, clarithromycin, clofibrate, hormonal contraceptives (patients should be advised to use nonhormonal methods of birth control during rifampin therapy), corticosteroids, cyclosporine, dapsone, diazepam, doxycycline, enalapril, fluoroquinolones, haloperidol, oral hypoglycemic agents, levothyroxine, methadone, narcotic analgesics, nonnucleoside reverse transcriptase inhibitors, nortriptyline, progestins, protease inhibitors, quinine, sulfapyridine, tacrolimus, theophylline, tricyclic antidepressants, and zidovudine.

Rifabutin levels may increase when it is coadministered with atovaquone, probenecid, and cotrimoxazole, and may decrease when given with ketoconazole and antacids (give rifampin at least 1 hour before the ingestion of antacids).

When rifabutin is given concomitantly with either halothane or isoniazid, the potential for hepatotoxicity is increased, and concomitant use of rifabutin and halothane should be avoided.

Drug/laboratory interactions:

Cross-reactivity and false-positive urine screening tests for opiates have been reported in patients receiving rifabutin.

Therapeutic levels of rifabutin have been shown to inhibit standard microbiological assays for serum folate and vitamin B12.

Dosage adjustment is frequently necessary with antiretroviral drugs, and updated recommendations may be found at http://aidsinfo.nih.gov.htm. Current recommendations are as follows:

Rifabutin	***Antiretroviral Drugs***
450 mg/day to 600 mg/day or 600 mg three times per week	Efavirenz: usual dosage
300 mg/day or 300 mg three times per week	Nevirapine: usual dosage
150 mg/day or 300 mg three times per week	Fosamprenavir: usual dosage Indinavir: 1000 mg three times per day Nelfinavir: 1250 mg twice a day
150 mg every other day or three times per week	Atazanavir: usual dosage Ritonavir: usual dosage Lopinavir plus ritonavir: usual dosage Ritonavir (any dosage) booster with saquinavir, indinavir, fosamprenavir, atazanavir, or darunavir: usual dosage
Usual dosage	Maraviroc: usual dosage
Usual dosage	Raltegravir: usual dosage

DOSING

Rifabutin is supplied as 150-mg tablets. Standard dosage is 300 mg daily. For intermittent dosing, the same dose can be given twice or thrice weekly.

SPECIAL POPULATIONS

RENAL IMPAIRMENT: If Creatinine clearance is less than 30 mL/min, decrease dosage by 50%.

HEPATIC DYSFUNCTION: Patients with impaired liver function should be given rifabutin only in cases of necessity and then with caution and monitoring of liver function.

PEDIATRIC PATIENTS: Not studied; however, 5 mg/kg/day to 10 mg/kg/day is used.

PREGNANCY: Category B.

BREASTFEEDING: Rifabutin can be used in the breastfeeding mother if the benefit outweighs the risk.

THE ART OF ANTIMICROBIAL THERAPY

Clinical Pearls

1. Rifabutin should never be used as monotherapy for prophylaxis of MAC in the setting of active tuberculosis, because resistance may develop.
2. Liver function tests and symptoms of gastrointestinal intolerance should be monitored in all patients receiving rifabutin.
3. Rifabutin is a potent inducer of the P450 cytochrome system, and coadministered medications may require discontinuation or monitoring for possible dosage adjustment. However, the interactions are less than those seen with rifampin.
4. Rifabutin can enhance the metabolism of endogenous substrates including adrenal hormones, thyroid hormones, and vitamin D.
5. Soft contact lenses can be permanently stained when a patient takes rifabutin.

RIFAMPIN (Rifadin, Rifadin IV)

Note: Also available combined with isoniazid as Rifamate and combined with isoniazid plus pyrazinamide as Rifater.

BASIC CHARACTERISTICS

Class: Rifamycin

Mechanisms of Action: Rifampin inhibits DNA-dependent RNA polymerase activity in susceptible cells.

Mechanisms of Resistance: Resistance occurs as single-step mutations of the DNA-dependent RNA polymerase.

Metabolic Route: Rifampin is rapidly eliminated in the bile and undergoes progressive deacetylation and elimination. However, up to 30% of a dose is excreted in the urine, with about half of this being unchanged drug.

FDA-APPROVED INDICATIONS

FDA-Approved Indications: Treatment of all forms of tuberculosis, and treatment of asymptomatic carriers of *Neisseria meningitidis* to eliminate meningococci from the nasopharynx.

Also Used for: Treatment of latent tuberculosis, combination therapy for *Staphylococcus aureus* infections, combination therapy for prosthetic valve endocarditis caused by coagulase-negative staphylococci, and other foreign body infections in combination with tetracyclines and fluoroquinolones.

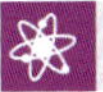

SIDE EFFECTS/TOXICITY

Rifampin is **contraindicated** in patients with a history of hypersensitivity to any of the rifamycins.

Side effects/toxicities include anaphylaxis; liver dysfunction; reddish coloration of the urine, sweat, sputum, and tears; "flu syndrome" (fever, chills, and malaise); rash; flushing; epigastric distress; anorexia; nausea; vomiting; flatulence; *Clostridium difficile*–associated diarrhea; disseminated intravascular coagulation; visual disturbances; adrenal insufficiency; confusion; renal insufficiency; elevations in serum uric acid; thrombocytopenia; leukopenia; and hemolytic anemia.

DRUG INTERACTIONS/FOOD INTERACTIONS

Absorption of rifampin is reduced when the drug is ingested with food, but absorption is usually adequate, and ingestion with food reduces gastrointestinal intolerance.

Rifampin is known to induce certain cytochrome P450 enzymes. Administration of rifampin with drugs that undergo biotransformation through these metabolic pathways may accelerate elimination and decrease the therapeutic effect of these coadministered drugs, many of which require monitoring and possible adjustment during and following coadministration with rifampin. The list of drugs so affected includes the following drugs/classes: antiarrhythmics, oral anticoagulants, anticonvulsants, antifungals, barbiturates, β-blockers, calcium channel blockers, cardiac glycoside preparations, CCR5 inhibitors, chloramphenicol, clarithromycin, clofibrate, hormonal contraceptives (patients should be advised to use nonhormonal methods of birth control during rifampin therapy), corticosteroids, cyclosporine, dapsone, diazepam, doxycycline, enalapril, fluoroquinolones, haloperidol, oral hypoglycemic agents, levothyroxine, methadone, narcotic analgesics, nortriptyline, progestins, protease inhibitors, quinine, sulfapyridine, tacrolimus, theophylline, tricyclic antidepressants, NNRTIs, and zidovudine.

Rifampin levels may increase when it is coadministered with atovaquone, probenecid, and cotrimoxazole, and may decrease when given with ketoconazole and antacids (give rifampin at least 1 hour before the ingestion of antacids).

When rifampin is given concomitantly with either halothane or isoniazid, the potential for hepatotoxicity is increased, and concomitant use of rifampin and halothane should be avoided.

Drug/laboratory interactions:

Cross-reactivity and false-positive urine screening tests for opiates have been reported in patients receiving rifampin.

Therapeutic levels of rifampin have been shown to inhibit standard microbiological assays for serum folate and vitamin B12.

DOSING

Rifampin is supplied as 150-mg and 300-mg tablets. It can also be administered intravenously.

Tuberculosis: 10 mg/kg, in a single daily administration up to 600 mg/day, oral or IV; the same dosage can be given twice or thrice weekly

Meningococcal carriers: 600 mg rifampin administered twice daily for 2 days

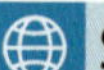

SPECIAL POPULATIONS

RENAL IMPAIRMENT: No dosage adjustment is necessary.

HEPATIC DYSFUNCTION: Patients with impaired liver function should be given rifampin only in cases of necessity and then with caution and monitoring of liver function.

PEDIATRIC PATIENTS:

Tuberculosis: 10 mg/kg to 20 mg/kg, not to exceed 600 mg/day, oral or IV

Meningococcal carriers aged 1 month or older: 10 mg/kg (not to exceed 600 mg per dose) every 12 hours for 2 days; those aged younger than 1 month: 5 mg/kg every 12 hours for 2 days

PREGNANCY: Category C.

BREASTFEEDING: Patients may breastfeed if benefit outweighs risk; small amounts of rifampin are secreted in breastmilk, though the levels are not adequate to treat tuberculosis in the infant.

THE ART OF ANTIMICROBIAL THERAPY

Clinical Pearls

1. Rifampin should never be used alone in the treatment of active tuberculosis because resistance may develop.
2. Liver function tests, symptoms of gastrointestinal intolerance, and complete blood count should be monitored at least monthly in all patients receiving rifampin.
3. Rifampin is a potent inducer of the P450 cytochrome system, and coadministered medications may require discontinuation or monitoring for possible dosage adjustment.
4. Rifampin penetrates foreign material well and is often used in synergy with tetracyclines and fluoroquinolones for foreign body infections (off-label use).
5. Some of the hypersensitivity-related toxicity seen with rifampin (e.g., flulike illness and thrombocytopenia) may be more frequent with intermittent administration.

RIFAMPIN PLUS ISONIAZID (Rifamate)

Note: Also available in combination with pyrazinamide as Rifater.

BASIC CHARACTERISTICS

Class: Rifamycin plus isonicotinic acid hydrazide

Mechanisms of Action: Rifampin inhibits DNA-dependent RNA polymerase activity in susceptible cells. Isoniazid inhibits the synthesis of mycolic acid, a constituent of the cell wall, and inhibits catalase-peroxidase.

Mechanisms of Resistance: Resistance to rifampin occurs as single-step mutations of the DNA-dependent RNA polymerase. Resistance to isoniazid occurs as point mutations in the catalase-peroxidase gene and the regulatory genes involved in mycolic acid synthesis.

Metabolic Route: Rifampin is rapidly eliminated in the bile and undergoes progressive deacetylation and elimination. However, up to 30% of a dose is excreted in the urine, with about half of this being unchanged drug. Isoniazid is metabolized by acetylation and dehydrazination. The rate of acetylation is genetically determined.

FDA FDA-APPROVED INDICATIONS

FDA-Approved Indications: Treatment of pulmonary tuberculosis in which organisms are susceptible, and when the patient has been titrated on the individual components and it has, therefore, been established that this fixed dosage is therapeutically effective.

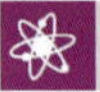

SIDE EFFECTS/TOXICITY

> **WARNING:** Severe and sometimes fatal hepatitis associated with isoniazid therapy may occur and may develop even after many months of treatment.

Rifampin plus isoniazid is **contraindicated** in patients with a history of hypersensitivity to any of the rifamycins or isoniazid.

Side effects/toxicities include anaphylaxis; liver dysfunction; reddish coloration of the urine, sweat, sputum, and tears; "flu syndrome" (fever, chills, and malaise); rash; flushing; epigastric distress; anorexia; nausea; vomiting; flatulence; *Clostridium difficile*–associated diarrhea; disseminated intravascular coagulation; visual disturbances; adrenal insufficiency; confusion; renal insufficiency; elevations in serum uric acid; thrombocytopenia; leukopenia; hemolytic anemia; peripheral neuropathy; hypersensitivity; fever; skin eruptions; vasculitis; a systemic lupus erythematosus–like syndrome; nausea; vomiting; epigastric distress; seizures; encephalopathy; metabolic acidosis; optic neuritis; arthralgias; agranulocytosis; hemolytic or sideroblastic anemia; and thrombocytopenia.

Foods rich in histamine (e.g., cheese, wine, tuna) or tyramine (e.g., cured meats, soybeans, aged cheese) may produce flushing and headache because of the isoniazid component.

Rifampin plus isoniazid can enhance the metabolism of endogenous substrates including adrenal hormones, thyroid hormones, and vitamin D.

 DRUG INTERACTIONS/FOOD INTERACTIONS

Absorption of rifampin plus isoniazid is reduced when the drug is ingested with food, but absorption is usually adequate, and ingestion with food reduces gastrointestinal intolerance.

Rifampin is known to induce certain cytochrome P450 enzymes. Administration of rifampin with drugs that undergo biotransformation through these metabolic pathways may accelerate elimination and decrease the therapeutic effect of these coadministered drugs, many of which require monitoring and possible adjustment during and following coadministration with rifampin. The list of drugs so affected includes the following drugs/classes: antiarrhythmics, oral anticoagulants, anticonvulsants, antifungals, barbiturates, β-blockers, calcium channel blockers, cardiac glycoside preparations, CCR5 inhibitors, chloramphenicol, clarithromycin, clofibrate, hormonal contraceptives (patients should be advised to use nonhormonal methods of birth control during rifampin therapy), corticosteroids, cyclosporine, dapsone, diazepam, doxycycline, enalapril, fluoroquinolones, haloperidol, oral hypoglycemic agents, levothyroxine, methadone, narcotic analgesics, nonnucleoside reverse transcriptase inhibitors, nortriptyline, progestins, protease inhibitors, quinine, sulfapyridine, tacrolimus, theophylline, tricyclic antidepressants, and zidovudine.

Rifampin plus isoniazid levels may increase when it is coadministered with atovaquone, probenecid, and cotrimoxazole, and may decrease when given with ketoconazole and antacids (give rifampin plus isoniazid at least 1 hour before the ingestion of antacids).

When rifampin plus isoniazid is given concomitantly with halothane, the potential for hepatotoxicity is increased, and concomitant use of rifampin plus isoniazid and halothane should be avoided.

Acetaminophen and alcohol should be avoided, as they may increase hepatotoxicity, as should disulfiram, enflurane, stavudine, and vincristine,

Drug/laboratory interactions:

Cross-reactivity and false-positive urine screening tests for opiates have been reported in patients receiving rifampin plus isoniazid.

Therapeutic levels of rifampin plus isoniazid have been shown to inhibit standard microbiological assays for serum folate and vitamin B12.

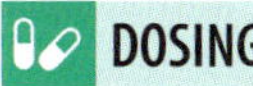 DOSING

Rifamate contains 300 mg of rifampin and 150 mg of isoniazid. Treatment usually consists of two Rifamate capsules once daily; for intermittent therapy, dosage is two capsules of Rifamate plus two 300-mg tablets of isoniazid given twice weekly by directly observed therapy. Tolerance of Rifamate is improved if taken with food.

SPECIAL POPULATIONS

RENAL IMPAIRMENT: No dosage adjustment is necessary.

HEPATIC DYSFUNCTION: Patients with impaired liver function should be given rifampin plus isoniazid only in cases of necessity and then with caution and monitoring of liver function.

PEDIATRIC PATIENTS: Not recommended for children or adolescents aged younger than 15 years.

PREGNANCY: Category C.

BREASTFEEDING: Patients may breastfeed while taking Rifamate; the small amounts of isoniazid and rifampin in breastmilk are not likely to be toxic to the infant but are too small to treat active or latent infection in the infant. Mother and infant should receive supplementary pyridoxine.

THE ART OF ANTIMICROBIAL THERAPY

Clinical Pearls

1. When possible, Rifamate should be used for tuberculosis after the individual components have been started and have been shown to be tolerated.
2. Rifamate is helpful when DOT is not possible, as it minimizes inadvertent monotherapy and subsequent risk of acquired drug resistance.
3. Fixed-dose combinations such as rifampin plus isoniazid may decrease the patient's pill burden.
4. Liver function tests and symptoms of gastrointestinal intolerance should be monitored in all patients receiving rifampin plus isoniazid.
5. Rifampin is a potent inducer of the P450 cytochrome system, and coadministered medications may require discontinuation or monitoring for possible dosage adjustment.
6. Pyridoxine (25 mg/day) should be given to prevent B6 deficiency in those patients at risk for peripheral neuropathy, such as those with nutritional deficiency, diabetes, HIV infection, renal failure, or alcoholism, and in pregnancy and in breastfeeding mothers.
7. Soft contact lenses may be permanently stained during treatment with rifampin plus isoniazid.

RIFAMPIN PLUS ISONIAZID PLUS PYRAZINAMIDE (Rifater)

BASIC CHARACTERISTICS

Class: Rifamycin plus isonicotinic acid hydrazide plus pyrazine analogue of nicotinamide, respectively.

Mechanisms of Action: Rifampin inhibits DNA-dependent RNA polymerase activity in susceptible cells. Isoniazid inhibits the synthesis of mycolic acid, a constituent of the cell wall, and inhibits catalase-peroxidase. Pyrazinamide's mechanism of action is unknown.

Mechanisms of Resistance: Resistance to rifampin occurs as single-step mutations of the DNA-dependent RNA polymerase. Resistance to isoniazid occurs as point mutations in the catalase-peroxidase gene and the regulatory genes involved in mycolic acid synthesis. Resistance to pyrazinamide occurs as point mutations in the pyrazinamidase gene.

Metabolic Route: Rifampin is rapidly eliminated in the bile and undergoes progressive deacetylation and elimination. However, up to 30% of a dose is excreted in the urine, with about half of this being unchanged drug. Isoniazid is metabolized by acetylation and dehydrazination. The rate of acetylation is genetically determined. Pyrazinamide is hydrolyzed in the liver and excreted in the urine.

FDA-APPROVED INDICATIONS

FDA-Approved Indications: Rifater is indicated in the initial phase of the short-course treatment of pulmonary tuberculosis. During this phase, which should last 2 months, Rifater should be administered on a daily, continuous basis.

SIDE EFFECTS/TOXICITY

WARNING: Severe and sometimes fatal hepatitis associated with isoniazid therapy may occur and may develop even after many months of treatment.

Rifater is **contraindicated** in patients with a history of hypersensitivity to any of the rifamycins or pyrazinamide isoniazid.

Side effects/toxicities include peripheral neuropathy, hypersensitivity, fever, vasculitis, a systemic lupus erythematosus–like syndrome, seizures, encephalopathy, metabolic acidosis, optic neuritis, arthralgias, agranulocytosis, hemolytic or sideroblastic anemia, and thrombocytopenia.

Rifater inhibits renal excretion of urates, leading to hyperuricemea or gout; more commonly, it produces nongouty polyarthralgias. Also seen: anorexia; nausea; vomiting; diarrhea; flatulence; hepatitis, cutaneous flushing; porphyria; dysuria; reddish coloration of the urine, sweat, sputum, and tears; "flu syndrome" (fever, chills, and malaise); rash;

Clostridium difficile–associated diarrhea; disseminated intravascular coagulation, confusion, and renal insufficiency. Rifampin can enhance the metabolism of endogenous substrates including adrenal hormones, thyroid hormones, and vitamin D.

DRUG INTERACTIONS/FOOD INTERACTIONS

Absorption of Rifater is reduced when the drug is ingested with food, but absorption is usually adequate, and ingestion with food reduces gastrointestinal intolerance.

Foods rich in histamine (e.g., cheese, wine, tuna) or tyramine (e.g., cured meats, soybeans, aged cheese) may produce flushing and headache. Antacids may impair absorption and should be separated from isoniazid ingestion by 2 hours.

Isoniazid inhibits the metabolism of many drugs, potentially increasing their serum levels; patients on anticoagulants, anticonvulsants, benzodiazepines, haloperidol, theophylline, and cycloserine should be monitored for toxic effects; levels of carbamazepine, phenytoin, and valproate should be measured. Acetaminophen and alcohol should be avoided, as they may increase hepatotoxicity, as should disulfiram, enflurane, stavudine, and vincristine.

Rifampin is known to induce certain cytochrome P450 enzymes. Administration of Rifater with drugs that undergo biotransformation through these metabolic pathways may accelerate elimination and decrease the therapeutic effect of these coadministered drugs, many of which require monitoring and possible adjustment during and following coadministration with Rifater. The list of drugs so affected includes the following drugs/classes: antiarrhythmics, oral anticoagulants, anticonvulsants, antifungals, barbiturates, β-blockers, calcium channel blockers, cardiac glycoside preparations, CCR5 inhibitors, chloramphenicol, clarithromycin, clofibrate, hormonal contraceptives (patients should be advised to use nonhormonal methods of birth control during Rifater therapy), corticosteroids, cyclosporine, dapsone, diazepam, doxycycline, enalapril, fluoroquinolones, haloperidol, oral hypoglycemic agents, levothyroxine, methadone, narcotic analgesics, nonnucleoside reverse transcriptase inhibitors, nortriptyline, progestins, protease inhibitors, quinine, sulfapyridine, tacrolimus, theophylline, tricyclic antidepressants, and zidovudine.

Rifampin levels may increase when it is coadministered with atovaquone, probenecid, and cotrimoxazole, and may decrease when given with ketoconazole and antacids (give Rifater at least 1 hour before the ingestion of antacids).

When Rifater is given concomitantly with halothane, the potential for hepatotoxicity is increased, and concomitant use of Rifater and halothane should be avoided.

Drug/laboratory interactions:

Cross-reactivity and false-positive urine screening tests for opiates have been reported in patients receiving rifampin or rifater.

Therapeutic levels of Rifater have been shown to inhibit standard microbiological assays for serum folate and vitamin B12.

Rifater may interfere with Ketostix and Acetest, producing a brown color,

DOSING

Rifater contains 120 mg rifampin, 50 mg isoniazid, and 300 mg pyrazinamide. Treatment is weight-based as follows:

- Patients weighing ≤ 44 kg: four tablets daily
- Patients weighing between 45 kg and 54 kg: five tablets daily
- Patients weighing ≥ 55 kg: six tablets daily

To obtain an adequate dosage of pyrazinamide in persons heavier than 90 kg, additional pyrazinamide tablets must be given.

SPECIAL POPULATIONS

RENAL IMPAIRMENT: Rifater should not be used because of the potential need to adjust pyrazinamide dosage.

HEPATIC DYSFUNCTION: Patients with impaired liver function should be given Rifater only in cases of necessity and then with caution and monitoring of liver function.

PEDIATRIC PATIENTS: Not recommended for children or adolescents younger than 15 years.

PREGNANCY: Category C. In the United States, pyrazinamide is generally avoided in pregnant patients, so Rifater should not be used. However, pyrazinamide is used during pregnancy in much of the world.

BREASTFEEDING: Patients may breastfeed if benefit outweighs risk. Mother and child should receive pyridoxine.

THE ART OF ANTIMICROBIAL THERAPY

Clinical Pearls

1. Rifater should be used for the induction phase of tuberculosis therapy.
2. Liver function tests and symptoms of gastrointestinal intolerance should be monitored in all patients receiving Rifater.
3. Rifampin is a potent inducer of the P450 cytochrome system, and coadministered medications may require discontinuation or monitoring for possible dosage adjustment.
4. Pyridoxine (25 mg/day) should be given to prevent isoniazid-related B6 deficiency in those at risk for peripheral neuropathy, such as those with nutritional

deficiency, diabetes, HIV infection, renal failure, or alcoholism, and in pregnancy and in breastfeeding mothers.

5. Patients with acute gout should not receive any medication containing pyrazinamide.
6. Fixed-dose combinations such as Rifater minimize inadvertent monotherapy and the subsequent risk of acquired drug resistance. They should be used when possible if therapy can not be given via directly observed therapy.
7. Soft contact lenses may be permanently stained during Rifater therapy.

RIFAPENTINE (Priftin)

BASIC CHARACTERISTICS

Class: Rifamycin

Mechanism of Action: Inhibits DNA-dependent RNA polymerase activity in susceptible cells.

Mechanisms of Resistance: Resistance occurs as single-step mutations of the DNA-dependent RNA polymerase.

Metabolic Route: Rifapentine is rapidly eliminated in the bile and undergoes progressive deacetylation and elimination. However, up to 30% of a dose is excreted in the urine, half of it as unchanged drug.

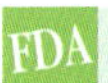

FDA-APPROVED INDICATIONS

FDA-Approved Indications: Rifapentine is indicated in the treatment of pulmonary tuberculosis. Multiple limitations in its use are described in Clinical Pearls.

SIDE EFFECTS/TOXICITY

Rifapentine is **contraindicated** in patients with a history of hypersensitivity to any of the rifamycins.

It is assumed that rifapentine's toxicity will resemble that of rifampin.

Side effects/toxicities include anaphylaxis; liver dysfunction; reddish coloration of the urine, sweat, sputum, and tears; "flu syndrome" (fever, chills, and malaise); rash; flushing; epigastric distress; anorexia; nausea; vomiting; flatulence; *Clostridium difficile*–associated diarrhea; disseminated intravascular coagulation; visual disturbances; confusion; renal insufficiency; elevations in serum uric acid; thrombocytopenia; leukopenia; hemolytic anemia; and enhanced metabolism of endogenous substrates including adrenal hormones, thyroid hormones, and vitamin D.

DRUG INTERACTIONS/FOOD INTERACTIONS

Absorption of rifapentine is reduced when the drug is ingested with food, but absorption is usually adequate, and ingestion with food reduces gastrointestinal intolerance.

It is assumed that rifapentine's drug interactions resemble those of rifampin.

Rifampin is known to induce certain cytochrome P450 enzymes. Administration of rifampin with drugs that undergo biotransformation through these metabolic pathways may accelerate elimination and decrease the therapeutic effect of these coadministered drugs, many of which require monitoring and possible adjustment during and following coadministration with rifampin. The list of drugs so affected includes the following drugs/classes: antiarrhythmics, oral anticoagulants, anticonvulsants, antifungals, barbiturates, β-blockers, calcium channel blockers, cardiac glycoside preparations, CCR5 inhibitors, chloramphenicol, clarithromycin, clofibrate, hormonal contraceptives (patients should be advised to use nonhormonal methods of birth control during rifampin therapy), corticosteroids, cyclosporine, dapsone, diazepam, doxycycline, enalapril, fluoroquinolones, haloperidol, oral hypoglycemic agents, levothyroxine, methadone, narcotic analgesics, nonnucleoside reverse transcriptase inhibitors, nortriptyline, progestins, protease inhibitors, quinine, sulfapyridine, tacrolimus, theophylline, tricyclic antidepressants, and zidovudine.

Rifampin levels may increase when it is coadministered with atovaquone, probenecid, and cotrimoxazole, and may decrease when it is given with ketoconazole and antacids (give rifampin at least 1 hour before the ingestion of antacids).

When rifampin is given concomitantly with either halothane or isoniazid, the potential for hepatotoxicity is increased, and concomitant use of rifampin and halothane should be avoided.

Drug/laboratory interactions:

Cross-reactivity and false-positive urine screening tests for opiates have been reported in patients receiving rifampin.

Therapeutic levels of rifampin have been shown to inhibit standard microbiological assays for serum folate and vitamin B12.

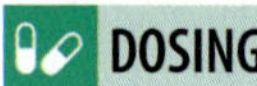

DOSING

Rifapentine is supplied as 150-mg tablets. Dosage is 10 mg/kg, (with a maximum dose of 600 mg) given once weekly.

SPECIAL POPULATIONS

RENAL IMPAIRMENT: Not studied in patients with renal impairment.

HEPATIC DYSFUNCTION: Patients with impaired liver function should be given rifapentine only in cases of necessity and then with caution and monitoring of liver function.

PEDIATRIC PATIENTS:

Not studied in children aged younger than 12 years.

For children aged 12 years and older:

- 600 mg for those who weigh ≥ 45 kg
- 450 mg for those < 45 kg

PREGNANCY: Category C.

BREASTFEEDING: It is not recommended to administer rifapentine to breastfeeding mothers.

THE ART OF ANTIMICROBIAL THERAPY

Clinical Pearls

1. Rifapentine is used in the continuation phase of therapy for tuberculosis (after the first 2 months), and is used **only** for selected patients: those who are HIV-negative, who have noncavitary pulmonary tuberculosis, and whose sputum smears are negative after 2 months of therapy.
2. Rifapentine is given once weekly, with isoniazid, by directly observed therapy.
3. If the culture at 2 months is positive, the continuation phase of weekly isoniazid and rifapentine should be extended to 7 months instead of 4 months.
4. Liver function tests and symptoms of gastrointestinal intolerance should be monitored in all patients receiving rifapentine.
5. Rifapentine is a potent inducer of the P450 cytochrome system, and coadministered medications may require discontinuation or monitoring for possible dosage adjustment.

BASIC CHARACTERISTICS

Class: Analogue of rifampin

Mechanism of Action: Rifaximin acts by binding to the β-subunit of bacterial DNA-dependent RNA polymerase resulting in inhibition of bacterial RNA synthesis.

Metabolic Route: Rifaximin is excreted in the feces.

FDA-APPROVED INDICATIONS

FDA-Approved Indications: Treatment of patients aged 12 years and older with travelers' diarrhea caused by noninvasive strains of *Escherichia coli.*

Also Used for: Prophylaxis of travelers' diarrhea, treatment of *Clostridium difficile*, and treatment of hepatic encephalopathy.

SIDE EFFECTS/TOXICITY

Contraindicated in patients with hypersensitivity to any of the rifamycins.

Side effects/toxicities include hypersensitivity reactions including exfoliative dermatitis, rash, angioneurotic edema, urticaria, flushing, sunburn, neck pain, ear pain, gingival disorder, dry throat, anorexia, loss of taste, abdominal distension, diarrhea, blood in stool, nasopharyngitis, respiratory tract infection, chest pain, dyspnea, fatigue, malaise, dehydration, arthralgia, myalgia, abnormal dreams, dizziness, motion sickness, tinnitus, migraine, syncope, insomnia, dysuria, hematuria, polyuria, proteinuria, urinary frequency, hot flashes, lymphocytosis, monocytosis, neutropenia, and aspartate aminotransferase increase.

DRUG INTERACTIONS/FOOD INTERACTIONS

Rifaximin can be administered with or without food. No significant drug interactions have been reported.

DOSING

Rifaximin is supplied as 200-mg tablets. The usual dosage is one tablet taken three times a day for 3 days.

SPECIAL POPULATIONS

RENAL IMPAIRMENT: No dosage adjustment is necessary.

HEPATIC DYSFUNCTION: No dosage adjustment is necessary.

PEDIATRIC PATIENTS: The safety and effectiveness of rifaximin in patients aged younger than 12 years have not been established.

PREGNANCY: Category C.

BREASTFEEDING: A decision should be made whether to discontinue breastfeeding or to discontinue the drug.

THE ART OF ANTIMICROBIAL THERAPY

Clinical Pearls

1. Rifaximin has no known significant interactions with other medications.
2. Rifaximin is not effective in patients with diarrhea complicated by fever and/or blood in the stool or diarrhea caused by pathogens other than *E. coli.*
3. Rifaximin is not suitable for treating systemic bacterial infections because less than 0.4% of the drug is absorbed after oral administration.
4. Pseudomembranous colitis has been reported with nearly all antibacterial agents; it is important to consider this diagnosis in patients who present with diarrhea subsequent to the administration of antibacterial agents, including rifaximin.

RIMANTADINE (Flumadine)

BASIC CHARACTERISTICS

Class: Adamantanamine

Mechanisms of Action:

1. Inhibits the ion channels of the M2 protein of influenza A and
2. inhibits viral uncoating during endocytosis.

Mechanism of Resistance: Mutations in the transmembrane region of the M2 protein lead to high-level resistance.

Metabolic Route: Rimantadine is well absorbed orally and is metabolized in the liver.

FDA FDA-APPROVED INDICATIONS

FDA-Approved Indications: Prophylaxis of influenza A in adults and children, and treatment of influenza A in adults.

SIDE EFFECTS/TOXICITY

Most frequent side effects/toxicities include nausea, dizziness, and insomnia. Also seen: depression, anxiety, irritability, seizures, congestive heart failure, taste loss, tinnitus, dry mouth, constipation, dry nose, and urinary retention.

DRUG INTERACTIONS/FOOD INTERACTIONS

Rimantadine is well absorbed orally, with or without food.

Cimetidine reduces the renal clearance of rimantadine.

DOSING

Rimantadine is supplied in 100-mg tablets and in a purplish-red, raspberry-flavored syrup containing 50 mg of rimantadine hydrochloride per teaspoonful.

The dosage for prophylaxis and treatment is 100 mg twice a day.

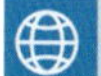

SPECIAL POPULATIONS

RENAL IMPAIRMENT: In patients with severe renal failure (creatinine clearance ≤ 10 mL/min) a dosage reduction to 100 mg daily is recommended.

HEPATIC DYSFUNCTION: In patients with severe hepatic dysfunction, a dosage reduction to 100 mg daily is recommended.

PEDIATRIC PATIENTS: In children aged younger than 10 years, rimantadine should be administered once a day, at a dosage of 5 mg/kg but not exceeding 150 mg. For children aged 10 years or older, use the adult dosage.

GERIATRIC PATIENTS: In elderly patients, a dosage reduction to 100 mg daily is recommended.

PREGNANCY: Category C.

BREASTFEEDING: The use of rimantadine is not recommended for breastfeeding mothers.

THE ART OF ANTIMICROBIAL THERAPY

Clinical Pearls

1. Rimantadine does not have activity against influenza B or novel H1N1 influenza.
2. Viruses resistant to amantadine are also resistant to rimantadine.
3. Patients with a history of epilepsy may be at increased risk for seizures while taking rimantadine.

RITONAVIR (Norvir)

BASIC CHARACTERISTICS

Class: Protease inhibitor

Mechanism of Action: Reversibly binds the active site of the enzyme protease. Inhibition of protease prevents cleavage of the *gag* and *gag-pol* polyprotein resulting in the production of immature, noninfectious virus.

Mechanism of Resistance: Development of mutations on the enzyme protease causes a conformational change that prevents ritonavir from binding the active site, allowing protease activity to continue. The most frequent resistance mutations include 46I, 71V, 82A, and 84V.

Metabolic Route: Ritonavir is metabolized by the liver.

FDA-APPROVED INDICATIONS

FDA-Approved Indications: Treatment of HIV-1 in combinations with other antiretroviral agents.

SIDE EFFECTS/TOXICITY

> **WARNING:** Coadministration of ritonavir with certain nonsedating antihistamines, sedative hypnotics, antiarrhythmics, or ergot alkaloid preparations may result in potentially serious and/or life-threatening adverse events because of possible effects of ritonavir on the hepatic metabolism of certain drugs.

Other side effects/toxicities include diarrhea; new-onset diabetes mellitus; exacerbation of preexisting diabetes mellitus, hyperglycemia; increased bleeding, including spontaneous skin hematomas and hemarthrosis, in patients with hemophilia type A or B; redistribution/accumulation of body fat including central obesity, dorsocervical fat enlargement (buffalo hump), peripheral wasting, facial wasting, and breast enlargement; cushingoid appearance; immune reconstitution syndrome; QTc prolongation; torsade de pointes; abdominal pain; headache; anorexia; dyspepsia; epigastric pain; hepatitis; mouth ulceration; pancreatitis; vomiting; anemia; leukopenia; thrombocytopenia; increases in alkaline phosphatase, amylase, creatine phosphokinase, lactic dehydrogenase, SGOT, SGPT, and γ glutamyl transpeptidase; hyperlipemia; hyperuricemia; hypoglycemia; and dehydration.

DRUG INTERACTIONS/FOOD INTERACTIONS

Ritonavir tablets should be taken with a meal; ritonavir capsules may be taken with or without meals.

Drugs that **should not be coadministered** with ritonavir include amiodarone, quinidine, flecainide, propafenone, alfuzosin, astemizole, terfenadine, ergot derivatives, Saint-John's-wort, HMG-CoA reductase inhibitors simvastatin or lovastatin, pimozide, cisapride, benzodiazepines, and rifampin.

Ritonavir is an inhibitor of the CYP3A enzyme; coadministration of ritonavir and drugs primarily metabolized by CYP3A may result in increased plasma concentrations of the other drug that could increase or prolong its therapeutic and adverse effects.

Ritonavir is metabolized by CYP3A and CYP2C19; coadministration of ritonavir and drugs that induce CYP3A or CYP2C19 may decrease ritonavir plasma concentrations and reduce its therapeutic effect. Coadministration of ritonavir and drugs that inhibit CYP3A or CYP2C19 may increase ritonavir plasma concentrations. Because of these metabolic effects, potential drug interactions that may require dosage change or clinical/laboratory monitoring are listed below:

Medication	*Adjustment or Action*
Itraconazole	Monitor for toxicity
Ketoconazole	Use with caution
Voriconazole	Monitor for toxicity
Rifabutin	Decrease rifabutin to 150 mg every other day or thrice weekly
Hormonal contraceptives	Use alternative or additional method
Atorvastatin or rosuvastatin	Use lowest possible dosage with close monitoring
Phenobarbital, phenytoin or carbamazepine	Monitor anticonvulsant level; consider alternative to anticonvulsant
Methadone	Monitor; may require higher methadone dosage
Sildenafil	25 mg every 48 hours
Tadalafil	5 mg, no more than 10 mg in 72 hours
Vardenafil	No more than 2.5 mg in 24 hours

DOSING

Ritonavir is supplied as a 100-mg capsule, 100-mg tablet, and a liquid containing 600 mg/7.5 mL. Although the recommended dosage of ritonavir is 600 mg twice daily by mouth it is rarely used in this fashion. It is primarily dosed as a booster of the other protease inhibitors as follows:

Other Protease Inhibitors	*Dosing Options*
Atazanavir	Atazanavir 300 mg daily + ritonavir 100 mg daily
Darunavir	Darunavir 600 mg twice daily + ritonavir 100 mg twice daily or Darunavir 800 mg daily + ritonavir 100 mg daily (naïve)
Fosamprenavir	Fosamprenavir 700 mg twice daily + ritonavir 100 mg twice daily or Fosamprenavir 1400 mg daily + ritonavir 100 mg daily or 200 mg daily (naive)
Indinavir	Indinavir 800 mg twice daily + ritonavir 100 mg twice daily
Nelfinavir	Not recommended
Saquinavir	Saquinavir 1000 mg twice daily + ritonavir 100 mg twice daily
Tipranavir	Tipranavir 500 mg twice daily + ritonavir 200 mg twice daily

SPECIAL POPULATIONS

RENAL IMPAIRMENT: There is no dosage adjustment needed.

HEPATIC DYSFUNCTION: In patients with known or suspected history of hepatitis B or C infection and in patients treated with other medications associated with liver toxicity, monitoring of liver enzymes is recommended.

PEDIATRIC PATIENTS: In children aged 2 years and older, the recommended oral dosage of ritonavir is 45 mg/kg to 55 mg/kg twice daily or 25 mg/kg to 35 mg/kg three times daily. All doses should be taken with a meal.

PREGNANCY: Category B.

BREASTFEEDING: It is recommended that HIV-positive mothers not breastfeed their children, to decrease mother-to-child transmission of HIV.

THE ART OF ANTIMICROBIAL THERAPY

Clinical Pearls

1. Ritonavir should always be used in combination with other antiretrovirals.
2. Ritonavir should be taken with food to decrease side effects.
3. Ritonavir is mainly used as a booster of other protease inhibitors except nelfinavir.
4. The protease inhibitors saquinavir, darunavir, and tipranavir **must** be administered with ritonavir.

5. Whenever initiating ritonavir, one should make sure to review all medications the patient is receiving to minimize drug interactions.
6. Ritonavir capsules must be refrigerated; the tablets can stay at room temperature.
7. Ritonavir tablets lead to higher systemic levels than the capsule and can result in more gastrointestinal side effects.

SAQUINAVIR (Invirase)

BASIC CHARACTERISTICS

Class: Protease inhibitor

Mechanism of Action: Saquinavir reversibly binds the active site of the enzyme protease. Inhibition of protease prevents cleavage of the *gag* and *gag-pol* polyprotein resulting in the production of immature, noninfectious virus.

Mechanism of Resistance: Development of mutations on the enzyme protease causes a conformational change that prevents saquinavir from binding the active site, allowing protease activity to continue. The most frequent resistance mutations include G48V and L90M. However, other combinations of mutations can lead to resistance to saquinavir.

Metabolic Route: Saquinavir is metabolized by the liver and excreted in the feces.

FDA-APPROVED INDICATIONS

FDA-Approved Indications: Treatment of HIV-1 in combinations with other antiretroviral agents.

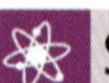

SIDE EFFECTS/TOXICITY

Side effects/toxicities include diarrhea; new-onset diabetes mellitus; exacerbation of preexisting diabetes mellitus; hyperglycemia; increased bleeding, including spontaneous skin hematomas and hemarthrosis, in patients with hemophilia type A or B; redistribution/accumulation of body fat including central obesity, dorsocervical fat enlargement (buffalo hump), peripheral wasting, facial wasting, and breast enlargement; cushingoid appearance; immune reconstitution syndrome; QTc prolongation; torsade de pointes; abdominal pain; headache; anorexia; dyspepsia; epigastric pain; hepatitis; mouth ulceration; pancreatitis; vomiting; anemia; leukopenia; thrombocytopenia; increases in alkaline phosphatase, amylase, creatine phosphokinase, lactic dehydrogenase, SGOT, SGPT, and γ glutamyl transpeptidase; hyperlipemia; hyperuricemia; hypoglycemia; and dehydration.

DRUG INTERACTIONS/FOOD INTERACTIONS

Saquinavir must be given with ritonavir and must be given within 2 hours of a meal.

Saquinavir **should not be administered** concurrently with amiodarone, bepridil, flecainide, propafenone, quinidine, astemizole, terfenadine, cisapride, pimozide, triazolam, midazolam, ergot derivatives, rifampin, fluticasone, Saint-John's-wort, HMG-CoA reductase inhibitors simvastatin or lovastatin, benzodiazepines, darunavir, or tipranavir.

Saquinavir inhibits the CYP3A enzyme; coadministration of saquinavir and drugs primarily metabolized by CYP3A may result in increased plasma concentrations of the other drug that could increase or prolong its therapeutic and adverse effects.

Saquinavir is metabolized by CYP3A and CYP2C19; coadministration of saquinavir and drugs that induce CYP3A or CYP2C19 may decrease saquinavir plasma concentrations and reduce its therapeutic effect. Coadministration of saquinavir and drugs that inhibit CYP3A or CYP2C19 may increase saquinavir plasma concentrations. Because of these metabolic effects, potential drug interactions that may require dosage change or clinical/laboratory monitoring are:

Medication/Food	*Adjustment or Action*
Itraconazole	Decrease itraconazole; monitor drug level
Voriconazole	Monitor for toxicity
Rifabutin	Decrease rifabutin to 150 mg every other day or thrice weekly
Atorvastatin	Use lowest possible dosage with close monitoring
Phenobarbital, phenytoin, or carbamazepine	Monitor anticonvulsant level; consider alternative
Methadone	Monitor; may require higher methadone dose
Sildenafil	25 mg every 48 hours
Tadalafil	5 mg, no more than 10 mg in 72 hours
Vardenafil	2.5 mg in 24 hours
Grapefruit juice	Increases levels of saquinavir; monitor
Dexamethasone	Decreases levels of saquinavir; monitor
Maraviroc	Decrease maraviroc to 150 mg twice daily

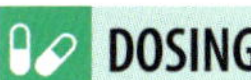

DOSING

Saquinavir 1000 mg twice daily (five 200-mg capsules or two 500-mg tablets) in combination with ritonavir 100 mg twice daily.

SPECIAL POPULATIONS

RENAL IMPAIRMENT: There is no dosage adjustment needed.

HEPATIC DYSFUNCTION: Caution should be exercised.

PEDIATRIC PATIENTS: Saquinavir is not recommended for children aged younger than 16 years.

PREGNANCY: Category B.

BREASTFEEDING: It is recommended that HIV-positive mothers not breastfeed their children, to decrease mother-to-child transmission of HIV.

THE ART OF ANTIMICROBIAL THERAPY

Clinical Pearls:

1. Saquinavir should always be used in combination with other antiretrovirals.
2. Saquinavir **must** be given at the same time as ritonavir to achieve adequate levels.
3. When one is evaluating resistance to ritonavir-boosted protease inhibitors, phenotypic resistance testing is extremely helpful.
4. Although not FDA-approved, an alternative dosage of 2000 mg of saquinavir with 100 mg of ritonavir has been used.
5. Whenever initiating saquinavir, one should make sure to review all medications the patient is receiving to minimize drug interactions.

SPECTINOMYCIN HYDROCHLORIDE (Trobicin)

BASIC CHARACTERISTICS

Class: Aminocyclitol antibiotic

Mechanism of Action: Inhibits protein synthesis in the bacterial cell; the site of action is the 30S ribosomal subunit.

Metabolic Route: Spectinomycin is excreted unchanged in the urine.

FDA-APPROVED INDICATIONS

FDA-Approved Indications: Treatment of acute gonorrheal urethritis and proctitis in men and acute gonorrheal cervicitis and proctitis in women.

SIDE EFFECTS/TOXICITY

Contains benzyl alcohol. Benzyl alcohol has been reported to be associated with a fatal "gasping syndrome" in premature infants and an increased incidence of neurologic and other complications.

Other side effects/toxicities: anaphylaxis; soreness at the injection site; urticaria; dizziness; nausea; chills; fever; insomnia; a decrease in hemoglobin, hematocrit, and creatinine clearance; and elevation of alkaline phosphatase, BUN, and SGPT.

DRUG INTERACTIONS/FOOD INTERACTIONS

None reported.

DOSING

2-g dose administered intramuscularly.

In geographic areas where antibiotic resistance is known to be prevalent, initial treatment with 4 g intramuscularly is preferred.

SPECIAL POPULATIONS

RENAL IMPAIRMENT: No dosage adjustment is necessary.

HEPATIC DYSFUNCTION: No dosage adjustment is necessary.

PEDIATRIC PATIENTS: Safety and effectiveness in the pediatric population have not been established.

PREGNANCY: Category B.

BREASTFEEDING: Caution should be exercised.

THE ART OF ANTIMICROBIAL THERAPY

Clinical Pearls:

1. Spectinomycin hydrochloride is not effective in the treatment of syphilis.
2. The 4-g dose contains 10 mL and may be divided into two intramuscular (gluteal) sites.

SPIRAMYCIN (Rovamycine)

BASIC CHARACTERISTICS

Class: Macrolide

Mechanism of Action: Binds to the 50S subunit of bacterial ribosomes, resulting in blockage of the transpeptidation or translocation reactions.

Mechanisms of Resistance: Unknown.

Metabolic Route: Metabolized in the liver and excreted in the bile.

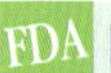

FDA-APPROVED INDICATIONS

Not FDA-approved, but used for prevention of congenital toxoplasmosis, alternative for treatment of toxoplasmosis during pregnancy, treatment of cryptosporidiosis in immunocompromised patients, and second-line therapy for bacterial infections.

SIDE EFFECTS/TOXICITY

Patients with hypersensitivity reactions to other macrolides may also have hypersensitivity to spiramycin.

Side effects/toxicities include hypersensitivity reactions, anaphylaxis, urticaria, pruritus, rash, nausea, vomiting, diarrhea, abdominal pain, esophagitis, hepatitis, pseudomembranous colitis, QT prolongation, ventricular arrhythmias, neuromuscular blockade, paresthesias, and thrombocytopenia.

DRUG INTERACTIONS/FOOD INTERACTIONS

Spiramycin may be taken with or without food.

Spiramycin decreases carbidopa absorption and levodopa concentrations. There is an increased risk of ventricular arrhythmias when spiramycin is used with astemizole, cisapride, and terfenadine. Increased risk of dystonia when spiramycin is used with fluphenazine.

DOSING

Spiramycin is administered as tablets, capsules, intravenously, or by rectal suppositories.

Bacterial infections:

- **Oral:** 1 g to 2 g twice daily or 500 mg to 1 g thrice daily; for severe infections, the dosage may be increased to 2 g to 2.5 g twice daily.
- **IV:** 500 mg every 8 hours; for severe infections, 1 g every 8 hours.
- **Rectal:** two or three 750-mg suppositories every 24 hours.

Toxoplasmosis in pregnancy: 3 g per day, divided into three or four doses.

SPECIAL POPULATIONS

RENAL IMPAIRMENT: No dosage adjustment is necessary.

HEPATIC DYSFUNCTION: Biliary obstruction or hepatic function impairment may decrease the elimination of spiramycin.

PEDIATRIC PATIENTS: The intravenous formulation is not recommended for children.

Oral Formulation:

- **Antibacterial:** Children who weigh 20 kg and more: 25 mg/kg two times a day or 16.7 mg/kg three times a day.
- **For subclinical congenital infection caused by toxoplasmosis:** 0.5 mg/kg/day to 1 mg/kg/day of pyrimethamine in combination with 50 mg/kg/day to 100 mg/kg/day of sulfadiazine for 4 weeks, alternating with 50 mg/kg to 100 mg/kg of spiramycin for 6 weeks; these dosing courses are repeated for 1 year.
- **Overt congenital infection:** 0.5 mg/kg/day to 1 mg/kg/day of pyrimethamine in combination with 50 mg/kg/day to 100 mg/kg/day of sulfadiazine and folinic acid 5 mg every 3 days for 6 months, alternating with 50 mg/kg to 100 mg/kg of spiramycin in combination with pyrimethamine and sulfadiazine for 4 weeks; these dosing courses are repeated until the child is aged 18 months.

Rectal Suppositories:

- **Newborns:** One 250-mg suppository per 5 kg every 24 hours.
- **Children aged younger than 12 years:** Two or three 500-mg suppositories every 24 hours.
- **Children aged 12 years and older:** The usual adult dosage.

PREGNANCY: Safe to use in pregnancy.

BREASTFEEDING: Caution should be used when one is administering spiramycin to a breastfeeding mother.

THE ART OF ANTIMICROBIAL THERAPY

Clinical Pearls:

1. Spiramycin is not commercially available in the US. However, physicians who wish to use spiramycin should contact the FDA's Division of Anti-Infective Drug Products (301-443-4310).
2. Spiramycin is an alternative agent for the treatment of toxoplasmosis in the pregnant woman.

3. For prevention of congenital toxoplasmosis, women who develop toxoplasmosis during the first trimester of pregnancy should be treated with spiramycin (3 g/day to 4 g/day). After the first trimester, if there is no documented transmission to the fetus, spiramycin can be continued until delivery. If fetal transmission is documented, therapy with pyrimethamine and sulfadiazine should be started, but only after the first trimester because of pyrimethamine's teratogenicity.
4. Although spiramycin is a macrolide, it is considered second-line therapy for bacterial infections.

STAVUDINE (Zerit)

BASIC CHARACTERISTICS

Class: Nucleoside reverse transcriptase inhibitor.

Mechanism of Action: Converted by cellular enzymes to its active drug stavudine triphosphate, an analogue of thymidine triphosphate. The stavudine triphosphate competes with the naturally occurring nucleotide for incorporation in newly forming HIV DNA. Because stavudine triphosphate does not have a terminal hydroxyl group, it halts transcription and replication of the virus.

Mechanism of Resistance: Changes in the structure of HIV reverse transcriptase leads to preferred incorporation of thymidine triphosphate and decreased incorporation of stavudine triphosphate, which allows transcription of DNA to continue. Resistance mutations include the "TAMS": 41L, 67N, 70R, 210W, 215F, and 219E.

Metabolic Route: Forty percent of stavudine is cleared unchanged in the urine, and the remainder is metabolized by endogenous mechanisms.

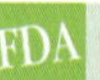

FDA-APPROVED INDICATIONS

FDA-Approved Indications: Treatment of HIV infection in combination with other antiretrovirals.

SIDE EFFECTS/TOXICITY

WARNING: Lactic acidosis and severe hepatomegaly with steatosis, including fatal cases, have been reported with the use of nucleoside analogues alone or in combination, including stavudine and other antiretrovirals.

Fatal lactic acidosis has been reported in pregnant women who received the combination of stavudine and didanosine with other antiretroviral agents.

The combination of stavudine and didanosine should be used with caution during pregnancy and is recommended only if the potential benefit clearly outweighs the potential risk.

Fatal and nonfatal pancreatitis have occurred during therapy when stavudine was part of a combination regimen that included didanosine, with or without hydroxyurea, in both treatment-naïve and treatment-experienced patients, regardless of degree of immunosuppression.

Other side effects/toxicities include immune reconstitution inflammatory syndrome; fat redistribution including central obesity and dorsocervical fat enlargement, peripheral wasting, facial wasting, and breast enlargement; liver function abnormalities; motor weakness; peripheral neuropathy.

 DRUG INTERACTIONS/FOOD INTERACTIONS

Stavudine can be taken with or without food and is unaffected by pH.

Stavudine should not be administered with either didanosine or ribavirin.

Stavudine should not be administered with any medication containing zidovudine, including Retrovir, Combivir, or Trizivir.

 DOSING

The dosing for stavudine is 40 mg twice daily for patients who weigh 60 kg or more and 30 mg twice daily for patients who weigh less than 60 kg.

 SPECIAL POPULATIONS

RENAL IMPAIRMENT: The dosage of stavudine should be adjusted as follows:

CrCl Measurement or Hemodialysis	*Body Weight ≥ 60 kg*	*Body Weight < 60 kg*
> 50 mL/min	40 mg twice daily	30 mg twice daily
26 mL/min to 50 mL/min	20 mg twice daily	15 mg twice daily
10 mL/min to 25 mL/min or hemodialysis	20 mg once daily	15 mg once daily

CrCl = Creatinine Clearance.

HEPATIC DYSFUNCTION: No dosage adjustment is necessary.

PEDIATRIC PATIENTS: The recommended dosage for newborns from birth to 13 days old is 0.5 mg/kg/dose given every 12 hours. The recommended dosage for pediatric patients aged at least 14 days and weighing less than 30 kg is 1 mg/kg/dose, given every 12 hours. Pediatric patients weighing 30 kg or greater should receive the recommended adult dosage.

PREGNANCY: Class C.

BREASTFEEDING: It is recommended that HIV-positive mothers not breastfeed their children, to decrease mother-to-child transmission of HIV.

 THE ART OF ANTIMICROBIAL THERAPY

Clinical Pearls:

1. Stavudine should always be used in combination with other antiretroviral agents.
2. Stavudine should not be given with zidovudine-containing medications, including Combivir, Retrovir, and Trizivir.
3. Stavudine has been associated with peripheral neuropathy, lactic acidosis, and severe lipoatrophy and is, therefore, not frequently used.

STIBOGLUCONATE (Pentostam)

BASIC CHARACTERISTICS

Class: Organometallic pentavalent antimonial

Mechanism of Action: Inhibits DNA topoisomerase, glycolytic enzymes, and fatty acid oxidation.

Metabolic Route: Stibogluconate is eliminated rapidly, mainly via the urine.

FDA-APPROVED INDICATIONS

Not FDA-approved, but active against all *Leishmania* species.

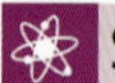

SIDE EFFECTS/TOXICITY

Side effects/toxicities include hepatitis, arthralgias, myalgias, thrombophlebitis, headache, anorexia, abdominal pain, nausea, vomiting, pancreatitis, metallic taste, pruritus, arrhythmias and prolongation of QT interval, elevated serum amylase, thrombocytopenia, and leukopenia.

DRUG INTERACTIONS/FOOD INTERACTIONS

No interactions are known, but drugs that may impair renal function or prolong the QT interval should be used with caution.

DOSING

The recommended daily dosage by is 20 mg/kg/day; however, twice-daily or thrice-daily dosages of 10 mg/kg have been used. It is given by slow intravenous infusion; intramuscular administration is painful, and oral absorption is inadequate.

Cutaneous leishmaniasis is treated for 20 days.

Visceral leishmaniasis is treated for 28 to 30 days.

Mucocutaneous leishmaniasis is treated for 28 days.

SPECIAL POPULATIONS

RENAL IMPAIRMENT: An alternative drug such as liposomal amphotericin B should be used in patients with renal impairment.

HEPATIC DYSFUNCTION: No dosage adjustment is necessary.

PEDIATRIC PATIENTS: The dosage is 20 mg/kg with an upper daily dose limit of 850 mg/day.

PREGNANCY: Do not use.

BREASTFEEDING: Should be safe.

THE ART OF ANTIMICROBIAL THERAPY

Clinical Pearls:

1. Antimonials are more toxic in HIV-infected patients.
2. Children tolerate antimonials better than adults do.
3. Alcohol should be avoided during therapy with stibogluconate.
4. Electrocardiography should be monitored and treatment interrupted for significant QTc prolongation.
5. Stibogluconate is available from the CDC Drug Service, Centers for Disease Control and Prevention, Atlanta, Georgia 30333: Parasitic Diseases Drug Service, 770-488-7775.

BASIC CHARACTERISTICS

Class: Aminoglycoside

Mechanism of Action: Binds the 30S subunit of the bacterial ribosome, which terminates protein synthesis.

Mechanisms of Resistance:

1. Gram-negative bacteria inactivate aminoglycosides by acetylation,
2. some bacteria alter the 30S ribosomal subunit, which prevents streptomycin's interference with protein synthesis, and
3. low-level resistance may result from inhibition of streptomycin uptake by the bacteria.

Metabolic Route: Streptomycin is excreted unchanged in the urine.

FDA

FDA-APPROVED INDICATIONS

FDA-Approved Indications: Treatment of *Mycobacterium tuberculosis;* infections caused by *Yersinia pestis, Franciscella tularensis, Brucella* species, *Calymmatobacterium granulomatis, Haemophilus ducreyi, Haemophilus influenzae, Klebsiella pneumoniae, Escherichia coli, Proteus* species, *Enterobacter aerogenes, Enterococcus faecalis* in urinary tract infections, and gram-negative bacillary bacteremia (concomitantly with another antibacterial agent); and in synergy with penicillin to treat endocardial infections with viridans streptococci and *E. faecalis.*

SIDE EFFECTS/TOXICITY

WARNINGS: Ototoxicity: vestibular toxicity and auditory ototoxicity, especially in patients with renal damage, those treated with higher doses, and those with prolonged treatment. Avoid use with potent diuretics such as ethacrynic acid because of additive ototoxicity.

Nephrotoxicity: especially in patients with impaired renal function and those treated with higher doses or prolonged treatment. Avoid concurrent use with other nephrotoxic agents and potent diuretics, which can cause dehydration.

Neuromuscular blockade: especially in those receiving anesthetics, neuromuscular blocking agents, or massive transfusions.

Additional neurotoxicity includes optic nerve dysfunction, peripheral neuritis, arachnoiditis, and encephalopathy. Other side effects/toxicities include nausea, vomiting, rash, fever, pancytopenia, and hemolytic anemia.

DRUG INTERACTIONS

Streptomycin should not be administered with other medications that are nephrotoxic or ototoxic.

DOSING

Intramuscular only.

Tuberculosis (all doses once daily)**:** 15 mg/kg/day up to 1 g, given daily at first, then two or three times per week. For patients aged older than 59 years, 10 mg/kg/dose (maximum 750 mg).

Tularemia: 1 g to 2 g daily in divided doses for 7 to 14 days until the patient is afebrile for 5 to 7 days.

Plague: 2 g streptomycin daily in two divided doses should be administered intramuscularly. A minimum of 10 days of therapy is recommended.

Bacterial endocarditis:

- **Streptococcal endocarditis:** 1 g twice daily for the first week, and 500 mg twice daily for the second week. If the patient is 60 years or older, the dosage should be 500 mg twice daily for the entire 2-week period in combination with penicillin.
- **Enterococcal endocarditis:** 1 g twice daily for 2 weeks and 500 mg twice daily for an additional 4 weeks in combination with penicillin.

SPECIAL POPULATIONS

RENAL IMPAIRMENT: In patients with renal impairment, the usual dosage is administered; however, the interval is increased as described in the following table. Streptomycin levels should be measured.

CrCl or Hemodialysis	*Dosage*
> 50 mL/min	Usual dosage
10 mL/min to 50 mL/min	Increase interval to three times usual interval
< 10 mL/min	Increase interval to four times usual interval
Hemodialysis	Administer half the usual dosage after dialysis
Continuous renal replacement therapy	Increase interval to three times usual interval

Note: CrCl = Creatinine Clearance.

HEPATIC DYSFUNCTION: No adjustment necessary.

PEDIATRIC PATIENTS: 20 mg/kg/day to 40 mg/kg/day, up to 1 g a day for tuberculosis as well as the severe bacterial infections.

PREGNANCY: Category D.

BREASTFEEDING: It is not known if streptomycin is secreted in human milk.

THE ART OF ANTIMICROBIAL THERAPY

Clinical Pearls:

1. Streptomycin is administered by intramuscular injection only.
2. When streptomycin must be given for prolonged periods of time, alkalinization of the urine may minimize or prevent renal damage.
3. Although streptomycin is recommended as a fourth agent for routine treatment of tuberculosis, ethambutol is usually used in its place, because of increased resistance to streptomycin and generally less toxicity with ethambutol.
4. If treating tuberculosis, one should never use streptomycin alone.
5. The peak concentration of streptomycin should be between 35 μg/mL and 45 μg/mL.
6. Streptomycin is considered a second-line agent for the treatment of gram-negative bacillary bacteremia, meningitis, and pneumonia; brucellosis; granuloma inguinale; chancroid; and urinary tract infection.
7. Monitor renal function, hearing, and vestibular function during streptomycin therapy.
8. When dosing aminoglycosides, use ideal body weight, not true body weight.

SULFADIAZINE

 BASIC CHARACTERISTICS

Class: Sulfonamide

Mechanism of Action: Sulfonamides competitively inhibit the incorporation of para-aminobenzoic acid into dihydropteroic acid.

Mechanisms of Resistance:

1. Overproduction of para-aminobenzoic acid, and
2. structural change in dihydropteroate synthesis.

Metabolic Route: Sulfadiazine is excreted in the urine.

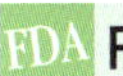 FDA-APPROVED INDICATIONS

FDA-Approved Indications: Chancroid, trachoma, inclusion conjunctivitis, nocardiosis, urinary tract infections, toxoplasmosis encephalitis as adjunctive therapy with pyrimethamine, malaria caused by chloroquine-resistant strains of *Plasmodium falciparum* when used as adjunctive therapy, prophylaxis of meningococcal meningitis for sulfa-sensitive group A strains, treatment of meningococcal meningitis, acute otitis media, prophylaxis against recurrences of rheumatic fever as an alternative to penicillin, and *Haemophilus influenzae* meningitis as adjunctive therapy with parenteral streptomycin.

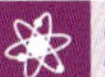 SIDE EFFECTS/TOXICITY

Contraindicated in patients with hypersensitivity to sulfonamides, infants aged younger than 2 months (except as adjunctive therapy with pyrimethamine in the treatment of congenital toxoplasmosis), in pregnancy at term, and during the breast-feeding period, because sulfonamides cross the placenta and are secreted in breast-milk and may cause kernicterus.

Side effects/toxicities include hypersensitivity reactions including fever and rash (erythema multiforme, Stevens-Johnson syndrome), generalized skin eruptions, epidermal necrolysis, urticaria, serum sickness, pruritus, and exfoliative dermatitis; nausea, emesis, abdominal pains, hepatitis, diarrhea, pancreatitis, stomatitis; renal failure, stone formation; headache; peripheral neuritis, depression, convulsions, ataxia, hallucinations, tinnitus, vertigo; goiter; diuresis; hypoglycemia; aplastic anemia, thrombocytopenia, leukopenia, hemolytic anemia, purpura, hypoprothrombinemia; methemoglobinemia, and hemolysis in individuals deficient in glucose-6-phosphate dehydrogenase.

DRUG INTERACTIONS/FOOD INTERACTIONS

Sulfadiazine can be taken with or without food.

Administration of a sulfonamide may increase the effect of oral anticoagulants, sulfonylurea hypoglycemic agents, thiazide diuretics, uricosuric agents, and methotrexate.

Agents such as indomethacin, probenecid, and salicylates may displace sulfonamides from plasma albumin and increase the concentrations of free drug in plasma.

DOSING

Sulfadiazine is administered in 500-mg tablets.

Loading dose of 2 g to 4 g followed by 2 g to 4 g, divided into three to six doses daily.

SPECIAL POPULATIONS

RENAL IMPAIRMENT: Use with caution.

HEPATIC DYSFUNCTION: Use with caution.

RENAL AND HEPATIC FAILURE: Should measure levels of sulfadiazine.

PEDIATRIC PATIENTS: Sulfadiazine is contraindicated in infants aged younger than 2 months except as adjunctive therapy with pyrimethamine in the treatment of congenital toxoplasmosis.

For those 2 months and over: A loading dose of one half the 24-hour dosage followed by a maintenance dosage of 150 mg/kg or 4 g/m^2, divided into four to six doses, every 24 hours, with a maximum of 6 g every 24 hours.

Rheumatic fever prophylaxis, for those who weigh less than 30 kg: 500 mg every 24 hours; 30 kg or more, 1 g every 24 hours.

PREGNANCY: Category C.

BREASTFEEDING: Mothers should stop breastfeeding before starting sulfadiazine.

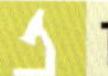

THE ART OF ANTIMICROBIAL THERAPY

Clinical Pearls:

1. Complete blood counts and urinalyses with careful microscopic examinations should be done frequently in patients receiving sulfonamides.
2. Patients taking sulfadiazine should drink adequate amounts of water to decrease the likelihood of crystalluria and stone formation.
3. Systemic sulfonamides are contraindicated in infants aged younger than 2 months except as adjunctive therapy with pyrimethamine in the treatment of congenital toxoplasmosis.
4. The sulfonamides should **not** be used for the **treatment** of group A β-hemolytic streptococcal infections; in an established infection, they will not eradicate the streptococci.

SURAMIN SODIUM (Germanin)

BASIC CHARACTERISTICS

Class: Hexasulphated naphthylamide

Mechanism of Action: Binds to several enzymes in the trypanosomes; however, the mechanism is not fully understood.

Mechanisms of Resistance: Data incomplete.

Metabolic Route: Suramin sodium is excreted in the urine unchanged.

FDA-APPROVED INDICATIONS

Not FDA-approved, but used for treatment of *Trypanosoma brucei gambiense* (West African trypanosomiasis) and *Trypanosoma brucei rhodesiense* (East African trypanosomiasis).

SIDE EFFECTS/TOXICITY

Side effects/toxicities include shock after first dose (rare), fever, renal failure, skin reactions including fatal toxic epidermal necrolysis, polyneuropathy, optic atrophy, corneal deposits, coagulopathy, adrenal insufficiency, liver function test anomalies, proteinuria, thrombocytopenia, and neutropenia.

DRUG INTERACTIONS/FOOD INTERACTIONS

Data incomplete.

DOSING

A test dose of 5 mg/kg (maximum of 200 mg) should be given for 1 to 2 days followed by 20 mg/kg (up to 1 g) on days 1, 3, 7, 14, and 21.

SPECIAL POPULATIONS

RENAL IMPAIRMENT: Dosage should be reduced or alternative agent should be used.

HEPATIC DYSFUNCTION: No dosage adjustment is necessary.

PEDIATRIC PATIENTS: Same dosage as adults.

PREGNANCY: Has been used in the past with no significant problems.

BREASTFEEDING: Data incomplete.

THE ART OF ANTIMICROBIAL THERAPY

Clinical Pearls:

1. Suramin can be obtained from the Centers for Disease Control and Prevention Parasitic Diseases Drug Service, 770-488-7775.

2. Suramin is considered the drug of choice for *T. brucei gambiense* and *T. brucei rhodesiense.*
3. Patients with concomitant onchocerciasis may show aggravation of ocular lesions and hypersensitivity, and such patients should be pretreated with ivermectin, if possible, before receiving suramin.
4. Because of poor cerebrospinal fluid penetration, suramin monotherapy should be avoided in patients with central nervous system trypanosomiasis.

TEICOPLANIN (Targocid)

 BASIC CHARACTERISTICS

Class: Glycopeptide

Mechanism of Action: Inhibits synthesis and assembly of the cell wall peptidoglycan polymers by complexing with their d-alanyl-d-alanine precursor, preventing its binding to the peptidoglycan terminus. Teicoplanin may impair RNA synthesis and injure protoplasts by altering the permeability of their cytoplasmic membrane.

Mechanisms of Resistance: The main mechanisms of resistance are carried by gene complex VanA mainly found in vancomycin-resistant enterococci (VRE) and they also have been found in staphylococci, including vancomycin-resistant *Staphylococcus aureus* (VRSA). VanA is plasmid mediated. It is the most common type of resistance and results in the synthesis of peptidoglycan cell wall precursors containing a pentapeptide ending with D-alanine-D-lactate.

Metabolic Route: Teicoplanin is excreted in the urine.

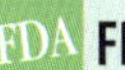 FDA-APPROVED INDICATIONS

Not FDA-approved, but used for treatment of the following serious infections caused by staphylococci or streptococci, which cannot be treated satisfactorily with less-toxic agents, including β-lactam antibiotics: osteomyelitis, septic arthritis, noncardiac bacteremia, and scpticemia.

 SIDE EFFECTS/TOXICITY

Contraindicated in patients with known hypersensitivity to the drug.

Teicoplanin should be administered with caution in patients known to be hypersensitive to vancomycin because cross-hypersensitivity may occur.

Side effects/toxicities include infusion-related events, fever, rigors, pruritus, rash (toxic epidermal necrolysis, erythema multiforme, Stevens-Johnson syndrome, and rare reports of exfoliative dermatitis), nausea, vomiting, diarrhea, increased transaminases and/or alkaline phosphatase, renal failure, dizziness, headache, hearing loss, tinnitus, vertigo and other vestibular disorders, eosinophilia, thrombocytopenia, leukopenia, and neutropenia.

 DRUG INTERACTIONS/FOOD INTERACTIONS

Teicoplanin should be administered with caution in patients receiving concurrent nephrotoxic or ototoxic drugs, such as aminoglycosides, amphotericin B, cyclosporine, and furosemide.

 DOSING

Intravenous dosing may be by slow injection over 5 minutes or by infusion over 30 minutes. Maintenance dosage is once daily; however, initially, a loading dose regimen of three doses at 12-hour intervals is recommended for rapid attainment of steady-state plasma levels.

An intramuscular injection of teicoplanin should not exceed 400 mg at a single site.

Septicemia/bacteremia, acute or chronic osteomyelitis: Treatment should be started with 400 mg to 800 mg (or 6 mg/kg to 12 mg/kg) by the intravenous route every 12 hours for three doses then the daily maintenance dose should be 400 mg (or 6 mg/kg).

Septic arthritis: Patients with septic arthritis should receive 800 mg (or 12 mg/kg), intravenously, every 12 hours for three doses, then a daily maintenance dose of 800 mg (or 12 mg/kg).

SPECIAL POPULATIONS

RENAL IMPAIRMENT: For patients with impaired renal function, reduction of dosage is not required until the fourth day of teicoplanin treatment.

CrCl Measurement or Hemodialysis	*Dosage*
10 mL/min to 50 mL/min	Usual dose every 48 hours
<10 mL/min	Usual dose every 72 hours
Hemodialysis	Usual dose every 72 hours
Chronic ambulatory peritoneal dialysis	Usual dose every 72 hours
Continuous renal replacement therapy	Usual dose every 48 hours

CrCl = Creatinine Clearance.

Trough plasma teicoplanin concentrations should be monitored periodically after the first week of therapy and the dosage adjusted to prevent through concentrations exceeding 30 μg/mL in patients with septic arthritis or 15 μg/mL in other cases.

HEPATIC DYSFUNCTION: No dosage adjustment is necessary.

PEDIATRIC PATIENTS: Not studied in pediatric patients.

PREGNANCY: Category B.

BREASTFEEDING: Caution should be exercised.

THE ART OF ANTIMICROBIAL THERAPY

Clinical Pearls:

1. Teicoplanin-related infusion toxicity is not related to concentration or rate of infusion.
2. Cross-sensitivity to vancomycin may be seen.
3. Seizures have been seen with intraventricular use of teicoplanin.

TELAVANCIN (Vibativ)

BASIC CHARACTERISTICS

Class: Lipoglycopeptide

Mechanisms of Action: Inhibits bacterial cell wall synthesis by interfering with the polymerization and cross-linking of peptidoglycan. Binds to the bacterial membrane and disrupts membrane barrier function.

Mechanisms of Resistance: Unknown.

Metabolic Route: Excreted unchanged in the urine.

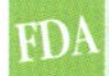

FDA-APPROVED INDICATIONS

FDA-Approved Indications: Treatment of complicated skin and skin structure infections caused by susceptible gram-positive organisms.

SIDE EFFECTS/TOXICITY

> **WARNING:** Women of childbearing potential should have a serum pregnancy test prior to administration of telavancin. Avoid use of telavancin during pregnancy unless the potential benefit to the patient outweighs the potential developmental risk to the fetus.

Side effects/toxicities include increases in serum creatinine, red-man syndrome, *Clostridium difficile*–associated diarrhea, prolongation of QTc interval, nausea, vomiting, taste disturbance, and foamy urine.

DRUG INTERACTIONS/FOOD INTERACTIONS

Elevations in the test results for prothrombin time, international normalized ratio, activated partial thromboplastin time, activated clotting time, and coagulation-based factor Xa tests. D-dimer, bleeding time, and whole blood clotting time are not affected.

DOSING

Telavancin dosing is 10 mg/kg daily.

SPECIAL POPULATIONS

RENAL IMPAIRMENT:

CrCl Measurement or Hemodialysis	*Telavancin Dosage Regimen*
> 50 mL/min	10 mg/kg every 24 hours
30 mL/min to 50 mL/min	7.5 mg/kg every 24 hours

CrCl Measurement or Hemodialysis	*Telavancin Dosage Regimen*
10 mL/min to 29 mL/min	10 mg/kg every 48 hours
<10	Not recommended

Note: CrCl = Creatinine Clearance.

HEPATIC DYSFUNCTION: No dosage adjustment is necessary.

PEDIATRIC PATIENTS: Safety and efficacy in patients aged younger than 18 years have not been established.

PREGNANCY: Category C.

BREASTFEEDING: Telavancin should be used with caution in breastfeeding mothers.

THE ART OF ANTIMICROBIAL THERAPY

Clinical Pearls:

1. Dosage of telavancin should be adjusted in patients with renal impairment.
2. Women of childbearing potential should have a serum pregnancy test before telavancin administration.
3. Telavancin may cause false elevation of prothrombin time and international normalized ratio results.
4. Telavancin is not active against vancomycin-resistant enterococci.

BASIC CHARACTERISTICS

Class: Nucleoside reverse transcriptase inhibitor.

Mechanism of Action: Telbivudine is a synthetic thymidine nucleoside analogue with activity against hepatitis B virus (HBV). It is phosphorylated by cellular kinases to the active triphosphate form that inhibits HBV DNA polymerase (reverse transcriptase) by competing with the natural substrate, thymidine 5′-triphosphate. Incorporation of telbivudine 5′-triphosphate into viral DNA causes DNA chain termination.

Mechanism of Resistance: Mutations rtM204I/V with or without rtL180M on HBV DNA polymerase lead to decreased incorporation of telbivudine triphosphate.

Metabolic Route: Telbivudine is excreted unchanged in the urine.

FDA FDA-APPROVED INDICATIONS

FDA-Approved Indications: Treatment of chronic HBV in adult patients (aged 16 years or older) with evidence of viral replication and either persistent elevations in serum aminotransferases or histologically active disease.

SIDE EFFECTS/TOXICITY

> **WARNING: Lactic acidosis and severe hepatomegaly with steatosis**, including fatal cases, have been reported with the use of nucleoside analogues alone or in combination with antiretrovirals.
>
> **Severe acute exacerbations of HBV** have been reported in patients who have discontinued anti-HBV therapy, including telbivudine. Hepatic function should be monitored closely with both clinical and laboratory follow-up for at least several months in patients who discontinue anti-HBV therapy.

Other side effects/toxicities include cases of myopathy/myositis several weeks to months after starting therapy, myalgia, peripheral neuropathy (risk for which is increased with concomitant interferon administration), fever, rash, fatigue, insomnia, headache, cough, nausea, diarrhea, fatigue, arthralgia, increased ALT, and increased creatinine kinase.

DRUG INTERACTIONS/FOOD INTERACTIONS

Telbivudine can be taken with or without food. Because telbivudine is eliminated primarily by renal excretion, coadministration of telbivudine with drugs that alter renal function may alter plasma concentrations of telbivudine.

TELBIVUDINE (Tyzeka)

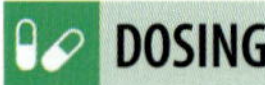

DOSING

Telbivudine is supplied as 600-mg tablets and a solution containing 100 mg/5 mL. The recommended dosage of telbivudine for the treatment of chronic HBV is 600 mg once daily.

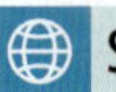

SPECIAL POPULATIONS

RENAL IMPAIRMENT:

CrCl Measurement or Hemodialysis	*Dosage*
≥50 mL/min	600 mg daily
30 mL/min to 49 mL/min	600 mg every 48 hours
< 30 mL/min	600 mg every 72 hours
Hemodialysis	600 mg every 96 hours (if on hemodialysis day, administer after hemodialysis)

Note: CrCl = Creatinine Clearance.

HEPATIC DYSFUNCTION: No adjustment to the recommended dosage of telbivudine is necessary in patients with hepatic impairment.

PEDIATRIC PATIENTS: Telbivudine is not recommended to be used in children.

PREGNANCY: Category B.

BREASTFEEDING: The use of telbivudine is not recommended for breastfeeding mothers.

THE ART OF ANTIMICROBIAL THERAPY

Clinical Pearls:

1. Telbivudine should be used with caution in patients with HBV who are coinfected with HIV, hepatitis C virus, or hepatitis D virus, as it has not been investigated in patients with these coinfections.
2. Telbivudine may be taken with or without food.
3. Resistance mutations are similar between entecavir and telbivudine.

TENOFOVIR DISOPROXIL FUMARATE (Viread)

Note: Also available combined with emtricitabine as Truvada and with both emtricitabine and efavirenz as Atripla.

BASIC CHARACTERISTICS

Class: Nucleotide reverse transcriptase inhibitor (NRTI)

Mechanism of Action: Converted by cellular enzymes to its active drug tenofovir biphosphate, an analogue of adenosine triphosphate. The tenofovir biphosphate competes with the naturally occurring nucleotides for incorporation in newly forming HIV DNA. Because tenofovir biphosphate does not have a terminal hydroxyl group, it halts transcription and replication of the virus.

Mechanism of Resistance: Changes in the structure of HIV reverse transcriptase lead to preferred incorporation of adenosine triphosphate and decreased incorporation of tenofovir biphosphate, which allows transcription of DNA to continue. Resistance mutations include K65R and TAMS.

Metabolic Route: Tenofovir is excreted in the urine unchanged.

FDA FDA-APPROVED INDICATIONS

FDA-Approved Indications: Treatment of HIV infection, in combinations with other antiretrovirals, and treatment of chronic hepatitis B in adults.

SIDE EFFECTS/TOXICITY

WARNING: Severe acute exacerbations of hepatitis have been reported in hepatitis B–infected patients who have discontinued anti–hepatitis B therapy, including tenofovir. Hepatic function should be monitored closely with both clinical and laboratory follow-up for at least several months in patients who discontinue anti–hepatitis B therapy, including tenofovir. If appropriate, resumption of anti–hepatitis B therapy may be warranted.

Lactic acidosis and hepatomegaly with steatosis have been reported with nucleoside analogues, including tenofovir. If this syndrome occurs, the drug should be discontinued.

Other side effects/toxicities: immune reconstitution inflammatory syndrome; fat redistribution including central obesity and dorsocervical fat enlargement, peripheral wasting, facial wasting, and breast enlargement; renal impairment, including cases of acute renal failure and Fanconi's syndrome; decreased bone mineral density; rash; nausea; diarrhea; headache; pain; depression; and asthenia.

DRUG INTERACTIONS/FOOD INTERACTIONS

Tenofovir should be administered with food.

Tenofovir should not be administered with adefovir.

Tenofovir should not be given with didanosine because of decreased CD4 counts in patients maintained on this regimen. If didanosine is given with tenofovir, the didanosine should be decreased to 250 mg daily.

Tenofovir decreases the levels of atazanavir. If the two drugs are given together, atazanavir must be given with ritonavir.

Tenofovir should not be administered with other medications containing tenofovir (i.e., Truvada and Atripla).

DOSING

Tenofovir is administered in a 300-mg tablet. The recommended adult dosage is 300 mg once daily.

SPECIAL POPULATIONS

RENAL IMPAIRMENT: Dosage of tenofovir should be adjusted based on renal function. For creatinine clearance 30 mL/min to 49 mL/min, tenofovir should be administered every 48 hours. For clearance less than 30 mL/min, it should be administered every 72 to 96 hours. For those on hemodialysis, it is administered once weekly.

HEPATIC DYSFUNCTION: No dosage adjustment is necessary.

PEDIATRIC PATIENTS: Tenofovir has not been studied in children.

PREGNANCY: Category B.

BREASTFEEDING: It is recommended that HIV-positive mothers not breastfeed their children, to decrease mother-to-child transmission of HIV. Mothers should be instructed not to breastfeed if they are receiving tenofovir.

THE ART OF ANTIMICROBIAL THERAPY

Clinical Pearls:

1. Tenofovir should be used in combination with other antiretroviral agents.
2. Tenofovir is present in three different medications: Viread, Truvada, and Atripla.
3. Patients with HIV should be tested for hepatitis B virus before initiating antiretroviral therapy with tenofovir.
4. Tenofovir and didanosine combinations should be administered with caution (see "DRUG INTERACTIONS/FOOD INTERACTIONS").
5. Atazanavir should be boosted with ritonavir if given with tenofovir.

TENOFOVIR PLUS EMTRICITABINE (Truvada)

Note: Also available with efavirenz as Atripla.

BASIC CHARACTERISTICS

Class: Nucleotide reverse transcriptase inhibitors (NRTI).

Mechanism of Action: Tenofovir and emtricitabine are converted by cellular enzymes to their active drugs tenofovir biphosphate (an analogue of adenosine triphosphate), and emtricitabine triphosphate (an analogue of cytosine triphosphate). These drugs compete with the naturally occurring nucleotides for incorporation in newly forming HIV DNA. Because they do not have a terminal hydroxyl group, they halt transcription and replication of the virus.

Mechanism of Resistance: Changes in the structure of HIV reverse transcriptase leads to preferred incorporation of adenosine triphosphate and decreased incorporation of tenofovir biphosphate, which allows transcription of DNA to continue. Resistance mutations include K65R, M184V, and "TAMS": 41L, 67N, 70R, 210W, 215F and 219E.

Metabolic Route: Tenofovir and emtricitabine are excreted in the urine unchanged.

FDA FDA-APPROVED INDICATIONS

FDA-Approved Indications: Treatment of HIV infection, in combinations with other antiretrovirals.

Also Used for: Active against hepatitis B.

SIDE EFFECTS/TOXICITY

WARNING: Severe acute exacerbations of hepatitis have been reported in hepatitis B–infected patients who have discontinued anti–hepatitis B therapy, including Truvada or any medications containing either tenofovir or emtricitabine. Hepatic function should be monitored closely with both clinical and laboratory follow-up for at least several months in patients who discontinue anti–hepatitis B therapy, including Truvada. If appropriate, resumption of anti–hepatitis B therapy may be warranted.

Lactic acidosis and hepatomegaly with steatosis have been reported with nucleoside analogues, including tenofovir. If this syndrome occurs, the drug should be discontinued.

Other side effects/toxicities: immune reconstitution inflammatory syndrome; fat redistribution including central obesity and dorsocervical fat enlargement, peripheral wasting, facial wasting, and breast enlargement; diarrhea; nausea; fatigue; headache; dizziness; depression; insomnia; abnormal dreams; rash; renal impairment, including acute renal failure and Fanconi's syndrome; and decreased bone mineral density.

DRUG INTERACTIONS/FOOD INTERACTIONS

Truvada should not be administered with adefovir.

Truvada should not be given with didanosine because of decreased CD4 counts in patients maintained on this regimen. If didanosine is given with Truvada or any medication containing tenofovir, the didanosine should be decreased to 250 mg daily.

Truvada or any medication containing tenofovir decreases the levels of atazanavir. If the two drugs are given together, atazanavir must be given with ritonavir.

Truvada should be administered with food.

Truvada should not be administered with any medication containing lamivudine because lamivudine and emtricitabine are both cytosine analogues and may be antagonistic.

Truvada should not be administered with Viread, Emtriva, or Atripla.

DOSING

Truvada is administered in a fixed-dose tablet containing 300 mg of tenofovir and 200 mg of emtricitabine. The recommended adult dosage is one tablet once daily.

SPECIAL POPULATIONS

RENAL IMPAIRMENT: Truvada should not be administered to those with renal insufficiency.

HEPATIC DYSFUNCTION: No dosage adjustment is necessary.

PEDIATRIC PATIENTS: Truvada has not been studied in children.

PREGNANCY: Category B.

BREASTFEEDING: It is recommended that HIV-positive mothers not breastfeed their children, to decrease mother-to-child transmission of HIV. Mothers should not breastfeed if they are receiving Truvada.

THE ART OF ANTIMICROBIAL THERAPY

Clinical Pearls:

1. Truvada should be used in combination with other antiretroviral agents.
2. Truvada contains both tenofovir and emtricitabine and should not be administered with Viread, Emtriva, or Atripla.
3. Patients with HIV should be tested for hepatitis B virus before initiating antiretroviral therapy with Truvada.
4. Truvada and didanosine combinations should be administered with caution.
5. Atazanavir should be boosted with ritonavir if given with Truvada.

TENOFOVIR PLUS EMTRICITABINE PLUS EFAVIRENZ (Atripla)

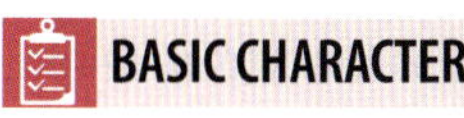

BASIC CHARACTERISTICS

Class: Combination of a nonnucleoside reverse transcriptase inhibitor (efavirenz), a nucleotide reverse transcriptase inhibitor (tenofovir), and a nucleoside reverse transcriptase inhibitor (emtricitabine).

Mechanisms of Action: Tenofovir and emtricitabine are converted by cellular enzymes to their active drugs tenofovir biphosphate (an analogue of adenosine triphosphate), and emtricitabine triphosphate (an analogue of cytosine triphosphate). These drugs compete with the naturally occurring nucleotides for incorporation in newly forming HIV DNA. Because they do not have a terminal hydroxyl group, they halt transcription and replication of the virus. Efavirenz inhibits reverse transcriptase activity by binding the enzyme.

Mechanisms of Resistance: Changes in the structure of HIV reverse transcriptase lead to the inability of efavirenz to bind the enzyme and allow transcription to continue. The most frequent resistance mutations include K103N and Y181C.

Changes in the structure of HIV reverse transcriptase leads to preferred incorporation of adenosine triphosphate and cytosine triphosphate and decreased incorporation of tenofovir biphosphate and emtricitabine triphosphate, which allows transcription of DNA to continue. Resistance mutations include K65R, M184V, and TAMS.

Metabolic Route: Efavirenz is metabolized by the cytochrome P450 system to hydroxylated metabolites with subsequent glucuronidation. Tenofovir and emtricitabine are excreted in the urine unchanged.

FDA-APPROVED INDICATIONS

FDA-Approved Indications: Treatment of HIV-1 as a single-regimen tablet.

SIDE EFFECTS/TOXICITY

WARNING: Lactic acidosis and severe hepatomegaly with steatosis, including fatal cases, have been reported with the use of nucleoside analogues, including tenofovir. Atripla is not approved for the treatment of chronic hepatitis B virus (HBV) infection. **Severe acute exacerbations of HBV** have been reported in patients coinfected with HBV and HIV-1 who have discontinued emtricitabine or tenofovir, which are components of Atripla. Hepatic function should be monitored closely in these patients. If appropriate, initiation of anti-HBV therapy may be warranted.

Other side effects/toxicities include serious psychiatric toxicity, including severe depression, suicidal ideation, nonfatal suicide attempts, aggressive behavior, paranoid reactions, manic reactions, insomnia, impaired concentration, somnolence, abnormal dreams, and hallucinations; headache; rash; diarrhea; nausea; abdominal pain; elevated liver enzymes; cough; rhinitis; convulsions; elevated cholesterol; immune reconstitution inflammatory syndrome; fat redistribution including central obesity and dorsocervical fat enlargement, peripheral wasting, facial wasting, and breast enlargement; and renal impairment, including acute renal failure and Fanconi's syndrome; decreased bone mineral density has been seen with tenofovir.

DRUG INTERACTIONS/FOOD INTERACTIONS

Atripla should be administered on an empty stomach.

Atripla should not be administered concurrently with astemizole, bepridil, cisapride, midazolam, pimozide, triazolam, ergot derivatives, Saint-John's-wort, voriconazole, etravirine, adefovir, tenofovir, emtricitabine, lamivudine, efavirenz, or Truvada. Atripla should not be administered with any medication containing lamivudine because lamivudine and emtricitabine are both cytosine analogues and may be antagonistic.

Atripla causes hepatic enzyme induction of CYP3A4; coadministration of efavirenz with drugs primarily metabolized by 2C9, 2C19, and 3A4 isozymes may result in altered plasma concentrations of the coadministered drug; Drugs that induce CYP3A4 activity would be expected to increase the clearance of efavirenz resulting in lowered plasma concentrations. Because of these metabolic activities, the following drug interactions warrant consideration of dosage adjustment and monitoring of clinical effects and serum levels of affected drugs:

Medication	*Adjustment or Action*
Clarithromycin	Consider alternative agent to clarithromycin
Rifabutin	Increase rifabutin to 450 mg to 600 mg per day or 600 mg thrice weekly
Rifampin	Consider adding efavirenz 200 mg/day to the Atripla
Hormonal contraceptives	Use alternative or additional method
Phenobarbitol, phenytoin, or carbamazepine	Monitor anticonvulsant level; consider alternative anticonvulsant
Methadone	Opiate withdrawal common; titrate methadone
Warfarin	Monitor international normalized ratio closely
Fosamprenavir	Fosamprenavir 1400 mg + ritonavir 300 mg daily or usual twice daily dosage
Darunavir	Monitor levels of Darunavir with normal dosing
Indinavir	Indinavir 800 mg twice daily + ritonavir 100 mg twice daily
Maraviroc	Maraviroc dosage should be 600 mg twice daily

Medication	*Adjustment or Action*
Didanosine	Decrease didanosine to 250 mg daily
Atazanavir	Atazanavir 300 mg + ritonavir 100 mg (treatment-naïve patients only)

DOSING

Each tablet contains 600 mg of efavirenz, 200 mg of emtricitabine, and 300 mg of tenofovir disoproxil fumarate. The recommended dosage is one tablet at bedtime.

SPECIAL POPULATIONS

RENAL IMPAIRMENT: It is not recommended to be administered in patients with renal insufficiency.

HEPATIC DYSFUNCTION: In patients with known or suspected history of hepatitis B or C infection and in patients treated with other medications associated with liver toxicity, monitoring of liver enzymes is recommended.

PEDIATRIC PATIENTS: Atripla should not be given to those aged younger than 18 years.

PREGNANCY: Category D.

BREASTFEEDING: It is recommended that HIV-positive mothers not breastfeed their children, to decrease mother-to-child transmission of HIV.

THE ART OF ANTIMICROBIAL THERAPY

Clinical Pearls:

1. Atripla is a stand-alone antiretroviral regimen.
2. Atripla should be dosed at bedtime to decrease the central nervous system adverse events.
3. If Atripla is given without food, less is absorbed and side effects can be decreased.
4. Women receiving Atripla should use two methods of birth control.
5. Atripla contains tenofovir, emtricitabine, and efavirenz. It should not be administered with Viread, Emtriva, Truvada, or Sustiva.
6. Patients with HIV-1 should be tested for HBV before initiating antiretroviral therapy with Atripla.
7. Atripla and didanosine combinations should be administered with caution.

TERBINAFINE (Lamisil)

BASIC CHARACTERISTICS

Class: Allylamine derivative

Mechanism of Action: Inhibits squalene epoxidase, blocking the biosynthesis of ergosterol, an essential component of fungal cell membranes.

Mechanism of Resistance: Not defined.

Metabolic Route: Eliminated in the urine.

FDA FDA-APPROVED INDICATIONS

FDA-Approved Indications: Tablet: Treatment of onychomycosis of the toenail or fingernail caused by dermatophytes (tinea unguium). Oral granules: Treatment of tinea capitis in patients aged 4 years and older.

SIDE EFFECTS/TOXICITY

Contraindicated in individuals with hypersensitivity to terbinafine or to any other ingredients of the formulation.

Side effects/toxicities include liver failure in individuals with and without preexisting liver disease, serious skin reactions (e.g., Stevens-Johnson syndrome and toxic epidermal necrolysis, psoriasisiform eruptions), precipitation and exacerbation of cutaneous and systemic lupus erythematosus, changes in the ocular lens and retina, reversible lymphopenia and neutropenia, malaise, fatigue, vomiting, arthralgia, myalgia, and hair loss.

DRUG INTERACTIONS

Terbinafine is an inhibitor of the CYP450 2D6 isozyme. Drugs predominantly metabolized by the CYP450 2D6 isozyme include tricyclic antidepressants, selective serotonin reuptake inhibitors, β-blockers, antiarrhythmics class 1C (e.g., flecainide and propafenone), and monoamine oxidase inhibitors type B. Coadministration of these drugs with terbinafine hydrochloride should be done with careful monitoring and may require a reduction in dosage of the 2D6-metabolized drug.

Terbinafine clearance is increased 100% by rifampin and decreased 33% by cimetidine.

DOSING

Tablets (250 mg):

- Fingernail onychomycosis: 250 mg once daily for 6 weeks
- Toenail onychomycosis: 250 mg once daily for 12 weeks

Oral granules (Available in 125 mg packets): Once a day for 6 weeks based upon body weight (see table). Sprinkle the contents of each packet on a spoonful of pudding or other soft, nonacidic food such as mashed potatoes and swallow the entire spoonful (without chewing); do not use applesauce or fruit-based foods. Take with food. If two packets (250 mg) are required with each dose, either the content of both packets may be sprinkled on one spoonful, or the contents of both packets may be sprinkled on two spoonfuls of nonacidic food as directed previously.

Body Weight	*Dosage of Oral Granules*
< 25 kg	125 mg/day
25 kg to 35 kg	187.5 mg/day
> 35 kg	250 mg/day

SPECIAL POPULATIONS

RENAL IMPAIRMENT: Not recommended in patients with creatinine clearance 50 mL/min or less.

HEPATIC DYSFUNCTION: Not recommended for patients with chronic or active liver disease.

PEDIATRIC PATIENTS: Safety and dosing have not been studied in children.

PREGNANCY: Category B.

BREASTFEEDING: Terbinafine is not recommended in breastfeeding mothers.

THE ART OF ANTIMICROBIAL THERAPY

Clinical Pearls:

1. Before treatment is initiated, a KOH preparation, fungal culture, or nail biopsy should be obtained to confirm the diagnosis of onychomycosis.
2. Hepatic and hematologic function should be monitored throughout therapy.

BASIC CHARACTERISTICS

Class: Tetracycline

Mechanism of Action: Reversibly binds the 30S ribosomal subunit preventing the addition of new amino acids into the growing peptide chain.

Mechanisms of Resistance: Decreased entry into the cell or increased excretion of the drug may occur. Rarely, the tetracyclines are inactivated.

Metabolic Route: Tetracyclines are concentrated by the liver in the bile, and excreted in the urine and feces at high concentrations and in a biologically active form.

FDA FDA-APPROVED INDICATIONS

FDA-Approved Indications: Treatment of serious infections caused by susceptible strains of microorganisms in the following conditions: respiratory tract infections; skin and skin structure infections; urinary tract infections; Rocky Mountain spotted fever; typhus group infections; Q fever; rickettsialpox; psittacosis; infections caused by *Chlamydia trachomatis* such as uncomplicated urethral, endocervical, or rectal infections, inclusion conjunctivitis, trachoma, and lymphogranuloma venereum; granuloma inguinale; relapsing fever; bartonellosis; chancroid; tularemia; plague; cholera; brucellosis; infections caused by *Campylobacter fetus*; amebiasis; acne; syphilis and yaws; Vincent's infection; infections caused by *Neisseria gonorrhoeae*; anthrax; listeriosis; actinomycosis; and infections caused by *Clostridium* species.

SIDE EFFECTS/TOXICITY

This drug is **contraindicated** in persons who have shown hypersensitivity to any of the tetracyclines.

Tetracyclines should not be used during pregnancy or in those aged younger than 8 years unless absolutely necessary and no reasonable alternative exists.

Side effects/toxicities include hypersensitivity reactions, including rash, anaphylaxis, urticaria, angioneurotic edema, serum sickness, photosensitivity, pericarditis, and exacerbation of systemic lupus erythematosus; nausea, vomiting, diarrhea, glossitis, esophagitis, hepatotoxicity, pseudomembranous colitis; bulging fontanels in infants and benign intracranial hypertension in adults; vertigo, pseudotumor cerebri, tinnitus and decreased hearing; dose-related rise in BUN, hemolytic anemia, thrombocytopenia, neutropenia, and eosinophilia.

DRUG INTERACTIONS/FOOD INTERACTIONS

Tetracycline hydrochloride tablets should be taken at least 1 hour before meals or 2 hours after meals.

Concurrent use of tetracycline may render oral contraceptives less effective.

Patients who are on anticoagulant therapy may require downward adjustment of their anticoagulant dosage.

It is advisable to avoid giving tetracycline-class drugs in conjunction with penicillin.

Absorption of oral tetracycline is impaired by antacids containing aluminum, calcium, or magnesium, and iron-containing preparations.

The concurrent use of tetracycline and methoxyflurane has resulted in fatal renal toxicity.

Pregnant women with renal disease may be more prone to develop tetracycline-associated liver failure.

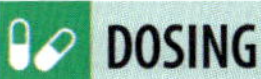

DOSING

Tetracycline is administered as 250-mg and 500-mg tablets. The **usual daily dosage** is 500 mg twice daily or 250 mg four times daily. Higher dosages such as 500 mg four times daily may be required for severe infections or for those infections that do not respond to the smaller doses. Therapy is usually continued for at least 24 to 48 hours after symptoms and fever have subsided.

Brucellosis: 500 mg four times daily for 3 weeks (in combination with other antibiotics)

Syphilis: 500 mg four times daily for 15 days for syphilis of less than 1 year's duration, and for 30 days for syphilis of more than 1 year's duration

Gonorrhea, chlamydial urogenital infection: 500 mg four times daily for 7 days

SPECIAL POPULATIONS

RENAL IMPAIRMENT:

CrCl Measurement or Hemodialysis	*Dosage*
10 mL/min to 50 mL/min	Usual dosage every 12 to 24 hours
< 10 mL/min	Usual dosage once daily
Hemodialysis, chronic ambulatory peritoneal dialysis, and continuous renal replacement therapy	Should not be used in dialysis patients

Note: CrCl = Creatinine Clearance.

HEPATIC DYSFUNCTION: Data incomplete.

PEDIATRIC PATIENTS: **For children aged 8 years and older:** The usual daily dosage is 10 mg/lb to 20 mg/lb (25 mg/kg to 50 mg/kg) body weight divided in four equal doses.

PREGNANCY: Category D.

BREASTFEEDING: Do not administer to breastfeeding mothers.

THE ART OF ANTIMICROBIAL THERAPY

Clinical Pearls:

1. To reduce the risk of esophageal irritation and ulceration, tetracycline should be taken with adequate amounts of fluid and should not be taken immediately before going to bed.
2. Tetracycline can cause fetal harm when administered to a pregnant woman.
3. The use of drugs of the tetracycline class during tooth development (last half of pregnancy, infancy, and childhood to the age of 8 years) may cause permanent discoloration of the teeth (yellow-gray-brown).
4. Tetracycline should not be administered with calcium or other cations.

THIABENDAZOLE (Mintezole)

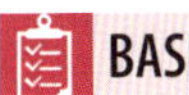

BASIC CHARACTERISTICS

Class: Broad-spectrum anthelminthic

Mechanism of Action: Inhibits the helminth-specific enzyme fumarate reductase. Thiabendazole also suppresses egg and/or larval production.

Metabolic Route: Thiabendazole is metabolized in the liver and excreted in the urine.

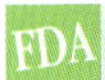

FDA-APPROVED INDICATIONS

FDA-Approved Indications: Treatment of strongyloidiasis (threadworm), cutaneous larva migrans (creeping eruption), and visceral larva migrans.

Also Used for: (when preferred regimens cannot be used): Treatment of hookworm (*Necator americanus* and *Ancylostoma duodenale*), whipworm (trichuriasis), roundworm (ascariasis), and trichinellosis.

SIDE EFFECTS/TOXICITY

Side effects/toxicities include erythema multiforme, Stevens-Johnson syndrome, dizziness, weariness, drowsiness, giddiness, headache, numbness, hyperirritability, convulsions, collapse, confusion, depression, floating sensation, weakness, lack of coordination, jaundice, cholestasis, parenchymal liver damage, anorexia, nausea, vomiting, diarrhea, epigastric distress, abdominal pain, tinnitus, abnormal sensation in eyes, xanthopsia, blurred vision, drying of mucous membranes, sicca syndrome, hypotension, hyperglycemia, leukopenia, hematuria, enuresis, malodorous urine, and crystalluria.

DRUG INTERACTIONS/FOOD INTERACTIONS

Thiabendazole should be given after meals if possible.

When concomitant use of thiabendazole and xanthine derivatives (theophylline) is anticipated, it may be necessary to monitor blood levels and/or reduce the dosage of such compounds.

DOSING

Administered as 500-mg chewable tablets or as a suspension containing 500 mg thiabendazole per 5 mL.

The recommended maximum daily dose is 3 g.

Tablets should be chewed before swallowing.

To determine the dosage, please see first table. For frequency and duration, see second table.

THIABENDAZOLE (Mintezole)

Thiabendazole Dosage by Body Weight:

Weight, lbs	*Tablet*	*Oral suspension*
30-49	250 mg (0.5 tablet)	2.5 mL
50-74	500 mg (1 tablet)	5 mL
75-99	750 mg (1.5 tablets)	7.5 mL
100-124	1000 mg (2 tablets)	10 mL
125-149	1250 (2.5 tablets)	12.5 mL
150 and over	1500 (3 tablets)	15 mL

Thiabendazole Dosage Frequency and Duration:

Indication	*Regimen*
Strongyloidiasis	Two doses per day for 2 days
Cutaneous larva migrans	Two doses per day for 2 days
Visceral larva migrans	Two doses per day for 7 days
Trichinellosis	Two doses per day for 2 to 4 days
Intestinal roundworms	Two doses per day for 2 days

SPECIAL POPULATIONS

RENAL IMPAIRMENT: There is no dosage adjustment for patients with renal insufficiency.

HEPATIC DYSFUNCTION: Monitoring of liver function tests is suggested if prolonged thiabendazole therapy is given.

PEDIATRIC PATIENTS: The safety and effectiveness of thiabendazole in pediatric patients weighing less than 30 lbs has been limited.

PREGNANCY: Category C.

BREASTFEEDING: A decision should be made whether to discontinue breastfeeding or to discontinue the drug.

THE ART OF ANTIMICROBIAL THERAPY

Clinical Pearls:

1. Thiabendazole should be used only in patients in whom susceptible worm infestation has been diagnosed and should not be used prophylactically.
2. Because central nervous system side effects may occur quite frequently with thiabendazole therapy, activities requiring mental alertness should be avoided.

 BASIC CHARACTERISTICS

Class: Carboxypenicillin

Mechanism of Action: Binds penicillin binding protein (PBP), disrupting cell wall synthesis.

Mechanisms of Resistance:

1. The PBP can be altered, with reduced affinity,
2. production of a β-lactamase resulting in hydrolysis of the β-lactam ring, and
3. decreased ability of the antibiotic to reach the PBP when bacteria decrease porin production, resulting in a decrease of the drug concentration within the cell.

Metabolic Route: Ticarcillin is excreted unchanged in the urine.

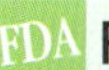 FDA-APPROVED INDICATIONS

FDA-Approved Indications: Ticarcillin is indicated in the treatment of infections caused by susceptible strains of microorganisms in the following conditions: bacterial septicemia, skin and skin structure infections, acute and chronic respiratory tract infections, genitourinary tract infections, intraabdominal infections, and infections of the female pelvis and genital tract.

 SIDE EFFECTS/TOXICITY

A history of allergic reaction to any of the penicillins is a **contraindication.**

Side effects/toxicities include *Clostridium difficile*–associated diarrhea, hypersensitivity reactions including anaphylaxis, rash including erythema multiforme and Stevens-Johnson syndrome, mucocutaneous candidiasis, nausea, vomiting, diarrhea, constipation, black hairy tongue, headache, arrhythmias, hyperactivity, seizures, confusion, hepatitis, renal dysfunction, anemia, thrombocytopenia, eosinophilia, leukopenia, hypernatremia, hypokalemia, and abnormalities of coagulation.

 DRUG INTERACTIONS/FOOD INTERACTIONS

Concurrent use of ticarcillin and probenecid may result in increased and prolonged blood levels of ticarcillin.

Chloramphenicol, macrolides, sulfonamides, and tetracyclines may interfere with the bactericidal effects of penicillins.

High urine concentrations of ticarcillin may result in false-positive reactions when one is testing for the presence of glucose in urine with Clinitest. It is recommended that glucose tests based on enzymatic glucose oxidase reactions (such as Clinistix) be used instead.

TICARCILLIN (Ticar)

DOSING

Bacterial septicemia: 200 mg/kg to 300 mg/kg divided every 4 to 6 hours

Respiratory tract infections: 3 g every 4 hours or 4 g every 6 hours

Skin and skin structure infections: 3 g every 4 hours or 4 g every 6 hours

Intraabdominal infections: 3 g every 4 hours or 4 g every 6 hours

Uncomplicated urinary tract infection: 1 g every 6 hours

Complicated urinary tract infection: 3 g every 6 hours

SPECIAL POPULATIONS

RENAL IMPAIRMENT:

CrCl Measurement or Hemodialysis	*Dosage*
30 mL/min to 60 mL/min	2 g every 4 hours
10 mL/min to 29 mL/min	2 g every 8 hours
< 10 mL/min	2 g every 12 hours
< 10 mL/min with hepatic impairment	2 g every 24 hours
Hemodialysis	2 g every 12 hours with 3 g after hemodialysis
Chronic ambulatory peritoneal dialysis	3 g every 12 hours
Continuous renal replacement therapy	2 g every 8 hours

Note: CrCl = Creatinine Clearance.

HEPATIC DYSFUNCTION: No dosage adjustment is necessary.

PEDIATRIC PATIENTS:

Bacterial septicemia: 200 mg/kg to 300 mg/kg divided every 4 to 6 hours

Respiratory tract infections: 200 mg/kg to 300 mg/kg divided every 4 to 6 hours

Skin and skin structure infections: 200 mg/kg to 300 mg/kg divided every 4 to 6 hours

Intraabdominal infections: 200 mg/kg to 300 mg/kg divided every 4 to 6 hours

Uncomplicated urinary tract infection: 50 mg/kg to 100 mg/kg divided every 6 to 8 hours

Complicated urinary tract infection: 150 mg/kg to 200 mg/kg divided every 4 to 6 hours

Neonate:

Infants Under 2000 g	*Body Weight*	*Infants 2000 g and Over*	*Body Weight*
Aged 0 to 7 days	75 mg/kg/ 12 hours	Aged 0 to 7 days	75 mg/kg/ 8 hours
Aged older than 7 days	75 mg/kg/ 8 hours	Aged older than 7 days	100 mg/kg/ 8 hours

PREGNANCY: Category B.

BREASTFEEDING: Ticarcillin should be used only with caution in breastfeeding mothers.

THE ART OF ANTIMICROBIAL THERAPY

Clinical Pearls:

1. Dosage of ticarcillin needs to be adjusted for patients with renal dysfunction.
2. Because the theoretical sodium content is 5.2 mEq (120 mg) per gram of ticarcillin, and the actual vial content can be as high as 6.5 mEq per gram, electrolyte and cardiac status should be monitored carefully.
3. In a few patients receiving intravenous ticarcillin, hypokalemia has been reported. Serum potassium should be measured periodically.

TICARCILLIN DISODIUM PLUS CLAVULANATE POTASSIUM (Timentin)

BASIC CHARACTERISTICS

Class: Carboxypenicillin plus β-lactamase inhibitor

Mechanism of Action: Binds penicillin-binding protein (PBP), disrupting cell wall synthesis.

Mechanisms of Resistance:

1. The PBP can be altered, with reduced affinity,
2. production of a β-lactamase resulting in hydrolysis of the β-lactam ring, and
3. decreased ability of the antibiotic to reach the PBP when bacteria decrease porin production, resulting in a decrease of the drug concentration within the cell.

Metabolic Route: The majority of ticarcillin and half of clavulanate are excreted unchanged in the urine.

FDA FDA-APPROVED INDICATIONS

FDA-Approved Indications: Ticarcillin plus clavulanate is indicated in the treatment of infections caused by susceptible strains of microorganisms in the following conditions: septicemia (including bacteremia), lower respiratory tract infections, bone and joint infections, skin and skin structure infections, urinary tract infections, gynecologic infections, and intraabdominal infections.

SIDE EFFECTS/TOXICITY

A history of allergic reaction to any of the penicillins is a **contraindication**.

Side effects/toxicities include *Clostridium difficile*–associated diarrhea, hypersensitivity reactions including anaphylaxis, rash including erythema multiforme and Stevens-Johnson syndrome, mucocutaneous candidiasis, nausea, vomiting, diarrhea, constipation, black hairy tongue, headache, arrhythmias, hyperactivity, seizures, confusion, hepatitis, renal dysfunction, anemia, thrombocytopenia, eosinophilia, leukopenia, hypernatremia, hypokalemia, and abnormalities of coagulation.

DRUG INTERACTIONS/FOOD INTERACTIONS

Concurrent use of ticarcillin plus clavulanate and probenecid may result in increased and prolonged blood levels of ticarcillin plus clavulanate.

High urine concentrations of ticarcillin may produce false-positive urine protein reactions, and false-positive Coombs' test.

Chloramphenicol, macrolides, sulfonamides, and tetracyclines may interfere with the bactericidal effects of penicillins.

High urine concentrations of ticarcillin may result in false-positive reactions when one is testing for the presence of glucose in urine with Clinitest. It is recommended that glucose tests based on enzymatic glucose oxidase reactions (such as Clinistix) be used instead.

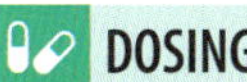

DOSING

The usual dosage for **systemic and urinary tract infections** is 3.1 g every 4 to 6 hours.

For **gynecologic infections**, **moderate infections**, 200 mg/kg/day in divided doses every 6 hours, and for **severe infections**, 300 mg/kg/day in divided doses every 4 hours.

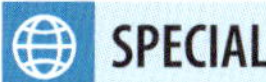

SPECIAL POPULATIONS

RENAL IMPAIRMENT:

CrCl Measurement or Hemodialysis	*Dosage*
30 mL/min to 60 mL/min	2 g every 4 hours
10 mL/min to 29 mL/min	2 g every 8 hours
< 10 mL/min	2 g every 12 hours
< 10 mL/min with hepatic dysfunction	2 g every 24 hours
Chronic ambulatory peritoneal dialysis	3.1 g every 12 hours
Hemodialysis	2 g every 12 hours with 3.1 g after dialysis
Continuous renal replacement therapy	Unknown

Note: CrCl = Creatinine Clearance.

HEPATIC DYSFUNCTION: No dosage adjustment is necessary.

PEDIATRIC PATIENTS: There are insufficient data to support the use of ticarcillin plus clavulanate in patients aged younger than 3 months.

Patients aged 3 months and older who weigh less than 60 kg: 50 mg/kg every 6 hours for mild to moderate infections and every 4 hours for severe infections.

For patients who weigh 60 kg or more: use the adult dosing recommendations.

PREGNANCY: Category B.

BREASTFEEDING: Ticarcillin plus clavulanate should be used only with caution in breastfeeding mothers.

THE ART OF ANTIMICROBIAL THERAPY

Clinical Pearls:

1. Dosage of ticarcillin plus clavulanate needs to be adjusted for patients with renal dysfunction.
2. The theoretical sodium content is 4.51 mEq (103.6 mg) per gram of ticarcillin plus clavulanate. This should be considered when one is treating patients who require restricted salt intake.
3. Treatment of *Pseudomonas* may be more successful with the addition of an aminoglycoside.

TIGECYCLINE (Tygacil)

BASIC CHARACTERISTICS

Class: Glycylcycline

Mechanism of Action: Inhibits protein translation in bacteria by binding to the 30S ribosomal subunit and blocking entry of amino-acyl tRNA molecules into the A site of the ribosome.

Mechanisms of Resistance: Tigecycline is not affected by the major tetracycline-resistance mechanism, ribosomal protection. Tigecycline resistance in some bacteria is associated with multidrug-resistant efflux pumps.

Metabolic Route: Tigecycline is excreted 60% in feces and the remainder in the urine.

FDA-APPROVED INDICATIONS

FDA-Approved Indications: Treatment of the following conditions caused by susceptible organisms: complicated skin and skin structure infections, complicated intraabdominal infections, and community-acquired bacterial pneumonia.

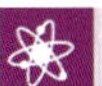

SIDE EFFECTS/TOXICITY

Contraindicated for use in patients who have known hypersensitivity to tigecycline.

Side effects/toxicities include anaphylaxis/anaphylactoid reactions, liver dysfunction and liver failure, fetal harm when administered to a pregnant woman, permanent discoloration of teeth (yellow-gray-brown) if administered during tooth development (last half of pregnancy, infancy, and childhood to the age of 8 years), nausea, vomiting, diarrhea, abdominal pain, *Clostridium difficile*–associated diarrhea, headache, hypocalcemia, hypoglycemia, hyponatremia, and thrombocytopenia.

Tigecycline is structurally similar to tetracycline-class antibiotics and may have similar adverse effects to those seen with tetracyclines, including photosensitivity, pseudotumor cerebri, pancreatitis, and antianabolic action (which has led to increased BUN, azotemia, acidosis, and hyperphosphatemia).

DRUG INTERACTIONS/FOOD INTERACTIONS

Prothrombin time should be monitored if tigecycline is administered with warfarin.

Concurrent use of antibacterial drugs with oral contraceptives may render oral contraceptives less effective.

DOSING

The recommended dosage regimen is an initial dose of 100 mg, followed by 50 mg every 12 hours.

 SPECIAL POPULATIONS

RENAL IMPAIRMENT: No dosage adjustment is necessary.

HEPATIC DYSFUNCTION: In patients with severe hepatic impairment (Child-Pugh class C), the initial dose of tigecycline should be 100 mg followed by a reduced maintenance dosage of 25 mg every 12 hours. Patients with severe hepatic impairment (Child-Pugh class C) should be treated with caution and monitored for treatment response.

PEDIATRIC PATIENTS: Safety and efficacy in patients aged younger than 18 years have not been established.

PREGNANCY: Category D.

BREASTFEEDING: Tigecycline should be used with caution in breastfeeding mothers.

 THE ART OF ANTIMICROBIAL THERAPY

Clinical Pearls:

1. Tigecycline can cause fetal harm when administered to a pregnant woman.
2. The use of drugs of the tetracycline class during tooth development (last half of pregnancy, infancy, and childhood to the age of 8 years) may cause permanent discoloration of the teeth (yellow-gray-brown).
3. Tigecycline is not active against *Pseudomonas* species.
4. Tigecycline is associated with poor outcomes in hospital-associated pneumonia.
5. Caution is urged in patients with known hypersensitivity to tetracyclines.

BASIC CHARACTERISTICS

Class: Nitroimidazole

Mechanism of Action: Data incomplete.

Metabolic Route: Tinidazole is mostly excreted unchanged in the urine.

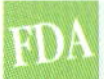

FDA-APPROVED INDICATIONS

FDA-Approved Indications: Treatment of trichomoniasis, giardiasis, intestinal amebiasis, amebic liver abscess, and bacterial vaginosis.

SIDE EFFECTS/TOXICITY

WARNING: Carcinogenicity has been seen in animals treated chronically with other nitroimidazole derivatives.

The use of tinidazole is **contraindicated** in patients with a previous history of hypersensitivity to tinidazole or other nitroimidazole derivatives, during the first trimester of pregnancy, and in breastfeeding mothers.

Side effects/toxicities include fever, hypersensitivity, angioedema, rash including Stevens-Johnson syndrome and erythema multiforme, seizures, coma, confusion, peripheral neuropathy, vertigo, ataxia, insomnia, depression, drowsiness, tongue discoloration, stomatitis, diarrhea, urticaria, pruritus, rash, flushing, sweating, dryness of mouth, thirst, salivation, darkened urine, palpitations, bronchospasm, *Candida* overgrowth, raised transaminase levels, arthralgias, arthritis, myalgias, neutropenia, leukopenia, and thrombocytopenia.

DRUG INTERACTIONS/FOOD INTERACTIONS

Tinidazole should be taken with food.

Do not administer tinidazole with alcoholic beverages, preparations containing ethanol or propylene glycol, disulfiram, fluorouracil, or cholestyramine.

Coadministered drugs may affect the level of tinidazole or of the coadministered drug, as follows; monitoring is recommended:

Coadministered Drug	*Effect*
Cimetidine	Increased levels of tinidazole
Cyclosporine	Increased effect of cyclosporine
Fosphenytoin	Decreased levels of tinidazole
Ketoconazole	Increased levels of tinidazole

Coadministered Drug	*Effect*
Lithium	Increased effect of lithium
Phenobarbitol	Decreased levels of tinidazole
Phenytoin	Decreased levels of tinidazole
Rifampin	Decreased levels of tinidazole
Tacrolimus	Increased effect of tacrolimus
Warfarin	Increased effect of warfarin

Tinidazole may interfere with determinations of serum chemistry values, such as AST, ALT, LDH, triglycerides, and hexokinase glucose.

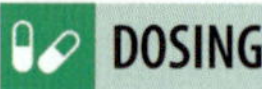

DOSING

Tinidazole is administered as 250-mg and 500-mg tablets.

Trichomoniasis: a single 2-g oral dose taken with food

Giardiasis: a single 2-g dose taken with food

Amebiasis:

- Intestinal: 2-g dose per day for 3 days taken with food
- Amebic liver abscess: 2-g dose per day for 3 to 5 days taken with food

Bacterial vaginosis: 2-g oral dose once daily for 2 days taken with food or a 1-g oral dose once daily for 5 days taken with food

SPECIAL POPULATIONS

RENAL IMPAIRMENT: If tinidazole is administered on the same day as and before hemodialysis, it is recommended that an additional dose of tinidazole equivalent to one half of the recommended dose be administered after the end of the hemodialysis.

HEPATIC DYSFUNCTION: Usual recommended doses of tinidazole should be administered cautiously in patients with hepatic dysfunction

PEDIATRIC PATIENTS:

Giardiasis: In pediatric patients aged older than 3 years, the recommended dosage is a single dose of 50 mg/kg (up to 2 g) with food.

Amebiasis:

- Intestinal: In pediatric patients aged older than 3 years, the recommended dosage is 50 mg/kg/day (up to 2 g per day) for 3 days with food.
- Amebic liver abscess: In pediatric patients aged older than 3 years, the recommended dosage is 50 mg/kg/day (up to 2 g per day) for 3 to 5 days with food. Children should be closely monitored when treatment durations exceed 3 days.

PREGNANCY: Category C; should not be used in the first trimester.

BREASTFEEDING: Interruption of breastfeeding is recommended during tinidazole therapy and for 3 days following the last dose.

THE ART OF ANTIMICROBIAL THERAPY

Clinical Pearls:

1. Ethanol should be avoided when taking tinidazole.
2. For those unable to swallow tablets, tinidazole tablets may be crushed in artificial cherry syrup to be taken with food.
3. Tinidazole should not be used in the first trimester of pregnancy.

TIPRANAVIR (Aptivus)

BASIC CHARACTERISTICS

Class: Protease inhibitor

Mechanism of Action: Reversibly binds the active site of the enzyme protease. Inhibition of protease prevents cleavage of the *gag* and *gag-pol* polyprotein resulting in the production of immature, noninfectious virus.

Mechanism of Resistance: Development of mutations on the enzyme protease causes a conformational change that prevents tipranavir from binding the active site, allowing protease activity to continue. There are more than 22 protease mutations identified for tipranavir, of which five are required to inhibit the activity of tipranavir.

Metabolic Route: Tipranavir is metabolized in the liver and excreted in the feces.

FDA FDA-APPROVED INDICATIONS

FDA-Approved Indications: Treatment of HIV-1 in combinations with other antiretroviral agents in patients who are treatment-experienced and infected with HIV-1 strains resistant to more than one protease inhibitor.

SIDE EFFECTS/TOXICITY

> **WARNING:** Clinical **hepatitis** and hepatic decompensation including some fatalities have been reported. Extra vigilance is warranted in patients with chronic hepatitis B or hepatitis C coinfection. Fatal and nonfatal **intracranial** hemorrhage have been reported.

Additional side effects/toxicities include new-onset diabetes mellitus; exacerbation of preexisting diabetes mellitus; hyperglycemia; increased bleeding, including spontaneous skin hematomas and hemarthrosis, in patients with hemophilia type A or B; redistribution/accumulation of body fat including central obesity, dorsocervical fat enlargement (buffalo hump), peripheral wasting, facial wasting, and breast enlargement; cushingoid appearance; immune reconstitution syndrome; hepatitis and hepatic decompensation; rash; elevations in total cholesterol and triglycerides; QTc prolongation; torsade de pointes; abdominal pain; diarrhea; headache; anorexia; dyspepsia; hepatitis; mouth ulceration; pancreatitis; vomiting; anemia; leukopenia; thrombocytopenia; increases in alkaline phosphatase, amylase, creatine phosphokinase, lactic dehydrogenase, SGOT, SGPT, and gamma glutamyl transpeptidase; hyperlipemia, hyperuricemia, hypoglycemia, and dehydration.

Tipranavir should be used with caution in patients who may be at risk of increased bleeding from trauma, surgery, or other medical conditions, or who are receiving medications known to increase the risk of bleeding such as antiplatelet agents and anticoagulants, or who are taking supplemental high doses of vitamin E.

DRUG INTERACTIONS/FOOD INTERACTIONS

Tipranavir can be taken with or without food.

Drugs that should not be coadministered with tipranavir include amiodarone, quinidine, flecainide, bepridil, propafenone, rifampin, ergot derivatives, Saint-John's-wort, HMG-CoA reductase inhibitors simvastatin or lovastatin, pimozide, proton pump inhibitors, cisapride, benzodiazepines, voriconazole, any protease inhibitor, or etravirine.

Tipranavir contains alcohol; therefore, disulfiram and metronidazole should be avoided.

Tipranavir is an inhibitor of the CYP3A enzyme; coadministration of tipranavir and drugs primarily metabolized by CYP3A may result in increased plasma concentrations of the other drug that could increase or prolong its therapeutic and adverse effects.

Tipranavir is metabolized by CYP3A; coadministration of tipranavir and drugs that induce CYP3A may decrease tipranavir plasma concentrations and reduce its therapeutic effect. Coadministration of tipranavir and drugs that inhibit CYP3A may increase tipranavir plasma concentrations. Because of these metabolic effects, potential drug interactions that may require dosage change or clinical/laboratory monitoring are listed below:

Medication	*Adjustment or Action*
Itraconazole	Do not exceed 200 mg/day of itraconazole
Ketoconazole	Do not exceed 200 mg/day of ketoconazole
Fluconazole	Do not exceed 200 mg/day of fluconazole
Clarithromycin	Decrease clarithromycin dose by 50% for patients with creatinine clearance 30 mL/min to 60 mL/min and reduce by 75% for patients with creatinine clearance < 30 mL/min
Rifabutin	Decrease rifabutin to 150 mg every other day or thrice weekly
Hormonal contraceptives	Use alternative or additional method
Atorvastatin or rosuvastatin	Use lowest possible dosage with close monitoring
Phenobarbital, phenytoin, or carbamazepine	Tipranavir may be less effective; monitor anticonvulsant level; consider alternative
Methadone	Monitor; may require higher methadone dosage
Sildenafil	No more than 25 mg every 48 hours
Tadalafil	5 mg, no more than 10 mg in 72 hours

Medication	*Adjustment or Action*
Vardenafil	No more than 2.5 mg in 72 hours
Antacids	Tipranavir should be given 2 hours before or 1 hour after
Didanosine	Tipranavir and didanosine should be separated by 2 hours
Valproic acid	Valproic acid may be less effective

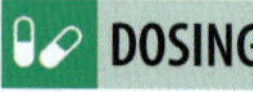 DOSING

Tipranavir is available in 250-mg tablets and a yellow, viscous clear liquid with a butter mint–butter toffee flavor that contains 100 mg/mL. The recommended adult dosage of tipranavir is 500 mg (two 250-mg capsules or 5 mL oral solution) coadministered with 200 mg of ritonavir, twice daily.

SPECIAL POPULATIONS

RENAL IMPAIRMENT: There is no dosage adjustment needed.

HEPATIC DYSFUNCTION: Tipranavir is contraindicated in patients with Child-Pugh class B or C hepatic impairment.

PEDIATRIC PATIENTS: The dosage of tipranavir is 14 mg/kg with 6 mg/kg ritonavir (or 375 mg/m^2 coadministered with ritonavir 150 mg/m^2) taken twice daily not to exceed a maximum dosage of tipranavir 500 mg coadministered with ritonavir 200 mg twice daily.

PREGNANCY: Category B.

BREASTFEEDING: It is recommended that HIV-positive mothers not breastfeed their children, to decrease mother-to-child transmission of HIV.

 THE ART OF ANTIMICROBIAL THERAPY

Clinical Pearls:

1. Tipranavir should always be used in combination with other antiretrovirals.
2. Tipranavir must be taken with ritonavir to achieve adequate systemic levels.
3. Even though tipranavir can be taken with or without food, it is likely that food may decrease gastrointestinal side effects.
4. Tipranavir has a sulfa moiety; use caution in patients with sulfa allergy.

5. Be cautious when using tipranavir in patients on medications that affect platelet function.
6. When one is assessing for resistance to tipranavir, a phenotype assay may be helpful.
7. Whenever initiating tipranavir, one should review all medications the patient is receiving to minimize drug interactions.
8. Tipranavir should be used with caution in patients with propensity for bleeding because of the risk of intracranial hemorrhage.

 BASIC CHARACTERISTICS

Class: Aminoglycoside

Mechanisms of Action:

1. Rearranges lipopolysaccharide in the outer membrane of the bacterial cell wall, resulting in disruption of the cell wall, and
2. binds the 30S subunit of the bacterial ribosome, which terminates protein synthesis.

Mechanisms of Resistance:

1. Gram-negative bacteria inactivate aminoglycosides by acetylation,
2. some bacteria alter the 30S ribosomal subunit, which prevents tobramycin's interference with protein synthesis, and
3. low-level resistance may result from inhibition of tobramycin uptake by the bacteria.

Metabolic Route: Tobramycin is excreted unchanged in the urine.

FDA FDA-APPROVED INDICATIONS

FDA-Approved Indications: Treatment of susceptible gram-negative bacteria causing bacteremia, pneumonia, osteomyelitis, arthritis, meningitis, skin and skin structure infection, intraabdominal infections, in burns and postoperative infections, and urinary tract infections.

Also Used for: Combination therapy with β-lactams for the treatment of gram-positive endovascular infections.

 SIDE EFFECTS/TOXICITY

WARNINGS: Ototoxicity: vestibular toxicity and auditory ototoxicity, especially in patients with renal damage, those treated with higher doses, and those with prolonged treatment. Avoid use with potent diuretics such as ethacrynic acid because of additive ototoxicity.

Nephrotoxicity: especially in patients with impaired renal function and those treated with higher doses or prolonged treatment. Avoid concurrent use with other nephrotoxic agents and potent diuretics, which can cause dehydration.

Neuromuscular blockade: especially in those receiving anesthetics, neuromuscular blocking agents, or massive transfusions.

Other side effects/toxicities include anemia, granulocytopenia, and thrombocytopenia; fever; rash; nausea; vomiting; diarrhea; confusion; abnormal liver function tests;

decreased serum calcium, magnesium, sodium, and potassium; leukopenia; and leukocytosis.

DRUG INTERACTIONS

Tobramycin should not be administered with other medications that are nephrotoxic or ototoxic.

DOSING

After a loading dose of 2 mg/kg, give 3 mg/kg/day to 5 mg/kg/day IM or IV divided every 8 hours; desired serum levels are peak 6 µg/mL to 12 µg/mL and trough less than 2 µg/mL. Can also be given once daily as 5 mg/kg to 7 mg/kg every 24 hours; desired serum levels are peak 16 µg/mL to 24 µg/mL, trough less than 1 µg/mL. Infuse over 60 minutes to avoid neuromuscular blockade.

Intrathecal dose: 4 mg to 8 mg per day.

SPECIAL POPULATIONS

RENAL IMPAIRMENT: Adjust dosage either by increased interval (serum creatinine multiplied by 8, or usual dose every 12 to 24 hours for creatinine clearance 10-50 and every 48 hours for CrCl 10 or less), or by lowering the dose by dividing the dose by the serum creatinine. With either approach, give an initial dose as for normal renal function, and then subsequent adjustments should be made by following serum assays. (See Dosing above for desired levels.)

- **Hemodialysis:** One-half of normal renal function dose after hemodialysis; follow serum assays.
- **Peritoneal dialysis**: 3-4 mg/L are removed in dialysate daily and should be replaced.
- **Continuous renal replacement therapy**: 3 mg/kg loading dose followed by 2 mg/kg every 24 to 48 hours

HEPATIC DYSFUNCTION: No dosage adjustment necessary.

PEDIATRIC PATIENTS: For patients older than 4 weeks: 3 mg/kg/day to 6 mg/kg/day; divide IV every 8 hours (newborn aged 0 to 7 days: < 4 mg/kg/day every 12 hours; newborn aged 1 to 4 weeks: 3 mg/kg/day to 5 mg/kg/day every 8 hours)

PREGNANCY: Category D.

BREASTFEEDING: It is not known if tobramycin is secreted in human milk.

THE ART OF ANTIMICROBIAL THERAPY

Clinical Pearls:

1. Aminoglycosides require oxygen to be active and, thus, are less effective in anaerobic environments such as an abscess or infected bone.
2. Aminoglycosides have decreased activity in low-pH environments such as respiratory secretions or abscesses.
3. When dosing aminoglycosides, use the ideal body weight, not true body weight.
4. Tobramycin has a postantibiotic effect that allows it to be used once daily.

TRIMETHOPRIM (Proloprim)

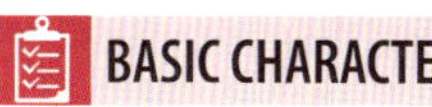

BASIC CHARACTERISTICS

Class: Antimetabolite

Mechanism of Action: Blocks the production of tetrahydrofolic acid from dihydrofolic acid by binding to and reversibly inhibiting the required enzyme, dihydrofolate reductase.

Mechanisms of Resistance: Plasmid-mediated alterations in dihydrofolate reductase and changes in cell permeability.

Metabolic Route: From 10% to 20% of trimethoprim is metabolized in the liver; the remainder is excreted unchanged in the urine.

FDA-APPROVED INDICATIONS

FDA-Approved Indications: Treatment of uncomplicated urinary tract infections caused by susceptible organisms.

Also Used for: Trimethoprim can be combined with dapsone for the treatment of *Pneumocystis jiroveci* pneumonia.

SIDE EFFECTS/TOXICITY

Contraindicated in individuals who are hypersensitive to trimethoprim and in those with documented megaloblastic anemia attributable to folate deficiency.

Side effects/toxicities include serious hypersensitivity reactions with anaphylaxis, exfoliative dermatitis, erythema multiforme, Stevens-Johnson syndrome, toxic epidermal necrolysis (Lyell syndrome), pruritus, phototoxicity, epigastric distress, nausea, vomiting, glossitis, aseptic meningitis, thrombocytopenia, leukopenia, neutropenia, megaloblastic anemia, methemoglobinemia, hyperkalemia, hyponatremia, and increases in BUN, serum creatinine, serum transaminase, and bilirubin.

DRUG INTERACTIONS/FOOD INTERACTIONS

Trimethoprim can be administered with or without food.

Trimethoprim increases phenytoin half-life.

Trimethoprim can interfere with a serum methotrexate assay and with the Jaffé alkaline picrate reaction assay for creatinine, resulting in overestimations of about 10% in the range of normal values.

DOSING

Trimethoprim is administered in 100-mg and 200-mg tablets.

The usual dosage is 100 mg every 12 hours or 200 mg every 24 hours, each for 10 days.

 SPECIAL POPULATIONS

RENAL IMPAIRMENT:

CrCl Measurement or Hemodialysis	*Dosage*
10 mL/min to 50 mL/min	Usual dosage every 18 hours
< 10 mL/min	Usual dosage every 24 hours
Hemodialysis	Usual dosage after dialysis only
Chronic ambulatory peritoneal dialysis	Usual dosage every 24 hours
Continuous renal replacement therapy	No data

Note: CrCl = Creatinine Clearance.

HEPATIC DYSFUNCTION: Use with caution.

PEDIATRIC PATIENTS: Safety and effectiveness in patients aged younger than 2 months have not been established. The effectiveness of trimethoprim as a single agent has not been established in patients aged younger than 12 years.

PREGNANCY: Category C.

BREAST FEEDING: Trimethoprim should be used only with caution in breastfeeding mothers.

 THE ART OF ANTIMICROBIAL THERAPY

Clinical Pearls:

1. Complete blood counts should be monitored and the drug should be discontinued if a significant reduction in the count of any formed blood element is found.
2. Trimethoprim should not be given to patients with documented megaloblastic anemia caused by folate deficiency.
3. It may be beneficial to measure levels of concomitantly administered phenytoin.

TRIMETHOPRIM PLUS SULFAMETHOXAZOLE (Bactrim, Bactrim DS, Septra, Septra DS)

BASIC CHARACTERISTICS

Class: Antimetabolite plus sulfonamide

Mechanism of Action: Sulfamethoxazole inhibits bacterial synthesis of dihydrofolic acid by competing with para-aminobenzoic acid. Trimethoprim blocks the production of tetrahydrofolic acid from dihydrofolic acid by binding to and reversibly inhibiting the required enzyme, dihydrofolate reductase.

Mechanisms of Resistance:

1. Plasmid-mediated alterations in dihydrofolate reductase and changes in cell permeability,
2. overproduction of para-aminobenzoic acid, and
3. structural change in dihydropteroate synthesis.

Metabolic Route: Both trimethoprim and sulfamethoxazole are excreted in the urine.

FDA FDA-APPROVED INDICATIONS

FDA-Approved Indications: Treatment of urinary tract infections, acute otitis media, acute exacerbations of chronic bronchitis in adults, shigellosis, *Pneumocystis jiroveci* pneumonia (treatment and prophylaxis), and travelers' diarrhea in adults.

Also Used for: Infections caused by *Listeria, Nocardia, Salmonella, Brucella, Paracoccidioides*, melioidosis, *Burkholderia, Stenotrophomonas, Cyclospora, Isospora;* Whipple's disease; an alternative therapy for toxoplasmosis; and community-acquired methicillin-resistant *Staphylococcus aureus* skin infections.

SIDE EFFECTS/TOXICITY

Contraindicated in patients with a known hypersensitivity to trimethoprim or sulfonamides, patients with a history of drug-induced immune thrombocytopenia with use of trimethoprim and/or sulfonamides, patients with documented megaloblastic anemia caused by folate deficiency, pregnant patients, breastfeeding mothers, pediatric patients aged less than 2 months, and patients with marked hepatic damage or with severe renal insufficiency when renal function status cannot be monitored.

Side effects/toxicities include Stevens-Johnson syndrome, toxic epidermal necrolysis, fulminant hepatic necrosis, stomatitis, glossitis, nausea, emesis, abdominal pain, pancreatitis, diarrhea, *Clostridium difficile*–associated diarrhea, anorexia, hepatitis, renal failure, interstitial nephritis, aseptic meningitis, convulsions, peripheral neuritis, ataxia, vertigo, tinnitus, headache, hallucinations, depression, apathy, nervousness, weakness, fatigue, insomnia, rhabdomyolysis, lung hypersensitivity reactions, diuresis, periarteritis, lupus, arthralgia, myalgias, hypoglycemia, hypoprothrombinemia, methemoglobinemia, eosinophilia, hypoglycemia, hyperkalemia, crystalluria, megaloblastic anemia, thrombocytopenia, agranulocytosis, aplastic anemia, and other blood dyscrasias.

DRUG INTERACTIONS/FOOD INTERACTIONS

Trimethoprim plus sulfamethoxazole can be given with or without food.

Reported interactions include thrombocytopenia with thiazides; increased effect of phenytoin, methotrexate, digoxin, oral hypoglycemics, and warfarin; increased sulfamethoxazole levels with indomethacin; decreased efficacy of tricyclic antidepressants; and hyperkalemia with ACE inhibitors.

DOSING

Trimethoprim plus sulfamethoxazole is in a fixed-dose ratio of 1:5.

Bactrim and Septra contain 400 mg sulfamethoxazole and 80 mg trimethoprim.

Bactrim DS and Septra DS (double-strength) contain 800 mg sulfamethoxazole and 160 mg trimethoprim.

Oral suspension contains 200 mg sulfamethoxazole and 40 mg trimethoprim per teaspoon.

Intravenous formulation contains 400 mg sulfamethoxazole and 80 mg trimethoprim per 5 mL.

Urinary tract infections, shigellosis, acute exacerbations of chronic bronchitis: The usual adult dosage in the treatment of urinary tract infections is one DS tablet, two single-strength tablets, four teaspoonfuls (20 mL), or 10 mL IV every 12 hours for 10 to 14 days.

***Pneumocystis jiroveci* pneumonia:**

- **Treatment:** 75 mg/kg to 100 mg/kg sulfamethoxazole and 15 mg/kg to 20 mg/kg trimethoprim per 24 hours given in equally divided doses every 6 hours for 14 to 21 days. Thus, a patient weighing 64 kg would take four single-strength tablets, two DS tablets, or 20 mL IV every 6 hours.
- **Prophylaxis:** The recommended dosage for prophylaxis in adults is one DS or single-strength tablet daily. Alternatively, one DS tablet every Monday, Wednesday, and Friday.
- **Travelers' diarrhea:** The usual adult dosage is one DS tablet, two single-strength tablets, or four teaspoonfuls (20 mL) every 12 hours for 5 days.

SPECIAL POPULATIONS

RENAL IMPAIRMENT:

Creatinine clearance 15 mL/min to 30 mL/min: use half the usual dose.

Creatinine clearance less than 15 mL/min, hemodialysis, chronic ambulatory peritoneal dialysis, and continuous renal replacement therapy: use not recommended.

HEPATIC DYSFUNCTION: No dosage adjustment is necessary.

PEDIATRIC PATIENTS: Trimethoprim plus sulfamethoxazole is not recommended for infants aged younger than 2 months.

Urinary tract infections or acute otitis media: 40 mg/kg sulfamethoxazole and 8 mg/kg trimethoprim per 24 hours, given in two divided doses every 12 hours for 10 days. An identical daily dosage is used for 5 days in the treatment of shigellosis.

***Pneumocystis jirovecii* pneumonia:**

- **Treatment:** 75 mg/kg to 100 mg/kg sulfamethoxazole and 15 mg/kg to 20 mg/kg trimethoprim per 24 hours given in equally divided doses every 6 hours for 14 to 21 days.
- **Prophylaxis:** 750 mg/m^2/day sulfamethoxazole with 150 mg/m^2/day trimethoprim given orally in equally divided doses twice a day, on three consecutive days per week. The total daily dose should not exceed 1600 mg sulfamethoxazole and 320 mg trimethoprim.

PREGNANCY: Category C.

BREASTFEEDING: Do not administer to breastfeeding mothers.

THE ART OF ANTIMICROBIAL THERAPY

Clinical Pearls:

1. Because sulfamethoxazole and trimethoprim may interfere with folic acid metabolism, it should be used during pregnancy only if the potential benefit justifies the potential risk to the fetus.
2. The sulfonamides should not be used for treatment of group A β-hemolytic streptococcal infections.
3. Although it is not an FDA-approved indication, the usual dosage of trimethoprim plus sulfamethoxazole for systemic infections caused by typical bacteria is 10 mg/kg/day of trimethoprim and 50 mg/kg/day of sulfamethoxazole.
4. Clinical signs such as rash, sore throat, fever, arthralgia, pallor, purpura, or jaundice may be early indications of serious reactions.
5. Patients taking trimethoprim plus sulfamethoxazole should drink adequate amounts of water to decrease the likelihood of crystalluria and stone formation.

TRIMETREXATE GLUCURONATE (Neutrexin)

BASIC CHARACTERISTICS

Class: Folate antagonist

Mechanism of Action: Synthetic inhibitor of the enzyme dihydrofolate reductase.

Metabolic Route: Trimetrexate glucuronate is metabolized into multiple products in the liver and excreted in the urine.

FDA-APPROVED INDICATIONS

FDA-Approved Indications: Along with concurrent leucovorin, indicated as an alternative therapy for the treatment of moderate-to-severe *Pneumocystis jiroveci* pneumonia (PCP) in immunocompromised patients, including patients with AIDS who are intolerant of, or are refractory to, trimethoprim plus sulfamethoxazole therapy or for whom trimethoprim plus sulfamethoxazole is contraindicated.

SIDE EFFECTS/TOXICITY

> **WARNING:** Trimetrexate glucuronate for injection **must be used with concurrent leucovorin** to avoid potentially serious or life-threatening toxicities.

Contraindicated in patients with clinically significant sensitivity to trimetrexate, leucovorin, or methotrexate.

Frequent side effects/toxicities: renal impairment, myelosuppression, stomatitis, mild elevations in transaminases and alkaline phosphatase, seizures, and hypersensitivity/allergic–type reactions including hypotension.

DRUG INTERACTIONS/FOOD INTERACTIONS

Because trimetrexate is metabolized by the P450 enzyme system, drugs that induce or inhibit this drug-metabolizing enzyme system may elicit important drug–drug interactions that may alter trimetrexate plasma concentrations; this would include drugs that could increase levels of trimetrexate, such as erythromycin, ketoconazole, and fluconazole, and drugs that could decrease levels of trimetrexate, such as rifampin and rifabutin.

Patients who require concomitant therapy with nephrotoxic, myelosuppressive, or hepatotoxic drugs should be treated with trimetrexate at the discretion of the physician and monitored carefully.

Treatment with zidovudine should be discontinued during trimetrexate therapy.

DOSING

Trimetrexate glucuronate is administered at a dosage of 45 mg/m^2 once daily by intravenous infusion over 60 minutes. Leucovorin must be administered daily during treatment and for 72 hours after the last dose. Leucovorin may be administered intravenously at a dose of 20 mg/m^2 over 5 to 10 minutes every 6 hours for a total daily dose of 80 mg/m^2, or orally as four doses of 20 mg/m^2 spaced equally throughout the day. The oral dosage should be rounded up to the next-higher 25-mg increment. The recommended course of therapy is 21 days of trimetrexate and 24 days of leucovorin.

Trimetrexate and leucovorin may alternatively be dosed by weight, as follows:

Body Weight	*Trimetrexate Dosage*	*Leucovorin Dosage*
<50 kg	1.5 mg/kg/day	0.6 mg/kg four times a day
50 kg to 80 kg	1.2 mg/kg/day	0.5 mg/kg four times a day
> 80 kg	1.0 mg/kg/day	0.5 mg/kg four times a day

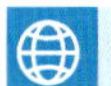

SPECIAL POPULATIONS

RENAL IMPAIRMENT: There is no dosage adjustment for renal impairment. However, interruption of therapy is advisable if serum creatinine levels increase to more than 2.5 mg/dL and the elevation is attributed to the trimetrexate.

HEPATIC DYSFUNCTION: There is no dosage adjustment for hepatic dysfunction. However, interruption of treatment is advisable if transaminase levels or alkaline phosphatase levels increase to more than five times the upper limit of normal range while on trimetrexate.

HEMATOLOGIC TOXICITY: DOSAGE ADJUSTMENTS

Toxicity Grade	*Neutrophils (Polys and Bands)*	*Platelets*	*Trimetrexate Dosage*	*Leucovorin Dosage*
1	> 1000/mm^3	> 75,000/mm^3	45 mg/m^2 once daily	20 mg/m^2 every 6 hours
2	750 to 1000/mm^3	50,000 to 75,000/mm^3	45 mg/m^2 once daily	40 mg/m^2 every 6 hours
3	500 to 749/mm^3	25,000-49,999/mm^3	22 mg/m^2 once daily	40 mg/m^2 every 6 hours
4	< 500/mm^3	< 25,000/mm^3	Days 1 through 9: discontinue Days 10 through 21: interrupt up to 96 hours	40 mg/m^2 every 6 hours

PEDIATRIC PATIENTS: The safety and effectiveness of trimetrexate for the treatment of PCP has not been established for patients aged younger than 18 years.

PREGNANCY: Category D.

BREASTFEEDING: It is recommended that breastfeeding be discontinued if the mother is treated with trimetrexate.

THE ART OF ANTIMICROBIAL THERAPY

Clinical Pearls:

1. Trimetrexate must be given with leucovorin.
2. Leucovorin should be continued for 72 hours after the trimetrexate.

VALACYCLOVIR HYDROCHLORIDE (Valtrex)

BASIC CHARACTERISTICS

Class: Nucleoside analogue

Mechanism of Action: Valacyclovir is the valine ester of the nucleoside analogue acyclovir. After hydrolysis, it is phosphorylated by thymidine kinase to the active triphosphate form. Acyclovir triphosphate stops replication of herpes viral DNA in three ways: (1) competitive inhibition of viral DNA polymerase, (2) incorporation into and termination of the growing viral DNA chain, and (3) inactivation of the viral DNA polymerase. The greater antiviral activity of acyclovir against herpes simplex virus (HSV) compared to varicella zoster virus (VZV) is because of its more efficient phosphorylation by the viral thymidine kinase.

Mechanism of Resistance: Resistance of HSV and VZV to valacyclovir can result from qualitative or quantitative changes in the viral thymidine kinase or DNA polymerase.

Metabolic Route: After oral administration, valacyclovir hydrochloride is rapidly absorbed from the gastrointestinal tract and nearly completely converted to acyclovir and *L*-valine by first-pass intestinal and/or hepatic metabolism. The acyclovir is metabolized to 9-[(carboxymethoxy)methyl]guanine and is excreted in the urine.

FDA FDA-APPROVED INDICATIONS

FDA-Approved Indications:

Valacyclovir is indicated for the treatment of herpes zoster, the treatment or suppression of genital herpes in immunocompetent individuals, suppression of recurrent genital herpes in HIV-infected individuals, and the treatment of cold sores (herpes labialis).

SIDE EFFECTS/TOXICITY

Thrombotic thrombocytopenic purpura/hemolytic uremic syndrome (TTP/HUS), has occurred in patients with advanced HIV disease and also in allogeneic bone marrow transplant and renal transplant recipients at doses of 8 g per day.

Nausea, vomiting, and diarrhea were the most common side effects in those receiving oral valacyclovir. Central nervous system side effects including confusion, ataxia, altered behavior, seizure, and coma have been seen, particularly in older adults or in patients with renal impairment. Precipitation of acyclovir in renal tubules may occur when the solubility (2.5 mg/mL) is exceeded in the intratubular fluid. This has resulted in elevated BUN and serum creatinine and subsequent renal failure. Excessive doses of valacyclovir have been associated with acute renal failure in patients with underlying renal disease.

Other reported side effects/toxicities include anaphylaxis, angioedema, fever, headache, peripheral edema, diarrhea, anemia, leukopenia, thrombocytopenia, hepatitis, rash including toxic epidermal necrolysis and Stevens-Johnson syndrome, and visual disturbances.

DRUG INTERACTIONS/FOOD INTERACTIONS

Valacyclovir can be administered orally with or without food.

There are no known drug interactions.

DOSING

Valacyclovir is dispensed in 500-mg tablets.

Herpes zoster: 1 g three times daily for 7 days

Initial treatment of genital herpetic ulcers: 1 g twice daily for 10 days

Recurrent episodes of genital herpetic ulcers: 500 mg twice daily for 3 days

Suppressive genital herpes therapy: 1 g once daily

Suppressive genital herpes therapy in patients with HIV: 500 mg twice daily

Reduction of herpes transmission: 500 mg once daily

Cold sores (herpes labialis): 2 g twice daily for 1 day

SPECIAL POPULATIONS

RENAL IMPAIRMENT:

Indication	*CrCl 30 mL/min to 49 mL/min*	*CrCl 10 mL/min to 29 mL/min*	*CrCl < 10 mL/min and Hemodialysis*
Herpes zoster	1 g every 12 hours	1 g every 24 hours	500 mg every 24 hours
Initial genital herpes	1 g every 12 hours	1 g every 24 hours	500 mg every 24 hours
Recurrent genital herpes	500 mg every 12 hours	500 mg every 24 hours	500 mg every 24 hours
Suppression of genital herpes	1 g every 24 hours	500 mg every 24 hours	500 mg every 24 hours
Suppression of genital herpes in HIV	500 mg every 12 hours	500 mg every 24 hours	500 mg every 24 hours
Herpes labialis	Two 1-g doses 12 hours apart	Two 500-mg doses 12 hours apart	500 mg one-time dose

Note: CrCl = Creatinine Clearance.

Peritoneal dialysis: Supplemental dosage is not required following peritoneal dialysis.

Continuous renal replacement therapy (CRRT): Dosage as for CrCl 30 mL/min to 49 mL/min in table; supplemental dosage following CRRT not required.

HEPATIC DYSFUNCTION: No dosage adjustment is needed.

PEDIATRICS: Valacyclovir has not been studied in pediatric patients. Use acyclovir.

PREGNANCY: Category B.

BREASTFEEDING: Valacyclovir may be administered with caution to breastfeeding mothers.

THE ART OF ANTIMICROBIAL THERAPY

Clinical Pearls:

1. Valacyclovir is effective against HSV and VZV. It has no activity against the other herpesviruses.
2. Valacyclovir is not recommended for children; acyclovir is recommended in this age group.
3. Valacyclovir can cause confusion or renal insufficiency, especially in the elderly.
4. Valacyclovir doses of 8 g a day have been associated with TTP/HUS in patients with AIDS and in transplant recipients.

▪ VALGANCICLOVIR (Valcyte)

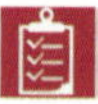

BASIC CHARACTERISTICS

Class: Nucleoside analogue

Mechanism of Action: Valganciclovir is a valyl ester of ganciclovir. After oral administration, valganciclovir is converted to ganciclovir, which is a synthetic guanine nucleoside analogue of 2′-deoxyguanosine that inhibits replication of herpesviruses. Ganciclovir is active against cytomegalovirus (CMV) and herpes simplex virus (HSV). Ganciclovir is phosphorylated and it inhibits viral DNA synthesis by (1) competitive inhibition of viral DNA polymerases, and (2) incorporation into viral DNA, resulting in eventual termination of viral DNA elongation.

Mechanism of Resistance: Resistance to ganciclovir in CMV is the decreased ability to form the active triphosphate moiety; resistant viruses have been described that contain mutations in the UL97 gene of CMV that controls phosphorylation of ganciclovir. Mutations in the viral DNA polymerase have also been reported to confer viral resistance to ganciclovir.

Metabolic Route: After oral administration, valganciclovir is converted to ganciclovir by intestinal and hepatic esterases. Ganciclovir is excreted in the urine.

FDA-APPROVED INDICATIONS

FDA-Approved Indications: Treatment of CMV retinitis in patients with AIDS. Also indicated for the prevention of CMV disease in kidney, heart, and kidney-pancreas transplant patients at high risk (donor CMV-seropositive/recipient CMV-seronegative).

Not indicated for use in patients with liver transplant.

SIDE EFFECTS/TOXICITY

WARNING: Granulocytopenia, anemia, and thrombocytopenia have been observed in patients treated with valganciclovir. Therefore, it should be used with caution in patients with preexisting cytopenias and should not be administered if the absolute neutrophil count is less than 500 cells/μL, the platelet count is less than 25,000/μL, or the hemoglobin is less than 8 g/dL. Granulocytopenia usually occurs during the first or second week of treatment but may occur at any time during treatment. Cell counts usually begin to recover within 3 to 7 days of discontinuing drug. Colony-stimulating factors have been shown to increase neutrophil and white blood cell counts in patients receiving valganciclovir.

Also, in animal studies ganciclovir (to which valganciclovir is metabolized) was carcinogenic, teratogenic, and caused aspermatogenesis.

Other side effects/toxicities include hepatic dysfunction, elevated creatinine, stomatitis, seizures, tinnitus, intestinal perforation, pancreatitis, pulmonary fibrosis, torsade de pointes, fever, diarrhea, vomiting, neuropathy, seizures, sweating, and pruritus.

DRUG INTERACTIONS/FOOD INTERACTIONS

Valganciclovir should be administered with food.

Both zidovudine and valganciclovir have the potential to cause neutropenia and anemia; some patients may not tolerate concomitant therapy with these drugs at full dosage. Generalized seizures have been reported in patients who received ganciclovir and imipenem plus cilastatin. These drugs should not be used concomitantly unless the potential benefits outweigh the risks.

Because of the possibility of additive toxicity, drugs such as dapsone, pentamidine, flucytosine, vincristine, vinblastine, adriamycin, amphotericin B, trimethoprim plus sulfamethoxazole combinations, or other nucleoside analogues, should be considered for concomitant use with valganciclovir only if the potential benefits are judged to outweigh the risks.

Increases in serum creatinine have been observed in patients treated with valganciclovir plus either cyclosporine or amphotericin B, drugs with known potential for nephrotoxicity.

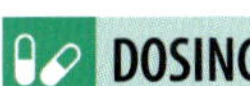

DOSING

Valganciclovir is administered in 450-mg tablets.

For treatment of CMV retinitis in patients with normal renal function:

- **Induction:** For patients with active CMV retinitis, the recommended dosage is 900 mg (two 450-mg tablets) twice a day for 21 days with food.
- **Maintenance:** Following induction treatment, or in patients with inactive CMV retinitis, the recommended dosage is 900 mg (two 450-mg tablets) once daily with food.

For the prevention of CMV disease in heart, kidney, and kidney-pancreas transplantation: The recommended dosage is 900 mg (two 450-mg tablets) once daily with food starting within 10 days of transplantation until 100 days posttransplantation.

SPECIAL POPULATIONS

RENAL IMPAIRMENT:

CrCl Measurement or Hemodialysis	*Induction Dosage*	*Maintenance Dosage*
≥60 mL/min	900 mg every 12 hours	900 mg daily

VALGANCICLOVIR (Valcyte)

CrCl Measurement or Hemodialysis	*Induction Dosage mg/kg*	*Maintenance Dosage mg/kg*
40 mL/min to 59 mL/min	450 mg every 12 hours	450 mg daily
25 mL/min to 39 mL/min	450 mg daily	450 mg every 2 days
10 mL/min to 24 mL/min	450 mg every 2 days	450 mg twice weekly
Hemodialysis	Do not administer	

Note: CrCl = Creatinine Clearance.

HEPATIC DYSFUNCTION: No dosage adjustment is needed.

PEDIATRIC PATIENTS: Valganciclovir has not been studied in pediatric patients.

PREGNANCY: Category C.

BREASTFEEDING: Mothers should be told to stop breastfeeding while receiving valganciclovir.

THE ART OF ANTIMICROBIAL THERAPY

Clinical Pearls:

1. Valganciclovir should not be administered if the absolute neutrophil count is less than 500 cells/μL or the platelet count is less than 25,000 cells/μL.
2. Valganciclovir is active against HSV, varicella zoster virus, and CMV. It may also have activity against Epstein-Barr virus and human herpesvirus 8, although its FDA-approved indications are for specific CMV infections, as detailed previously.
3. Valganciclovir is reliably absorbed and should be used instead of oral ganciclovir.

Note: For oral vancomycin, please see chapter on vancomycin-PO.

BASIC CHARACTERISTICS

Class: Glycopeptide

Mechanism of Action: Vancomycin inhibits synthesis and assembly of the cell wall peptidoglycan polymers by complexing with their D-alanyl-D-alanine precursor, preventing its binding to the peptidoglycan terminus. Vancomycin may impair RNA synthesis and injure protoplasts by altering the permeability of their cytoplasmic membrane.

Mechanisms of Resistance: The main mechanisms of resistance are carried by gene complexes (VanA, VanB, and VanC) mainly found in vancomycin-resistant enterococci (VRE) and have also been found in staphylococci, including vancomycin-resistant *Staphylococcus aureus* (VRSA):

1. VanA is plasmid-mediated. It is the most common type and results in the synthesis of peptidoglycan cell wall precursors containing a pentapeptide ending with D-alanine-D-lactate,
2. VanB is encoded on a transposon and leads to resistance, and
3. VanC is chromosomally encoded and leads to low-level resistance to vancomycin.

Intermediate resistance in staphylococci results when there is an abnormally thickened cell wall.

Metabolic Route: Vancomycin is excreted in the urine.

FDA-APPROVED INDICATIONS

FDA-Approved Indications: Treatment of serious or severe infections caused by susceptible strains of methicillin-resistant staphylococci in patients who cannot receive or who have failed to respond to other drugs (including penicillins or cephalosporins) and for infections caused by vancomycin-susceptible organisms that are resistant to other antimicrobial drugs. It is indicated for initial therapy when methicillin-resistant staphylococci are suspected, but after susceptibility data are available, therapy should be adjusted accordingly.

Also Used for: Treatment of staphylococcal endocarditis and other staphylococcal infections, including septicemia, osteomyelitis, pneumonia, and skin and skin structure infections. In addition, it is used for the treatment of enterococcal (in combination with aminoglycosides), streptococcal, and diphtheroid endocarditis. In combination with rifampin, an aminoglycoside, or both, vancomycin has been used in early-onset prosthetic valve endocarditis caused by *Staphylococcus epidermidis* or diphtheroids. Vancomycin has also been used for prophylaxis against bacterial endocarditis in penicillin-allergic patients.

VANCOMYCIN (intravenous only)

 SIDE EFFECTS/TOXICITY

Side effects/toxicities include pseudomembranous colitis, infusion-related toxicity (including anaphylactoid reactions, hypotension, wheezing, dyspnea, urticaria, or pruritus); rapid infusion may also cause flushing of the upper body (red-man syndrome) or pain and muscle spasm of the chest and back. Also seen are anaphylaxis, drug fever, chills, rash (including exfoliative dermatitis, linear IgA bullous dermatosis, Stevens-Johnson syndrome, toxic epidermal necrolysis, and vasculitis), **nephrotoxicity, ototoxicity** (including hearing loss, vertigo, dizziness, and tinnitus), neutropenia, and thrombocytopenia.

 DRUG INTERACTIONS/FOOD INTERACTIONS

Concomitant administration of vancomycin and anesthetic agents has been associated with erythema and histaminelike flushing and anaphylactoid reactions.

Concurrent and/or sequential systemic or topical use of other potentially neurotoxic and/or nephrotoxic drugs, such as amphotericin B, aminoglycosides, bacitracin, polymyxin B, colistin, viomycin, or cisplatin, when indicated, requires careful monitoring.

 DOSING

The usual daily intravenous dose is 2 g divided either as 500 mg every 6 hours or 1 g every 12 hours. Each dose should be administered at no more than 10 mg/min, or over a period of at least 60 minutes, whichever is longer.

 SPECIAL POPULATIONS

RENAL IMPAIRMENT: Dosage adjustment must be made in patients with impaired renal function.

CrCl Measurement or Hemodialysis	*Dosage*
50 mL/min to 80 mL/min	500 mg every 12 hours
10 mL/min to 49 mL/min	500 mg every 24 hours
0 mL/min to 9 mL/min	1 g weekly
Hemodialysis	1 g weekly
Chronic ambulatory peritoneal dialysis	1 g weekly
Continuous renal replacement therapy	1 g every 24 hours
Intrathecal dose	5 mg to 10 mg every 48 to 72 hours

Note: CrCl = Creatinine Clearance.

HEPATIC DYSFUNCTION: No dosage adjustment is necessary.

PEDIATRIC PATIENTS: The usual intravenous dosage of vancomycin is 10 mg/kg per dose given every 6 hours.

Infants and neonates: An initial dose of 15 mg/kg, followed by 10 mg/kg every 12 hours for the first week of life and every 8 hours thereafter up to the age of 1 month.

PREGNANCY: Category C.

BREASTFEEDING: Caution should be used.

THE ART OF ANTIMICROBIAL THERAPY

Clinical Pearls:

1. Red-man syndrome is not a true allergy; if a patient develops red-man syndrome, slowing the infusion, diluting the vancomycin, and administration of diphenhydramine may be of benefit.
2. Conventional dosage of vancomycin is 1 g every 12 hours; more recently, the dosage of 15 mg/kg every 12 hours has been suggested.
3. Although the cut-off for vancomycin susceptibility is 4 μg/mL, most experts believe that a minimum inhibitory concentration (MIC) of 2 μg/mL or greater is associated with failures of vancomycin.
4. Tolerance to vancomycin has been reported during the use of vancomycin (continued growth of *S. aureus* despite MICs suggesting it is still susceptible).
5. Vancomycin trough should be measured after four doses and 1 hour before the fifth dose. The recommended trough is 5 μg/mL to 12 μg/mL.
6. In patients with renal insufficiency, troughs should be monitored.
7. In patients on hemodialysis or peritoneal dialysis, levels of vancomycin should guide dosing, because patients metabolize vancomycin at different rates.

Note: For intravenous Vancomycin, please see chapter on Vancomycin (intravenous only)

BASIC CHARACTERISTICS

Class: Glycopeptide

Mechanism of Action: Inhibits synthesis and assembly of the cell wall peptidoglycan polymers by complexing with their D-alanyl-D-alanine precursor, preventing its binding to the peptidoglycan terminus. Vancomycin may impair RNA synthesis and injure protoplasts by altering the permeability of their cytoplasmic membrane.

Mechanisms of Resistance: The main mechanisms of resistance are carried by gene complexes (VanA, VanB, and Van C) mainly found in vancomycin-resistant enterococci (VRE) and have also been found in staphylococci, including vancomycin-resistant *Staphyloccus aureus* (VRSA):

1. VanA is plasmid-mediated. It is the most common type and results in the synthesis of peptidoglycan cell wall precursors containing a pentapeptide ending with D-alanine-D-lactate,
2. VanB is encoded on a transposon and leads to resistance, and
3. VanC is chromosomally encoded and leads to low-level resistance to vancomycin.

Intermediate resistance in staphylococci results when there is an abnormally thickened cell wall.

Metabolic Route: Oral vancomycin is poorly absorbed from the gastrointestinal tract.

FDA FDA-APPROVED INDICATIONS

FDA-Approved Indications: Treatment of enterocolitis caused by *Staphylococcus aureus* and antibiotic-associated pseudomembranous colitis caused by *Clostridium difficile.*

SIDE EFFECTS/TOXICITY

Some patients with inflammation of the intestinal mucosa may have significant systemic absorption of oral vancomycin and, therefore, may be at risk for the development of adverse reactions usually associated with parenteral vancomycin, e.g., ototoxicity, nephrotoxicity, neutropenia, thrombocytopenia, anaphylaxis, vasculitis, rash, and red-man syndrome (hypotension, urticaria, flushing, muscle spasm, dyspnea).

DRUG INTERACTIONS/FOOD INTERACTIONS

No known interactions.

DOSING

500 mg to 2 g administered orally in three or four divided doses for 7 to 10 days. Vancomycin is administered as 125-mg and 250-mg tablets.

SPECIAL POPULATIONS

RENAL IMPAIRMENT: No dosage adjustment is necessary.

HEPATIC DYSFUNCTION: No dosage adjustment is necessary.

PEDIATRIC PATIENTS: 40 mg/kg in three or four divided doses for 7 to 10 days. The total daily dosage should not exceed 2 g.

PREGNANCY: Category B.

BREASTFEEDING: Caution should be exercised.

THE ART OF ANTIMICROBIAL THERAPY

Clinical Pearls:

1. Oral vancomycin should not be used for any systemic infection because it is not well absorbed.
2. Intravenous vancomycin is not effective in treating *C. difficile* diarrhea.
3. Resin binders such as cholestyramine may bind oral vancomycin.

BASIC CHARACTERISTICS

Class: Triazole

Mechanism of Action: Inhibits lanosterol 14-a-demethylase, which is involved in the synthesis of ergosterol, an essential component of fungal cell membranes.

Mechanisms of Resistance:

1. Point mutations in the gene (*ERG11*) encoding for the target enzyme lead to an altered target with decreased affinity for azoles,
2. overexpression of *ERG11* results in the production of high concentrations of the target enzyme, creating the need for higher intracellular drug concentrations to inhibit all of the enzyme molecules in the cell, and
3. active efflux of itraconazole out of the cell through the activation of two types of multidrug efflux transporters.

Metabolic Route: Voriconazole is metabolized by cytochrome P450 CYP2C19, CYP2C9, and CYP3A4 and is excreted primarily in the urine.

FDA

FDA-APPROVED INDICATIONS

FDA-Approved Indications: Treatment of invasive aspergillosis; candidemia in nonneutropenic patients; disseminated *Candida* infections in skin, abdomen, kidney, bladder wall, and wounds; esophageal candidiasis; serious fungal infections caused by *Scedosporium apiospermum* (*Pseudoallescheria boydii*) and *Fusarium* species.

SIDE EFFECTS/TOXICITY

Voriconazole is contraindicated in patients with known hypersensitivity to voriconazole or its excipients. Caution should be used when one is prescribing voriconazole to patients with hypersensitivity to other azoles.

Side effects/toxicities include optic neuritis, papilledema, hepatotoxicity, fever, rash, photosensitivity, anaphylaxis, vomiting, nausea, diarrhea, headache, sepsis, peripheral edema, abdominal pain, respiratory disorder, adrenal insufficiency, diabetes insipidus, dysthyroidism, cardiac toxicity including QT prolongation and torsade de pointes, seizures, aplastic anemia, and electrolyte disturbances.

DRUG INTERACTIONS/FOOD INTERACTIONS

Oral voriconazole should be taken at least 1 hour before, or 1 hour following, a meal. Gastric pH does not affect drug levels.

Voriconazole is metabolized by the human hepatic cytochrome P450 enzymes CYP2C19, CYP2C9, and CYP3A4. Inhibitors or inducers of these enzymes may increase or decrease voriconazole plasma concentrations, respectively. In addition, voriconazole inhibits the metabolic activity of the cytochrome P450 enzymes CYP2C19, CYP2C9, and CYP3A, so that voriconazole may increase plasma concentrations of other drugs metabolized by these CYP450 enzymes, resulting in toxicity. The following list comprises significant drug interactions with voriconazole:

Coadministered Drug	*Interaction*
Alfentanil	Reduction in the dosage of alfentanil and other opiates metabolized by CYP3A4 (e.g., sufentanil) should be considered
Astemizole	**Contraindicated**
Barbiturates (long-acting)	**Contraindicated**
Benzodiazepines	Monitor for increased benzodiazepine effects
Calcium channel blockers	Monitor for increased calcium channel blocker effects
Carbamazepine	**Contraindicated**
Cisapride	**Contraindicated**
Cyclosporine	Reduce the cyclosporine dosage to one half of the starting dose and monitor cyclosporine blood levels.
Ergot alkaloids	**Contraindicated**
HMG-CoA reductase inhibitors (statins)	Monitor for increased statin effects
Methadone	Monitor; dosage reduction of methadone may be necessary
Nonnucleoside reverse transcriptase inhibitors (NNRTIs)	With efavirenz, voriconazole maintenance dosage should be increased to 400 mg every 12 hours and efavirenz should be decreased to 300 mg every 24 hours. With other NNRTIs, monitor for NNRTI toxicity and for elevated or decreased levels of voriconazole.
Omeprazole	When one is initiating therapy with voriconazole in patients who are already receiving omeprazole dosages of 40 mg or greater, reduce the omeprazole dosage by one half.
Oral contraceptives	Increased levels of both oral contraceptives and voriconazole. Monitor for adverse events related to both oral contraceptives and voriconazole.

Coadministered Drug	*Interaction*
Phenytoin	Monitor for phenytoin toxicity; increase voriconazole maintenance dosage from 4 mg/kg to 5 mg/kg IV every 12 hours or from 200 mg to 400 mg orally every 12 hours (100 mg to 200 mg orally every 12 hours in patients weighing less than 40 kg)
Pimozide	**Contraindicated**
Protease inhibitors	No interaction with indinavir; high-dose ritonavir (400 mg every 12 hours) is contraindicated, but low-dose ritonavir (100 mg every 12 hours) may be given if benefit outweighs risk; with other protease inhibitors, levels of both the protease inhibitor and voriconazole may be elevated
Quinidine	**Contraindicated**
Rifabutin	**Contraindicated**
Rifampin	**Contraindicated**
Saint-John's-wort	**Contraindicated**
Sulfonylurea oral hypoglycemics	Monitor for hypoglycemia
Tacrolimus	Reduce the tacrolimus dosage to one third of the starting dose and monitor tacrolimus blood levels
Terfenadine	**Contraindicated**
Vinca alkaloids	Monitor for increased vinca alkaloid effects
Warfarin	Monitor for increased warfarin effects

DOSING

Voriconazole is dispensed in 50-mg and 200-mg tablets, a powder for oral ingestion containing 45 mg/vial, and a powder for intravenous administration.

For treatment of aspergillosis, scedosporiosis, fusariosis, and invasive candidiasis: Loading dose of 6 mg/kg IV every 12 hours on the first day followed by 4 mg/kg every 12 hours, or 200 mg orally every 12 hours. Adult patients who weigh less than 40 kg should receive an oral maintenance dose of 100 mg every 12 hours.

For esophageal candidiasis: 200 mg orally every 12 hours.

SPECIAL POPULATIONS

RENAL IMPAIRMENT: In patients with creatinine clearance less than 50 mL/min, accumulation of the intravenous vehicle, SBECD (sulfobutylether-β-cyclodextrin), occurs. Oral voriconazole should be administered to these patients, unless an assessment of the benefit/risk to the patient justifies the use of intravenous voriconazole. There is no dosage adjustment for oral voriconazole in patients with renal impairment.

HEPATIC IMPAIRMENT: The maintenance dosage should be 100 mg every 12 hours in those with Child-Pugh class A and B. Voriconazole has not been studied in patients with severe cirrhosis (Child-Pugh class C). Patients with hepatic insufficiency must be carefully monitored for drug toxicity.

PEDIATRIC PATIENTS: Safety and effectiveness in patients aged younger than 12 years have not been established. In children aged 12 years and older, the maintenance dosage of 4 mg/kg every 12 hours can be given.

PREGNANCY: Category D.

BREASTFEEDING: The expected benefits of voriconazole therapy for the mother should be weighed against the potential risk from exposure of voriconazole to the infant.

THE ART OF ANTIMICROBIAL THERAPY

Clinical Pearls:

1. Voriconazole is active against most molds except *Zygomycetes* species.
2. Voriconazole should not be administered by IV route in patients with renal insufficiency; oral voriconazole is recommended instead.
3. Voriconazole is an inhibitor of cytochrome P450 and can enhance the activity of many commonly used drugs, including oral hypoglycemics and anticoagulants.
4. Voriconazole should be administered with caution to patients with potentially proarrhythmic conditions.

ZANAMIVIR (Relenza)

BASIC CHARACTERISTICS

Class: Neuraminidase inhibitor

Mechanism of Action: Inhibits influenza virus neuraminidase affecting release of viral particles.

Mechanism of Resistance: Mutations in the viral neuraminidase or viral hemagglutinin (or both).

Metabolic Route: Up to 17% of the inhaled compound is absorbed systemically. It is excreted unchanged in the urine.

FDA-APPROVED INDICATIONS

FDA-Approved Indications: Treatment of uncomplicated influenza A and B virus in adults and pediatric patients aged 7 years and older who have been symptomatic for no more than 2 days. Prophylaxis of influenza in adults and pediatric patients aged 5 years and older.

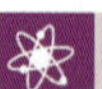

SIDE EFFECTS/TOXICITY

Zanamivir is not recommended for treatment or prophylaxis of influenza in individuals with underlying airways disease (such as asthma or chronic obstructive pulmonary disease). Serious cases of bronchospasm, including fatalities, have been reported in patients with and without underlying airways disease. Zanamivir should be discontinued in any patient who develops bronchospasm or decline in respiratory function.

Other adverse reactions include allergiclike reactions, such as oropharyngeal edema, serious skin rashes, and anaphylaxis; delirium; seizures and abnormal behavior; arrhythmias; syncope; seizures; rash; sinusitis; dizziness; fever; chills; and arthralgias.

DRUG INTERACTIONS/FOOD INTERACTIONS

Live attenuated influenza vaccine should not be administered within 2 weeks before or until 48 hours after administration of zanamivir.

DOSING

Administration to the respiratory tract by oral inhalation only, using the Diskhaler device provided. The recommended dosage of zanamivir for treatment of influenza in adults and pediatric patients aged 7 years and older is 10 mg twice daily (approximately 12 hours apart) for 5 days.

The recommended dosage of zanamivir for prophylaxis of influenza in adults and pediatric patients aged 5 years and older in a household setting is 10 mg once daily for 10 days.

The recommended dosage of zanamivir for prophylaxis of influenza in adults and adolescents in a community setting is 10 mg once daily for 28 days.

SPECIAL POPULATIONS

RENAL IMPAIRMENT: No dosage adjustment is recommended.

HEPATIC DYSFUNCTION: Zanamivir has not been studied in those with hepatic impairment.

PEDIATRIC PATIENTS: Used for treatment in children aged 7 years and older and for prophylaxis in children aged 5 years and older. The dosage is the same as for adults.

PREGNANCY: Category C.

BREASTFEEDING: Caution should be exercised when zanamivir is administered to a breastfeeding mother.

THE ART OF ANTIMICROBIAL THERAPY

Clinical Pearls:

1. Zanamivir has activity against both influenza A and B.
2. Zanamivir is active against avian H5N1 and novel H1N1 influenza.
3. Resistance in zanamivir leads to resistance in oseltamivir; however, zanamivir remains active against novel H1N1 in the presence of oseltamivir resistance.
4. Live attenuated influenza vaccine should not be administered within 2 weeks before or until 48 hours after administration of zanamivir.
5. Zanamivir is not recommended for treatment or prophylaxis of influenza in patients with underlying airways disease.
6. Zanamivir has not been proven effective for prophylaxis in nursing home residents.

Note: Also available combined with lamivudine as Combivir and with both lamivudine and abacavir as Trizivir.

BASIC CHARACTERISTICS

Class: Nucleoside reverse transcriptase inhibitor (NRTI).

Mechanism of Action: Converted by cellular enzymes to its active drug zidovudine triphosphate, an analogue of thymidine triphosphate. The zidovudine triphosphate competes with the naturally occurring nucleotide for incorporation in newly forming HIV DNA. Because zidovudine triphosphate does not have a terminal hydroxyl group, it halts transcription and replication of the virus.

Mechanism of Resistance: Changes in the structure of HIV reverse transcriptase leads to pyrophosphorolysis of the nucleoside analogues, which allows transcription of DNA to continue. Resistance mutations include the "TAMS": 41L, 67N, 70R, 210W, 215F, and 219E.

Metabolic Route: Zidovudine is primarily eliminated by hepatic metabolism. The major metabolite of zidovudine is 3′-azido-3′-deoxy-5′-*O*-β-*D*-glucopyranuronosylthymidine.

FDA-APPROVED INDICATIONS

FDA-Approved Indications: Treatment of HIV infection, in combinations with other antiretrovirals.

SIDE EFFECTS/TOXICITY

WARNING: Zidovudine is associated with **hematologic toxicity** including neutropenia and severe anemia particularly in patients with advanced HIV.

Prolonged use of zidovudine has been associated with symptomatic **myopathy.**

Lactic acidosis and severe hepatomegaly with steatosis, including fatal cases, have been reported with the use of nucleoside analogues alone or in combination, including zidovudine.

Other side effects/toxicities: immune reconstitution inflammatory syndrome; fat redistribution including central obesity and dorsocervical fat enlargement, peripheral wasting, facial wasting, and breast enlargement; fever; cough; headache; malaise; nausea; anorexia; and vomiting.

DRUG INTERACTIONS/FOOD INTERACTIONS

Zidovudine can be taken with or without food and is unaffected by pH.

Zidovudine should not be used with stavudine because they are both thymidine analogues and may be antagonistic.

Zidovudine should not be administered with ribavirin because of additive effects on anemia.

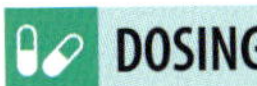

DOSING

Zidovudine is administered in 100-mg and 300-mg tablets, via intravenous injection or in a pale, strawberry-flavored liquid, which contains 50 mg/mL. The recommended adult dosage is 300 mg twice daily.

SPECIAL POPULATIONS

RENAL IMPAIRMENT: In patients on dialysis, the recommended dosage is 100 mg every 8 hours.

HEPATIC DYSFUNCTION: No dosage adjustment is necessary.

PEDIATRIC PATIENTS: The approved dosage is 160 mg/m^2 every 8 hours (480 mg/m^2/day up to a maximum of 200 mg every 8 hours).

PREGNANCY: Category C.

BREASTFEEDING: It is recommended that HIV-positive mothers not breastfeed their children, to decrease mother-to-child transmission of HIV.

THE ART OF ANTIMICROBIAL THERAPY

Clinical Pearls:

1. Zidovudine should be used in combination with other antiretroviral agents.
2. Zidovudine is present in three different medications: Retrovir, Trizivir, and Combivir.
3. Unlike other NRTIs, pharmacokinetic studies do not support once-daily dosing with zidovudine.

HELPFUL FORMULAS, EQUATIONS, AND DEFINITIONS

Child-Pugh Classification of Severity of Liver Disease
Estimating Creatinine Clearance
Estimating Ideal Body Weight in kg
Pregnancy Risk Categories
Continuous Renal Replacement Therapy (CRRT)
Body Surface Area (Mosteller Formula)

Child-Pugh Classification of Severity of Liver Disease

	Points Assigned		
Parameter	*1*	*2*	*3*
Ascites	Absent	Slight	Moderate
Bilirubin	<2 mg/dL (<34.2 micromol/liter)	2-3 mg/dL (34.2 to 51.3 micromol/liter)	>3 mg/dL (>51.3 micromol/liter)
Albumin	>3.5 g/dL (35 g/liter)	2.8-3.5 g/dL (28 to 35 g/liter)	<2.8 g/dL (<28 g/liter)
Prothrombin time			
Seconds over control	<4	4-6	>6
INR	<1.7	1.7-2.3	>2.3
Encephalopathy	None	Grade 1-2	Grade 3-4

Grading: A = 5-6 points; B = 7-9 points; C = 10-15 points

Estimating Creatinine Clearance (mL/min)

Cockcroft and Gault equation

$$CrCl = (140 - age) \times IBW/(Scr \times 72) \qquad (\times 0.85 \text{ for females})$$

Estimating Ideal Body Weight (IBW) in kg

Males: IBW = 50 kg + 2.3 kg for each inch over 5 feet
Females: IBW = 45.5 kg + 2.3 kg for each inch over 5 feet

Pregnancy Risk Categories

The FDA has established five categories (A, B, C, D, and X) to indicate a drug's potential for causing teratogenicity:

A - Controlled studies in women fail to demonstrate a risk to the fetus in the first trimester, and the possibility of fetal harm appears remote.

B - Animal studies do not indicate a risk to the fetus and there are no controlled human studies, or animal studies do show an adverse effect on the fetus but well-controlled studies in pregnant women have failed to demonstrate a risk to the fetus.

C - Studies have shown that the drug exerts animal teratogenic or embryocidal effects, but there are no controlled studies in women, or no studies are available in either animals or women.

D - Positive evidence of human fetal risk exists, but benefits in certain situations (e.g., life-threatening situations or serious diseases for which safer drugs cannot be used or are ineffective) may make the drug acceptable despite its risks.

X - Studies in animals or humans have demonstrated fetal abnormalities or there is evidence of fetal risk based on human experience, or both, and the risk clearly outweighs any possible benefit.

Continuous Renal Replacement Therapy (CRRT)

Continuous Renal Replacement Therapy (CRRT) is being used increasingly in patients with acute renal failure and comprises a variety of techniques, including continuous arteriovenous hemofiltration (CAVH), continuous venovenous hemofiltration (CVVH), continuous arteriovenous hemodialysis (CAVHD), continuous venovenous hemodialysis (CVVHD), and continuous venovenous hemodialfiltration (CVVHDF). For practical purposes of antibiotic administration, the arterial and venous samples can be assumed to be equal.

In general, CRRT produces a CrCl of approximately 30mL/min, though this is a rough estimate only, and, when possible, serum antibiotic assays should be monitored. Slow Extended Daily Dialysis (SLEDD) is a related modality that is used for 6-12 hours/day; antibiotic replacement in patients treated with SLEDD is in general similar to that used for patients receiving CRRT; for antimicrobial agents that experience significant removal during dialysis, those normally administered every 24 can be given after SLEDD each day, and those normally given every 12 hours should be given after SLEDD and 12 h later.

Body Surface Area (Mosteller formula)

$$\text{BSA (m}^2\text{)} = \sqrt{\frac{\text{Height (cm)} \times \text{Weight (kg)}}{3600}}$$

BIBLIOGRAPHY AND REFERENCES

Cunha, BA, ed. *Antibiotic Essentials.* Boston: Physician Press; 2009

Francis J. Curry National Tuberculosis Center and California Department of Public Health. *Drug-Resistant Tuberculosis: A Survival Guide for Clinicians,* Second Edition; 2008.

Gilbert B, Robbins P, Livornese LL, Jr. Use of Antibacterial

Agents in Renal Failure. *Infect Dis Clin N Am.* 2009;23:899–924.

Gilbert DN, Moellering RC, Eliopoulos GM, Chambers HF, Saag MS. *The Sanford Guide to Antimicrobial Therapy.* Sperryville, VA: Antimicrobial Therapy, Inc.; 2009.

Guerrant RL, Walker DH, Weller PF. *Tropical Infectious Diseases Principles, Pathogens and Practice,* Second Edition. Philadelphia, PA: Churchvill Livingstone; 2006.

Mandell GL, Bennett JE, Dolin R. *Principles and Practice of Infectious Diseases,* Seventh Edition. Philadelphia: Elsevier; 2010.

Schlossberg D, ed. *Clinical Infectious Disease.* London: Cambridge University Press; 2008.

The Medical Letter on Drugs and Therapeutics, Drugs For Parasitic Infections, February 2008

Yu VL, Edwards G, McKinnon P, Peloquin C, Morse GD. *Antimicrobial Therapy and Vaccines.* Pittsburgh, PA: ESun Technologies, LLC; 2005.

http://www.dailymed.nlm.nih.gov

http://www.accessdata.fda.gov/Scripts/cder/DrugsatFDA/

http://www.drugs.com/

http://www.rxlist.com/

http://www.PDR.net

http://labeldataplus.org

http://www.hiv-druginteractions.org/

http://www.aidsinfo.nih.gov/guidelines/

BRAND NAME INDEX

Abelcet (Amphotericin B lipid complex), 30
Albenza (Albendazole), 8
Alinia (Nitazoxanide), 308
Ambisome (Liposomal Amphotericin B), 22
Amikin (Amikacin), 12
Amoxil (Amoxicillin), 15
Amphotec (Amphotericin B Colloidal Dispersion [abcd]), 25
Ampicillin, 32
Ancef (Cefazolin), 72
Ancobon (Flucytosine), 197
Antiminth (Pyrantel pamoate), 353
Aptivus (Tipranavir), 446
Aralen (Chloroquine phosphate), 123
Artemether – see Artemisinin, 39
Artemisinin and its derivatives, 39
Artesunate – see Artemisinin, 39
Atabrine (Quinacrine HCl), 358
Atripla (Tenofovir/ emtricitabine/ efavirenz), 425
Augmentin (Amoxicillin-clavulanate), 18
Avelox (Moxifloxacin), 292
Azactam (Aztreonam), 57

Bactrim (Trimethoprim/Sulfamethoxazole), 453
Baraclude (Entecavir), 177
Benznidazole, 59
Biaxin (Clarithromycin), 133
Bicillin (Penicillin), 331
Biltricide (Praziquantel), 349
Bitin (Bithionol), 60

Cancidas (Caspofungin), 63
Capastat (Capreomycin), 61
Ceclor (Cefaclor), 65
Cedax (Ceftibuten), 107
Cefizox (Ceftizoxime), 109
Cefobid (Cefoperazone), 85
Cefotan (Cefotetan), 90
Cefrom (Cefpirome), 96
Ceftin (Cefuroxime axetil), 115
Cefzil (Cefprozil), 101
Chloromycetin (Chloramphenicol), 121
Cipro (Ciprofloxacin), 129
Claforan (Cefotaxime), 87
Cleocin (Clindamycin), 137
Coartem (Artemether/lumefantrine) – see Artemisinin, 39
Coly-Mycin (Colistimethate sodium), 142
Combivir (Zidovudine/lamivudine), 249
Copegus (Ribavirin), 368
Crixivan (Indinavir), 223
Cubicin (Daptomycin), 148
Cytovene (Ganciclovir), 208

Dapsone, 146
Daraprim (Pyrimethamine), 356
Dicloxacillin, 156
Diflucan (Fluconazole), 194
Dihydroartemisinin – v. Artemisinin, 39
Doribax (Doripenem), 163
Doryx (Doxycycline delayed release), 165
Duricef (Cefadroxil), 67
Dynacin (Minocycline), 289

Emtriva (Emtricitabine), 173
Epivir (Lamivudine), 243
Epzicom (Lamivudine/abacavir), 246
Eraxis (Anidulafungin), 37
Erythromycin, 182

Factive (Gemifloxacin), 212
Famvir (Famciclovir), 192

Flagyl (Metronidazole), 282
Floxin (Ofloxacin), 315
Flumadine (Rimantadine), 390
Fortaz (Ceftazidime), 104
Foscavir (Foscarnet), 203
Fungizone (Amphotericin B Deoxycholate), 27
Furadantin (Nitrofurantoin), 27
Furamide (Diloxanide furoate), 162
Furoxone (Furazolidone), 206
Fuzeon (Enfuvirtide), 175

Garamycin (Gentamicin), 214
Germanin (Suramin sodium), 413
Glucantime (Meglumine antimonite), 275
Grifulvin V (Griseofulvin), 217
Gris-Peg (Griseofulvin), 217

Halfan (Halofantrine), 219
Hepsera (Adefovir), 6
Hetrazan (Diethyl carbamazine), 160
Hydroxychloroquine, 123

Impavido (Miltefosine), 287
Infergen (Interferon alpha), 226
Intelence (Etravirine), 189
Invanz (Ertapenem), 179
Invirase (Saquinavir), 396
Isentress (Raltegravir), 366
Isoniazid, 230

Kaletra (Lopinavir/ritonavir), 262
Kantrex (Kanamycin), 238
Keflex (Cephalexin), 119
Ketoconazole, 240

Lamisil (Terbinafine), 428
Lampit (Nifurtimox), 307
Lamprene (Clofazimine), 140
Lariam (Mefloquine hydrochloride), 273
Levaquin (Levofloxacin), 255
Lexiva (Fosamprenavir), 199
Lorabid (Loracarbef), 265

Macrobid (Nitrofurantoin), 310
Macrodantin (Nitrofurantoin), 310
Malarone (Atovaquone/proguanil), 50
Mandokef (Cefamandole), 69
Mandol (Cefamandole), 69
Maxipime (Cefepime), 80
Mefoxin (Cefoxitin), 93
Melarsoprol B (Mel-B), 277
Mepron (Atovaquone), 48
Merrem (Meropenem), 279
Miltex (Miltefosine), 287
Minocin (Minocycline), 289
Mintezole (Thiabendazole), 433
Myambutol (Ethambutol), 185
Mycamine (Micafungin), 285
Mycobutin (Rifabutin), 372

Nafcillin, 295
NebuPent (Pentamidine), 337
Neo-Fradin (Neomycin), 300
Neutrexin (Trimetrexate glucuronate), 458
Noroxin (Norfloxacin), 312
Norvir (Ritonavir), 392
Noxafil (Posaconazole), 346

Omnicef (Cefdinir), 75
Ornidyl (Eflornithine), 171
Oxacillin, 320

Para-aminosalicylate Sodium (PASER), 323
Pegasys (Peginterferon alpha 2a), 325
Pegintron (Peginterferon alpha 2b), 328
Penicillin G (see Penicillin), 331

Penicillin G Benzathine – see Penicillin, 331
Penicillin G Procaine – see Penicillin, 331
Penicillin V – see Penicillin, 331
Pentam (Pentamidine), 339
Pentostam (Stibogluconate), 406
Permapen (Penicillin), 331
Piperazine citrate, 345
Pipracil (Piperacillin), 339
Prezista (Darunavir), 150
Priftin (Rifapentine), 385
Primaquine (Primaquine phosphate), 351
Primaxin (Imipenem-cilastatin), 320
Proloprim (Trimethoprim), 453
Pyrazinamide, 354

Qualaquin (Quinine sulfate), 361
Quinidine, 359

Rebetol (Ribavirin), 368
Relenza (Zanamivir), 476
Rescriptor (Delavirdine), 153
Retrovir (Zidovudine), 478
Reyataz (Atazanavir), 44
Ribasphere (Ribavirin), 368
Rifadin (Rifampin), 375
Rifamate (Rifampin/isoniazid), 378
Rifater (Rifampin/isoniazid/ pyrazinamide), 381
Rocephin (Ceftriaxone), 112
ROFERON-A (Interferon alpha), 226
Rovamycine (Spiramycin), 401

Selzentry (Maraviroc), 268
Septra (Trimethoprim/Sulfamethoxazole), 455
Seromycin (Cycloserine), 144
Spectracef (Cefditoren), 78
Sporanox (Itraconazole), 232
Streptomycin, 408
Stromectol (Ivermectin), 236
Sulfadiazine, 411
Suprax (Cefixime), 83
Sustiva (Efavirenz), 168
Symmetrel (Amantadine), 10
Synercid (Quinupristin-dalfopristin), 364

Tamiflu (Oseltamivir), 318
Targocid (Teicoplanin), 415
Tazicef (Ceftazidime), 104
Tetracycline Hydrochloride, 430
Ticar (Ticarcillin), 435
Tigacyl (Tigecycline), 441
Timentin (Ticarcillin-clavulanate), 438
Tindamax (Tinidazole), 443
Tobramycin, 450
Trecator (Ethionamide), 187
Trizivir (Zidovudine/lamivudine/ abacavir), 252
Trobicin (Spectinomycin), 399
Truvada (Tenofovir/emtricitabine), 421
Tyzeka (Telbivudine), 419

Unasyn (Ampicillin-sulbactam), 35

Valcyte (Valganciclovir), 464
Valtrex (Valacyclovir), 461
Vancocin (Vancomycin, oral), 470
Vancomycin (Vancomycin, IV), 467
Vansil (Oxamniquine), 322
Vantin (Cefpodoxime), 98
Vermox (Mebendazole), 271
Vfend (Voriconazole), 472
Vibativ (Telavancin), 417
Vibramycin (Doxycycline), 165
Videx EC (Didanosine), 158
Viracept (Nelfinavir), 297

Viramune (Nevirapine), 302
Virazole (Ribavirin, inhaled), 368
Viread (Tenofovir), 423
Vistide (Cidofovir), 126

Xifaxan (Rifaximin), 388

Yodoxin (Iodoquinol), 228
Yomesan (Niclosamide), 305

Zerit (Stavudine), 404
Ziagen (Abacavir), 1
Zinacef (Cefuroxime), 115
Zithromax (Azithromycin), 53
Zmax (Azithromycin), 53
Zosyn (Piperacillin-tazobactam), 342
Zovirax (Acyclovir), 3
Zyvox (Linezolid), 259